Respiratory Muscle Training

Content Strategist: *Rita Demetriou-Swanwick*
Content Development Specialist: *Carole McMurray*
Project Manager: *Shereen Jameel*
Designer/Design Direction: *Christian Bilbow*
Illustration Manager: *Jennifer Rose*
Illustrator: *Bruce Hogarth*

Respiratory Muscle Training
Theory and Practice

Alison McConnell PhD, FACSM, FBASES

Professor of Applied Physiology, Centre for Sports Medicine and Human Performance,
Brunel University, UK

Foreword by
Rik Gosselink PT, PhD

Professor of Rehabilitation Sciences,
Dean Faculty of Kinesiology and Rehabilitation Sciences, Respiratory Rehabilitation,
University of Leuven, Belgium

Illustrations by
Bruce Hogarth

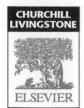

CHURCHILL LIVINGSTONE

ELSEVIER

Edinburgh London New York Oxford Philadelphia St Louis Sydney Toronto 2013

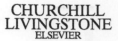

ISBN 978-0-7020-5020-6

British Library Cataloguing in Publication Data
A catalogue record for this book is available from the British Library

Library of Congress Cataloging in Publication Data
A catalog record for this book is available from the Library of Congress

Notices
Knowledge and best practice in this field are constantly changing. As new research and experience broaden our understanding, changes in research methods, professional practices, or medical treatment may become necessary.

Practitioners and researchers must always rely on their own experience and knowledge in evaluating and using any information, methods, compounds, or experiments described herein. In using such information or methods they should be mindful of their own safety and the safety of others, including parties for whom they have a professional responsibility.

With respect to any drug or pharmaceutical products identified, readers are advised to check the most current information provided (i) on procedures featured or (ii) by the manufacturer of each product to be administered, to verify the recommended dose or formula, the method and duration of administration, and contraindications. It is the responsibility of practitioners, relying on their own experience and knowledge of their patients, to make diagnoses, to determine dosages and the best treatment for each individual patient, and to take all appropriate safety precautions.

To the fullest extent of the law, neither the Publisher nor the authors, contributors, or editors, assume any liability for any injury and/or damage to persons or property as a matter of products liability, negligence or otherwise, or from any use or operation of any methods, products, instructions, or ideas contained in the material herein.

ELSEVIER your source for books, journals and multimedia in the health sciences

www.elsevierhealth.com

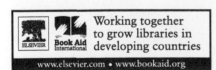

Working together to grow libraries in developing countries

www.elsevier.com • www.bookaid.org

The Publisher's policy is to use paper manufactured from sustainable forests

Contents

Contents

Part I: Theoretical basis of respiratory muscle training

Part II: Practical application of respiratory muscle training

Acknowledgements

There are so many people who have contributed directly and indirectly to this book. These include the academic colleagues and PhD students with whom I have worked over the years, as well as the many scientists whose research has provided the insights that have shaped my thinking – you are too numerous to mention individually, but you know who you are, and you have all made some contribution to the development of the ideas that have led to this book.

I have expressed my gratitude to two particularly influential individuals previously, and my appreciation of their contributions is no less heartfelt for being repeated here. In 1996, Professor Mike Caine and Claire Hodson joined me on my perilous journey to create an innovative product that people could use to train their breathing. Without Mike and Claire's faith and talent, the POWERbreathe® might never have seen the light of day, let alone commercial success. The insights on which this book are founded were made possible by the collective contribution that all three of us made to the creation of POWERbreathe® – thank you both (again).

I am also extremely grateful to Research Into Ageing (now part of Age UK), and its former Director, Elizabeth Mills. In 1990, the charity funded my original research on breathlessness in older people; that first step on my long journey could not have been made without the leap of faith required to give a junior lecturer her first research grant.

In terms of the creation of this book, I owe a special debt of gratitude to four individuals who provided invaluable feedback on my draft chapters. They are Professor Rik Gosselink, Cath O'Connor, Emma Hamilton and Dr Bernie Bissett. I'd also like to thank Drs Pete Brown and Graham Sharpe for debating the mechanisms underlying changes in blood lactate concentration after respiratory muscle training with me. Thank you all for your time, your insights, and for enabling me to keep to my submission timetable!

Writing any book is a time consuming journey requiring an obsessive focus that is difficult to achieve amidst one's normal daily routine. I am therefore grateful to Brunel University and to my colleagues for allowing me the time and thinking space to complete this journey.

I am also very grateful to my long-suffering photography model, Michèle Bonmati, who withstood two days of filming during a heat wave in Quebec. I am also enormously grateful to Physiotec (www.physiotec.ca), and in particular to Pierre Labonté, Jessica Babin and Alexandra Tétreault Ayotte for their assistance with the photography, and to POWERbreathe International Ltd. (www.powerbreathe.com) for donating the inspiratory muscle trainer, as well as for assisting with the production of the book jacket image. The principals at POWERbreathe also deserve a special mention – Harry and Anne Brar – thanks for your continued support, and for investing so much of yourselves in the slow, but steady process of making respiratory muscle training a mainstream clinical treatment.

This is my second book, but my first for a clinical audience, so thanks are due to the expert team at Elsevier for making it an excellent experience. In particular, I'd like to thank the individuals with whom I've worked directly – Rita Demetriou-Swanwick, Carole McMurray and Shereen Jameel.

Acknowledgements

I'm also grateful and honoured that Professor Rik Gosselink agreed to write the Foreword to *Respiratory Muscle Training: Theory and Practice*. Rik is a scientist whom I've admired for many years. Recently, I've finally had the pleasure and privilege of collaborating with him on a research project - as we say in Britain, Rik, 'you're a gentleman and a scholar'.

Last, but by no means least, I want to thank my partner Mel, who has yet again endured the obsession, bordering on mania, that accompanies my bouts of writing. Life can now return to some semblance of normality . . . until the next time.

Dedication

To my late father-in-law, Dr David Varvel, who was a truly exceptional human being. This is the book I dearly wish you could have seen David. . .

Foreword

The lungs do not move naturally of their own motion, but they follow the motion of the thorax and the dia-phragm. The lungs are not expanded because they are filled with air, but they are filled with air because they expand.

Francisci Deleboe Sylvii
Opera Medica, 1681

It is unthinkable to reflect on the physiology and pathophysiology of the circulation without taking into account the heart muscle as the driving force for blood transport. Cardiologists devote their expertise entirely to the heart and cardiac dysfunction in pathological conditions. However, when it comes to ventilation, a vital function as important as the circulation, the respiratory pump – the driving force for gas transport in the airways – was largely ignored or unknown to most clinicians. For many years the chest wall ('thorax' in Ancient Greek and including the rib cage, abdomen and respiratory muscles) was virtually neglected in respiratory medicine. It was only in the second part of the last century that our knowledge of respiratory muscle function and dysfunction grew. In 1985 and 1995 the hallmark of this evolution was the publication of the trilogy *The Thorax*, in the series *Lung Biology in Health and Disease*, with the late Professor Peter Macklem and Professor Charis Roussos as the editors. These standard works discuss extensively the physiology, applied physiology and disease of the chest wall. Interestingly, a chapter on respiratory muscle training was also included as a potential important part of rehabilitation in patients with respiratory disease. However, lack of scientific data at that point in time did not allow firm conclusions to be drawn on the effectiveness of this treatment.

Over the last decades much research has been published to substantiate the role of respiratory muscle dysfunction in the disability associated with a variety of health conditions. These conditions not only include respiratory diseases, such as asthma and chronic obstructive pulmonary disease (COPD), but also patients with cardiac, metabolic, neurological and orthopaedic disease. All patients with these conditions experience symptoms that originate from respiratory muscle weakness and/or increased work of breathing. These symptoms include dyspnoea, [nocturnal] hypoxaemia, hypercapnia, ineffective cough, exercise impairment, weaning failure and respiratory insufficiency. In the late 1970s, respiratory muscle training was explored for the first time in healthy people, patients with COPD, and patients with spinal cord injury. Research and clinical interest in respiratory muscle training has burgeoned over the last 30 years, in both patients and in athletes. In this respect, the publication of *Respiratory Muscle Training: Theory and Practice* is extremely timely, as there is no doubt that respiratory muscle training has finally come of age. The book provides theoretical insights into fundamental exercise physiology, respiratory physiology, pathology, exercise training and (respiratory) muscle training as well as describing in detail, the outcome of respiratory muscle training in various conditions. In addition to the solid theoretical background, practical issues on the assessment and training of respiratory muscles are also well set out.

The author of *Respiratory Muscle Training: Theory and Practice*, Professor Alison McConnell, is an internationally renowned expert in exercise physiology and specifically in respiratory muscle training. In this book she shares her extensive experience and knowledge of the concepts of muscle training and of the translation of this knowledge into respiratory muscle training for a variety of patient populations. *Respiratory Muscle Training: Theory and Practice* is the first scientific book that positions the training of the respiratory muscle pump firmly in the spotlight. I am convinced that the book will inspire, encourage and guide clinicians (physicians, physiotherapists, speech therapists, exercise physiologists) in the assessment and training of the respiratory muscles, which has become such an important component in the treatment of patients with a variety of disease conditions.

Rik Gosselink

Preface

Over the past decade, respiratory muscle training (RMT) has grown steadily in popularity, thanks to a burgeoning evidence base, and the support of a number of systematic reviews and meta-analyses. However, most healthcare professionals still have only a rudimentary knowledge of the theory and practice of RMT, and require guidance in order to implement the treatment effectively. This lack of knowledge results from the absence of RMT from the syllabi of physicians, physiotherapists and nurses. Similarly, the theory and practice of RMT is not typically taught at postgraduate level, except in specialist centres with 'resident' expertise in RMT. This is the gap that *Respiratory Muscle Training: Theory and Practice* is intended to bridge. The book will therefore be of interest to the following groups:

- Primary and secondary care physicians
- Physiotherapists
- Nurses
- Rehabilitation professionals
- Exercise scientists
- Academic clinical teachers
- Expert patients.

Respiratory Muscle Training: Theory and Practice is a distillation of 20 years of research and practical experience of RMT. It is an evidence-based compilation built upon current scientific knowledge, as well as personal experience at the cutting edge of respiratory training in a wide range of settings. The aim of the book is to give readers: (1) an introduction to respiratory physiology and exercise physiology, as well as training theory, (2) an understanding of how disease affects the respiratory muscles and the mechanics of breathing, (3) an insight into the disease-specific, evidence-based benefits of RMT, (4) advice on the application of RMT as a stand-alone treatment and as part of a rehabilitation programme, and (5) guidance on the application of functional training techniques to RMT.

The book will answer questions such as: why are patients without lung disease are limited by dyspnoea, why do certain breathing patterns exacerbate dyspnoea, what is the rationale for RMT in patients with heart failure, what are the disease-specific benefits of RMT, what is the best equipment to use, what are the evidence-based training regimens, how long does training take, how can RMT be incorporated into a programme of rehabilitation, how to ensure patients get results, how to monitor improvement, when will patients experience benefits and what will these be, how does RMT work, and how can RMT be optimized for activities of daily living?

Respiratory Muscle Training: Theory and Practice presents an exercise scientist's perspective on the application of RMT to the clinical setting. But how one might ask, does an exercise scientist become an expert on the respiratory muscles? My interest in respiratory muscles began in the late 1980s. As a PhD student at King's College Hospital, I studied the control of exercise hyperpnoea; later, as a post-doctoral researcher at the University of Birmingham, I examined the contribution of ventilatory control factors to the exercise hyperpnoea of healthy older people. The latter led me to an interest in the respiratory mechanics of healthy older people, who I had observed were more 'out of breath' during exercise than younger people. Further study led me to the respiratory muscles as a potential source of their breathlessness, since respiratory muscle strength declines with age (McConnell & Copestake, 1999) and weaker respiratory muscles intensify breathing effort (McConnell & Romer, 2004).

These insights led me to a very simple and easily testable hypothesis: 'strengthening the inspiratory muscles of otherwise healthy elderly people will reduce their exertional dyspnoea'. The hypothesis was confirmed in a preliminary study on older people (Copestake & McConnell, 1995), and subsequently in young athletes (Romer et al, 2002). The rest, as they say, is history, and I have experienced a 20-year journey during which my research progressed from the descriptive to the mechanistic. The journey has also resulted in numerous collaborations with clinicians, fellow exercise scientists, as well as professional athletes and coaches. The theoretical understanding that I have gained as a researcher, and the practical insights I have gained from both clinical and sports settings, are what this book is intended to share – in essence, *Respiratory Muscle Training: Theory and Practice* is my 'RMT brain dump'.

It's fair to say that RMT has had its share of detractors; in exercise science, the received wisdom is that healthy people exercising at sea level experience no breathing-related limitation to exercise tolerance. The received wisdom was based primarily on the observation that breathing does not limit oxygen diffusion at the lungs, which is true. However, this 'truth' fails to accommodate the fact that breathing is a 'muscular process', and that the exercise hyperpnoea exacts its own metabolic and perceptual costs upon us all. The magnitude of my heresy in questioning the basic premise of the received wisdom cannot be overstated, and the shift in thinking that has occurred over the past two decades has been nothing short of seismic. However, the role of breathing in exercise limitation is now well accepted (Chs 3 and 4) – so much so that the practice of RMT has become a mainstream activity practised by elite athletes and recreational exercisers alike. In 2011, I published my first book, which was a guide to inspiratory muscle training for sport ('Breathe strong, perform better'). Even before embarking on 'Breathe strong', I always planned to follow this 'consumer' book with a similar tome for a clinical audience; the result is what you see before you.

One would be forgiven for thinking that the reticence to accept the existence of a respiratory-related impairment to exercise might be less strong in a clinical setting than in the world of sport. However, even for conditions where the rationale for RMT appears clear (e.g., chronic lung disease), history tells a surprising story; scepticism has followed RMT wherever it has peeked over the parapet. In the context of chronic lung disease, the reasons for scepticism are primarily: (1) a misconception that respiratory muscles adapt to the disease and cannot, or need not, undertake any further training, (2) a flawed negative early meta-analysis that failed to exclude trials with inadequate training interventions, and (3) a focus upon exercise-induced contractile fatigue of the diaphragm as being the 'gold standard' indication for specific RMT. In spite of the sceptics, researchers from all corners of the world have drawn their own conclusions about RMT. There are now literally hundreds of peer-reviewed randomized controlled trials, which have included thousands of patients, with conditions as diverse as chronic lung disease and diabetes. The emerging systematic reviews and meta-analyses conclude that RMT generates a range of clinically meaningful outcomes for patients with conditions such as chronic obstructive pulmonary disease (Gosselink et al, 2011) and heart failure (Smart et al, 2012).

As its title suggests, this book is divided into two parts: theory and practice. Although these sections are inevitably interlinked, it is not essential to read the theory in order to benefit from the practice. The theory section (Part I) provides readers with access to the theoretical building blocks that support the practice (Part II). Accordingly, it can be dipped into and out of where readers' needs and interests dictate. For example, chest physicians (who are, quite correctly, inherently suspicious of snake oil sellers who peddle potions and gadgets claiming to improve a patient's condition) will no doubt wish to review the sections describing the peer-reviewed research that underpins the clinical benefits of inspiratory muscle training (Ch. 4).

The theoretical building blocks include aspects of the relevant anatomy and physiology of the respiratory system, and associated musculature, as well as an introduction to pertinent aspects of exercise physiology and training theory (Chs 1 and 2). The rationale for specific RMT is explored in Chapter 3, which describes disease-specific alterations in respiratory muscle function as well as disease-related changes to the demand for respiratory muscle work; together, these two factors define the 'demand/capacity' relationship of the respiratory muscles. The lesser-known, non-respiratory roles of the respiratory muscles are also described in Chapter 3. From rationale we move to evidence, and in Chapter 4 the evidence base for RMT is explored.

The practical section of the book (Part II) opens with a description of the different methods that have been used to train respiratory muscles, and their efficacy in terms of the specific changes in respiratory muscle function they elicit (Ch. 5). In Chapter 6, the reader is guided through the practical implementation of the most widely validated form of RMT, viz., inspiratory muscle resistance training (IMT). This chapter covers everything from the place of IMT in the treatment pathway and indications/contraindications, to the practicalities of implementation, monitoring progress and maintaining benefits. This chapter also includes advice on using RMT as a 'pre-habilitation' treatment and incorporating RMT into a rehabilitation programme; the chapter culminates with a case study. In describing the non-respiratory roles of the respiratory muscles, Chapter 3 also presents a rationale for adopting a more functional approach to IMT, and this is expanded in Chapter 7. In addition, this chapter suggests methods that can be used to identify load/capacity imbalance within the inspiratory muscles, as well as the quantification of the main symptom of inspiratory muscle overload, viz., dyspnoea. Finally, Chapter 7 describes over 100 'Functional' IMT exercises, which incorporate a stability and/or postural challenge, including exercises that address specific movements that provoke dyspnoea.

Respiratory Muscle Training: Theory and Practice is not intended to provide a recipe for IMT; rather, my intention has been to provide readers with the knowledge, insight and confidence to tailor IMT creatively to the specific needs of their patients. If, as a result, I have made myself obsolete as an expert on IMT then, as the saying goes, 'my work here is done'.

REFERENCES

Copestake, A.J., McConnell, A.K., 1995. Inspiratory muscle training reduces exertional breathlessness in healthy elderly men and women. In: International Conference on Physical Activity and Health in the Elderly. University of Sterling, Scotland, p. 150.

Gosselink, R., De Vos, J., van den Heuvel, S.P., et al., 2011. Impact of inspiratory muscle training in patients with COPD: what is the evidence? Eur. Respir. J. 37, 416–425.

McConnell, A.K., 2011. Breathe strong, perform better. Human Kinetics, Champaign, IL.

McConnell, A.K., Copestake, A.J., 1999. Maximum static respiratory pressures in healthy elderly men and women: issues of reproducibility and interpretation. Respiration 66, 251–258.

McConnell, A.K., Romer, L.M., 2004. Respiratory muscle training in healthy humans: resolving the controversy. Int. J. Sports Med. 25 (4), 284–293.

Romer, L.M., McConnell, A.K., Jones, D.A., 2002. Effects of inspiratory muscle training on time-trial performance in trained cyclists. J. Sports Sci. 20, 547–562.

Smart, N.A., Giallauria, F., Dieberg, G., 2012. Efficacy of inspiratory muscle training in chronic heart failure patients: a systematic review and meta-analysis. Int. J. Cardiol. (in press).

Part I

Theoretical basis of respiratory muscle training

Introduction to Part I

Part I of *Respiratory muscle training: theory and practice* consists of four chapters that provide the theoretical building blocks for the practical guidance on respiratory muscle training (RMT) that is provided in Part II. Although it is not essential to read Part I in order to put the guidance in Part II into practice, it provides information that will help empower readers with the knowledge to use Part II as a source of creative inspiration (no pun intended), rather than a recipe book that must be followed to the letter.

Chapter 1 provides an overview of the anatomy and physiology of the respiratory system, focussing on aspects that are revisited in later chapters, including respiratory mechanics and dyspnoea. In Chapter 2, some fundamental principles of exercise physiology and whole-body training are described in order that readers may understand how the normal physiology described therein interacts with pathology to influence exercise tolerance. Chapter 3 is dedicated to the respiratory muscles, and considers how disease influences breathing mechanics and respiratory muscle function to create imbalance in the demand/capacity relationship of these muscles. In addition, Chapter 3 describes respiratory muscle involvement in exercise limitation in health and disease, as well as the non-respiratory functions of the respiratory muscles, thereby establishing the rationale for RMT. In Chapter 4 the functional responses to RMT at both a muscle and whole-body level are considered in health and disease, thereby establishing the evidence base for RMT. This information establishes the rationale for the focus of Part II, which is the practical application of pressure threshold inspiratory muscle training.

Chapter | 1 |

Anatomy and physiology of the respiratory system

This chapter is not intended to provide a comprehensive description of the anatomy and physiology of the respiratory system; rather it is intended to provide a level of understanding that is required to underpin the remainder of this book. Readers wishing to gain a deeper insight into this interesting area are referred to the work of Davies & Moores (2010) and Lumb (2010).

THORACIC STRUCTURE AND FUNCTION

Introduction

This section will describe the principal structures whose physiology will be explored in subsequent sections of this, and other, chapters. It is not intended to provide a detailed description of thoracic structure and function; rather it is intended to provide a working knowledge to facilitate understanding of the applied aspects of this book.

The respiratory system is illustrated in Figure 1.1 and is made up of all the structures that guide air into the lungs (nose, mouth, and airways), plus the lungs themselves and the structures that surround the lungs (thoracic cavity, including the rib cage). The right lung comprises three lobes, whilst the left has two, which allows space for the heart to lie between the left lobes, sloping toward the left. The weight of both adult lungs is between 0.7 and 1.0 kg (1.5 and 2.2 pounds) when weighed at autopsy; however, in life they probably weigh twice this amount because the blood vessels within the lungs (pulmonary circulation) will be filled with about 0.9 litres of blood (weighing about 0.95 kg [2.1 pounds]). In other words, the adult human has about 2 kg (4.4 pounds) of lung tissue hanging inside the rib cage.

The airways

The airways branch a total of 23 times, creating a tree-like structure that ends in the alveoli, where the exchange of oxygen (O_2) and carbon dioxide (CO_2) takes place (Fig. 1.2). The branches follow an irregular, dichotomous pattern in which each airway gives rise to two 'daughter' airways. The structure is irregular because the daughter branches may not be of equal size. The number of airways (N) in each generation (Z) is given by the equation $N = Z^2$.

Air enters via the nose and mouth; then it travels into the pharynx, through the glottis and down the trachea. Next, the air travels into the right and left bronchi, and then through the branching structure of the remaining airways to the alveoli. The alveoli are collections of air sacs, similar to a bunch of grapes, which are surrounded by a dense network of capillaries (think of a bunch of grapes inside a net shopping bag; Fig. 1.1). The regions of the lung without alveoli (including the airways) are known as the conducting zone (branches 1–16), whilst the regions with alveoli are known as the respiratory zone (17–23), i.e., the zone where oxygen and carbon dioxide are exchanged (Fig. 1.2). From branch 17 onwards (respiratory bronchioles), the airways begin to display alveolar buds in their walls, and by branch 20 onwards virtually the entire airway is made up of alveoli (alveolar ducts). An important feature of the conducting airways is that the larger airways, such as the trachea, are reinforced with cartilage rings that help prevent collapse, whereas the walls of smaller airways contain no supporting skeleton. The small airways possess rings of smooth muscle that, when contracted, narrow the airways (bronchoconstriction). From branch 3 onwards, the airways are surrounded by lung parenchyma, and the elastic forces that operate to recoil the lung parenchyma help to tug the airways open during exhalation (airway tethering), with their radial traction (see section 'Mechanics of breathing: Airway resistance').

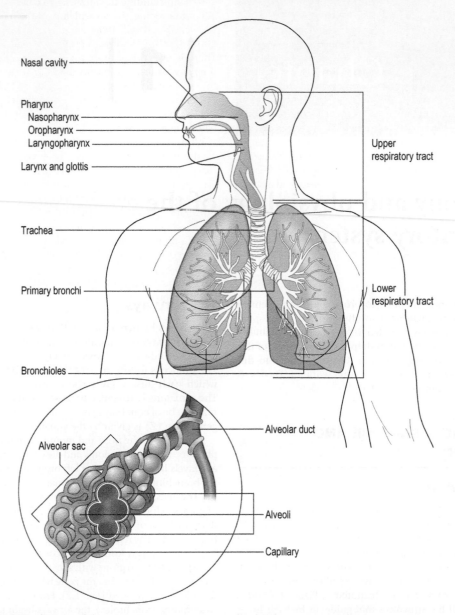

Figure 1.1 Schematic diagram of the respiratory system. See text for details.
(With permission from Thibodeau GA, Patton KT, 1996. Anatomy and physiology, 3rd edn. Mosby, St Louis.)

The alveoli

The branching structure of the lungs is an impressive work of evolution that has resulted in adult human lungs having a combined surface area of about 60 m² (646 square feet), which is about the same as a singles badminton court and about 40 times the area of the skin (see Fig. 1.23). Why the need for such a huge area? Like so much of evolution, the respiratory system is a slave to the laws of physics. As will be described in detail in the next section, the exchange of oxygen (O_2) and carbon dioxide (CO_2) between the 300 million alveoli and the capillaries surrounding them occurs via passive diffusion. For this process to keep pace with the metabolic needs of the average person, especially during exercise, a vast surface area (number of alveoli and capillaries) is required for diffusion.

However, this vast lung surface area would be of little use without the unique and intimate interrelationship that exists between the alveoli and their capillary network.

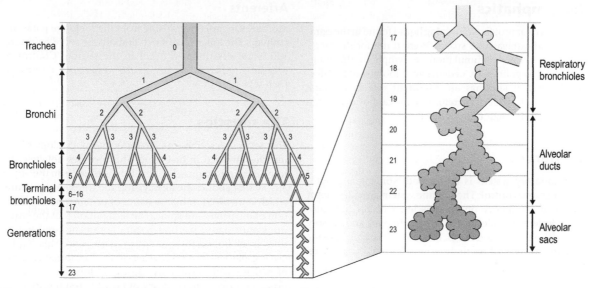

Figure 1.2 Diagram illustrating the branching structure of the lung airways.
(With permission from Davies A, Moores C, 2010. The respiratory system. Churchill Livingstone, London, p.15, Fig. 2.4.)

Figure 1.3 illustrates the key feature of this structure, i.e., the minimal distance separating the alveolar air from the capillary blood. Note that on one side of the capillary the alveolar and capillary cells fuse to form a very thin septum, whilst on the opposite side of the capillary the septum is thicker, providing stability and resisting collapse.

The epithelial junctions are sufficiently leaky to allow the passage of water and solutes between the plasma and interstitial fluid, but not larger molecules, whose osmotic potential would cause oedema. These leaks also facilitate the movement of macrophages into the alveolus, where they scavenge foreign bodies (both organic and inorganic). Lining the alveoli and conducting airways is a fluid layer containing surfactant; the importance of this layer for diffusion and normal lung mechanics is explained in subsequent sections. Suffice to say, at this point, dissolving in this layer is one of the sequential steps that O_2 and CO_2 must pass through on their journey.

The blood vessels

The lungs have two blood supplies. The first arises from the right ventricle and carries deoxygenated blood via the pulmonary artery to the pulmonary capillaries, and thence the pulmonary vein back to the left atrium. The vessels follow the airways in connective tissue sheaths. Unlike the systemic circulation, pulmonary arterioles have very little smooth muscle. The capillaries traverse a number of alveoli before combining to form venules and veins. The latter do not follow the same branching route as the arteries, but instead run along septa that separate segments of the lungs.

The second circulation in the lungs arises from the aorta as the bronchial arteries, which meet the metabolic requirements of the conducting airways by perfusing the walls of the airways as far as the respiratory bronchioles (after which O_2 requirements are met by alveolar gas exchange). Around one-quarter to one-third of the venous effluent from the bronchial circulation drains into the bronchial veins and thence to the right atrium. The remainder drains directly into the pulmonary veins via bronchopulmonary–arterial anastomoses, contributing to shunting of deoxygenated blood into the pulmonary veins. This shunt is the reason that the alveolar to arterial pressure difference for oxygen exists (see section 'Gas exchange, Diffusion' below).

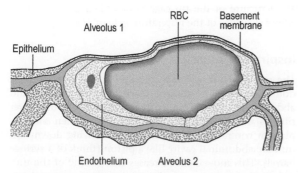

Figure 1.3 Drawing taken from an electron micrograph section of an alveolus showing the alveolar–capillary membrane. RBC = red blood cell.
(With permission from Davies A, Moores C, 2010. The respiratory system. Churchill Livingstone, London, p.18, Fig. 2.9.)

The lymphatics

Lymph is a clear protein-containing liquid found in the extracellular and extravascular spaces. Were it not for the lungs' lymphatic system, accumulation of lymph in the lungs would lead to pulmonary oedema and flooding of the alveoli. The system also has an important role in immune defence of the lungs. Lymph returns to the cardiovascular system through the right thoracic duct.

The nerves

The respiratory system is under both somatic and autonomic nervous control. The somatic system provides motor control of respiratory pump muscles, whereas the autonomic system provides both motor (efferent) and sensory (afferent) nerves to the lungs. For information on somatic nerve innervation of respiratory muscles see 'The muscles' (below).

Innervation of airways

The lungs are innervated exclusively by autonomic nerves, and there is no voluntary control of airway smooth muscle. Similarly, there is no sympathetic nervous control of airway smooth muscle; a sympathetic supply is present anatomically, but it appears to have no functional relevance for airway smooth muscle control. The only source of sympathetic bronchodilation is from circulating epinephrine (adrenaline) secreted by the adrenal gland, which acts on airway smooth muscle β_2-receptors. In contrast, the parasympathetic supply to airway smooth muscle is extremely important. It also innervates mucous glands and blood vessels. The release of acetylcholine from these parasympathetic cholinergic fibres stimulates smooth muscle contraction, leading to bronchoconstriction, or bronchospasm. There is a continuous basal tone within the system, which produces a small amount of basal bronchoconstriction. This can be eliminated by circulating adrenaline, and is the reason that airway calibre increases for a short time after exercise in healthy people.

Secretory cells respond to parasympathetic stimulation by increasing the production of mucous glycoproteins, making secretions thicker, whereas sympathetic stimulation makes them more watery.

Innervation of blood vessels

The blood vessels of the lungs are innervated by both branches of the autonomic nervous system. In contrast to the airway smooth muscle, the most important functional connection is the sympathetic branch, which induces vasoconstriction. However, this activation appears to be associated with a limited range of situations, e.g., 'fight or flight' and heavy exercise.

Afferents

Most sensory afferents arising from the lungs are parasympathetic. The lungs have a rich and diverse set of receptors, which are described in detail in the section 'Control of breathing, Afferent inputs to the respiratory controller' (below).

The muscles

This section describes the anatomy and physiology of the muscles involved in breathing. This includes not only the respiratory pump muscles, but also the muscles in the upper airway that abduct the airway, and the trunk musculature, which is involved in maintenance of posture and stabilization of the pelvis and spine. The recognition that the entire trunk musculature has both respiratory and non-respiratory roles is an important concept to grasp, since this 'multitasking' has a profound bearing on the functional capacity of patients with respiratory muscle dysfunction. This section will provide an overview of how the respiratory muscles function, and interact, during exercise. It will also consider how their function can be limited by factors such as lung volume and air-flow rate. This knowledge will help to establish the rationale for a functional approach to training of the respiratory and other trunk muscles.

Respiratory pump muscles

The respiratory pump muscles are a complex arrangement that form a semi-rigid bellows around the lungs. Essentially, all muscles that attach to the rib cage have the potential to generate a breathing action, but the principal muscles are shown in Figure 1.4. Muscles that expand the thoracic cavity are inspiratory muscles and induce inhalation, whereas those that compress the thoracic cavity are expiratory and induce exhalation. These muscles possess exactly the same basic structure as all other skeletal muscles, and they work in concert to expand or compress the thoracic cavity. The structure of the rib cage is described in the section 'Gross structure of the respiratory system' (below).

Inspiratory muscles

The principal muscle of inspiration is the diaphragm, a domed sheet of muscle that separates the thoracic and abdominal cavities. The diaphragm attaches to the lower ribs, as well as to the lumbar vertebrae. When the diaphragm contracts, the dome flattens, moving downward into the abdominal cavity like a piston (think of a syringe barrel). This movement increases the volume of the thoracic cavity, creating a negative pressure that is proportional to the extent of its movement, and thus, to the force of contraction. Diaphragm contraction also induces the lower ribs to move upward and forward, which also increases thoracic volume. The ribs move outward because the central

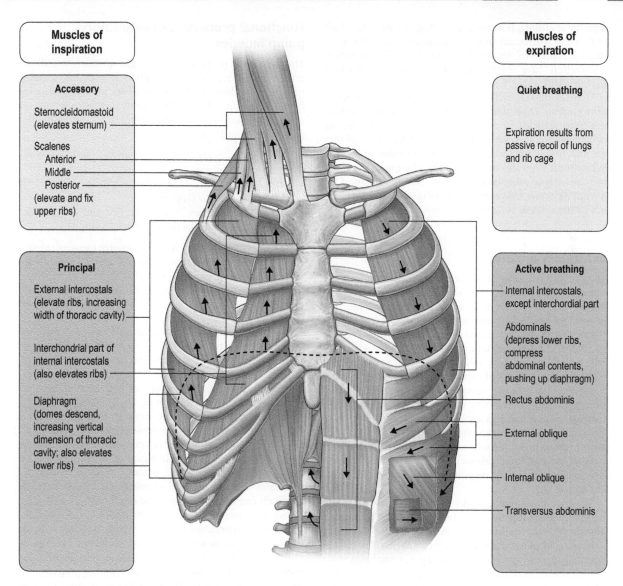

Muscles of inspiration

Accessory

Sternocleidomastoid (elevates sternum)

Scalenes
Anterior
Middle
Posterior
(elevate and fix upper ribs)

Principal

External intercostals (elevate ribs, increasing width of thoracic cavity)

Interchondrial part of internal intercostals (also elevates ribs)

Diaphragm (domes descend, increasing vertical dimension of thoracic cavity; also elevates lower ribs)

Muscles of expiration

Quiet breathing

Expiration results from passive recoil of lungs and rib cage

Active breathing

Internal intercostals, except interchordial part

Abdominals (depress lower ribs, compress abdominal contents, pushing up diaphragm)

Rectus abdominis

External oblique

Internal oblique

Transversus abdominis

Figure 1.4 The respiratory pump muscles.

tendon of the diaphragm (at the crown of the dome) pushes down onto the liver and stomach, which act as a fulcrum. This has the effect of raising the edges of the diaphragm, which are connected to the rib margins, forcing them upward and outward. When the diaphragm moves downward into the abdominal compartment, it also raises intra-abdominal pressure and assists the abdominal muscles in stabilizing the spine. Contraction of the diaphragm is controlled by a single nerve, the phrenic nerve, which originates from the 3rd to the 5th cervical vertebrae.

The muscles of the rib cage are known as the intercostal muscles because they are located in the space between adjacent ribs. Each space contains a layer of inspiratory and a layer of expiratory muscle fibres. The inspiratory intercostal muscles form the outer layer, and they slope downward and forward; contraction causes the ribs to move upward and outward, similar to the raising of a bucket handle. Contraction of these muscles also serves to stabilize the rib cage, making it more rigid, as well as bringing about flexing movements. The stiffening of the rib cage enables it to oppose the tendency to collapse slightly under the influence of the negative pressure generated by the movement of the diaphragm. Without this action, the rib cage would distort, and the action of the diaphragm would be less mechanically efficient, thus wasting energy. Intercostal muscle contraction also brings about stiffening of the rib cage during lifting, pushing and pulling movements, which makes the intercostal muscles important contributors to these actions. The nerves that control intercostal muscle contraction have their origin in the thoracic vertebrae (1st to 11th).

There are also muscles in the neck region with an inspiratory action. The scalene and sternocleidomastoid (sternomastoid) muscles are attached to the top of the sternum, upper two ribs and clavicle at one end; at the other end they are attached to the cervical vertebrae and mastoid process. When these muscles contract they lift the top of the chest, but the scalene muscles are also involved in flexion of the neck. The nerves that control these muscles have their origin in the cervical vertebrae.

Expiratory muscles

The principal muscles of expiration are those that form the muscular corset of the abdominal wall. The most well known and visible of these is the rectus abdominis; the other three muscles are less visible, but arguably more functionally important: the transversus abdominis and the internal and external oblique muscles. When these muscles contract, they pull the lower rib margins downwards and compress the abdominal compartment, raising its internal pressure. The pressure increase tends to push the diaphragm upwards into the thoracic cavity, inducing an increase in pressure and expiration. However, these muscles come into play as respiratory muscles only during exercise or forced-breathing manoeuvres; resting exhalation is a passive process brought about by the recoil of the lungs and rib cage at the end of inspiration (due to stored elastic energy).

The four abdominal muscles involved in breathing also have important functions as postural muscles: in rotating and flexing the trunk, and when coughing, speaking (or singing) and playing wind instruments. The compression and stiffening of the abdominal wall generated by contraction of the abdominal muscles also optimize the position of the diaphragm at the onset of inspiration. This also enhances spinal stability and postural control.

The rib cage also contains muscles with an expiratory action. These are the internal intercostal muscles, which slope backward; contraction causes the ribs to move downward and inward, similar to the lowering of a bucket handle. Both internal and external intercostal muscles are also involved in flexing and rotating of the trunk.

Other respiratory muscles

Theoretically, any of the muscles that attach to the rib cage have the potential to function as respiratory muscles. However, they do so only under extreme conditions such as after spinal injury, or during severe respiratory distress.

Functional properties of respiratory pump muscles

The functional properties of any given muscle are determined by the type of muscle fibres it contains. Human muscles have three main types of fibres, and most muscles contain a mixture of these, in differing proportions. The relative proportions of these three fibre types determine the properties of each muscle:

- *Type I:* Slow contracting and relatively weak, but very resistant to fatigue
- *Type IIA:* Moderately fast and strongly contracting, with high resistance to fatigue
- *Type IIX (also known as type IIB):* Fast and very strong, but with only moderate resistance to fatigue.

Type I and IIA fibres have a high oxidative capacity (ability to use oxygen to liberate energy) and a high to moderate density of blood capillaries (delivering oxygen). These fibres are also known as oxidative fibres, and they are capable of sustaining activity for prolonged periods without becoming fatigued.

It comes as no surprise to learn that the proportion of oxidative fibres (type I and type IIA) within the diaphragm and inspiratory intercostals is approximately 80% (Gollnick et al, 1972), whilst that of the expiratory intercostals is almost 100%. This compares with around 35–45% for limb muscles (Gollnick et al, 1972). The fibres of the abdominal muscles tend to be much more variable in their composition, reflecting the multiplicity of their roles. Another important factor determining muscle fatigue is its blood supply. Inadequate blood flow (ischaemia) not only limits oxygen delivery, it also limits the delivery of substrates and the removal of metabolic by-products, all of which can hasten fatigue. The diaphragm and rib cage muscles are supplied by numerous arteries. The diaphragm, for example, is perfused by three arteries, as well as benefiting from anastamoses that provide collateral sources of blood flow between arteries. The diaphragm also has an extremely dense capillary network and a capacity to increase its blood flow that exceeds that of limb muscles (Polla et al, 2004). The diaphragm maintains perfusion at contraction forces that occlude blood flow in limb muscles. This advantage derives from the fact that it is a thin sheet of muscle that produces a negative intrathoracic pressure during contraction; this pressure gradient maintains blood flow (Buchler et al, 1985). It has been suggested that this abundant and persistent arterial supply protects the diaphragm fibres from ischaemia (Hussain, 1996), providing resistance to fatigue.

In the past, the highly fatigue-resistant characteristics of the respiratory pump muscles contributed to a key assumption regarding the likelihood that the respiratory muscles contributed to exercise limitation. Physiologists assumed that the respiratory pump muscles, especially the diaphragm, were so well evolved from their continuous work that they were immune to fatigue. It wasn't until the 1990s that this myth was finally shattered, when exercise-induced diaphragm fatigue was measured in healthy young athletes (see Ch. 3, section 'Respiratory muscle involvement in exercise limitation, Healthy people').

Upper airway muscles

The first question to address is why upper airway muscles are relevant to breathing. The simple answer is that, without them, upper airway resistance would be intolerable. During normal resting breathing, the vocal folds abduct during inhalation in order to widen the laryngeal glottic opening, permitting unobstructed air flow through the larynx (Brancatisano et al, 1984). This occurs via reflex activation of the posterior cricoarytenoid (PCA) muscle. Without this activity, the vocal folds would collapse across that laryngeal opening, causing an increase in resistance to upper airway flow and leading to increased breathing effort and dyspnoea. The strength of contraction of the PCA muscles has been shown to be proportional to factors that are associated with increased levels of respiratory drive, as well as the negativity of intrathoracic pressure (Suzuki & Kirchner, 1969). During vigorous breathing the action of the PCA is supplemented by contraction of the cricothyroid (CT), which acts to tension the vocal folds, increasing the anteroposterior dimension of the larynx (Hoh, 2005). Active closure of the vocal folds (adduction) is performed by the lateral cricoarytenoid muscle (LCA), thyroarytenoid (TA) and interarytenoid (IA), but only the PCA is involved in resting breathing. However, during tidal breathing most of the closure is brought about by relaxation of the PCA rather than by activation of the adductor muscles (Murakami & Kirchner, 1972). Transient, reflex modulation of the area of the laryngeal portion of the airway plays an important role in controlling breathing frequency, duty cycle and end-expiratory lung volume, as narrowing of the airway provides an important braking effect during expiration. Active adduction is associated with activities such as vocalization, coughing and straining.

The fibre type of human laryngeal muscles has not been studied nearly so extensively as limb muscles, but a number of key observations have been made with respect to the vocal fold abductors (PCA and CT). The PCA and CT contain around 66% and 45% type I fibres, respectively. The type II fibres of these muscles are limited to IIA and IIX, but the latter are very few in number. In common with limb muscles, PCA and CT appear to contain no IIB fibres (Hoh, 2005). The proportion of fast IIX fibres appears to be larger in the adductor muscles (TA and LCA), which probably imparts a higher velocity of shortening. This may be functionally important in their role as protectors of the airway (Li et al, 2004).

Because of its role in vocalization, the LCA has been studied in relation to its fatigability. Intramuscular EMG (electromyography) suggests that prolonged, loud vocalization exercises result in changes within the EMG that are consistent with the development of muscle fatigue (Boucher et al, 2006). Thus, it is reasonable to suggest that under similarly challenging conditions for abduction (e.g., vigorous breathing) PCA and CT might be similarly susceptible to fatigue. This is discussed in relation to exercise intolerance in Chapter 3 (section 'Respiratory muscle involvement in exercise limitation').

Gross structure of the respiratory system

The respiratory system is housed within the thoracic cavity, which is formed by the rib cage, vertebrae, sternum and diaphragm. Within the thorax there are three further cavities: the left and right pleural cavities and the mediastinum (Fig. 1.5).

The arrangement and movements generated by the respiratory muscles are described above (in 'The muscles'). The skeletal structures that translate the muscle actions into movements are complex. The rib cage structure is such that the vertebral articulation of the ribs is higher than the sternal attachments; consequently, the ribs slope downwards anteriorly (Fig. 1.6).

All 12 ribs articulate with the vertebrae, but only the first six connect individually to the sternum. Ribs 7–10 articulate with the lower sternum via a common cartilage, whilst

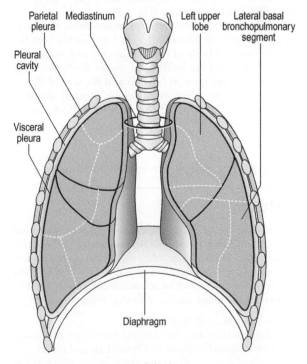

Figure 1.5 Gross anatomy of the lungs.
(With permission from Davies A, Moores C, 2010. The respiratory system. Churchill Livingstone, London, p. 21, Fig. 2.12.)

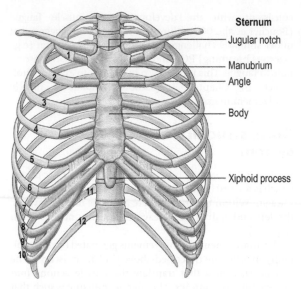

Figure 1.6 The rib cage.

ribs 11 and 12 have no anterior connections ('floating ribs'). The head of most ribs articulates with the bodies of two adjacent vertebrae, whilst their tubercles articulate with the transverse process of one of these vertebrae. Nerves and blood vessels run in a channel on the underside of the ribs called the costal groove (Fig. 1.7).

The sternum has three parts: the manubrium, body and xiphoid process (xiphisternum). The junction between the manubrium and body of the sternum (sternal angle) is a useful anatomical landmark as it marks the level of the bifurcation of the bronchi (carina) and the second rib.

The process by which breathing is brought about is described in the sections 'The muscles' and 'Mechanics of breathing'.

GAS EXCHANGE

Diffusion

Gas exchange is the process of transferring gases across the alveolar and capillary membranes and it requires both diffusion of gas and perfusion of blood. Diffusion is a passive process, and it is for this reason that the lungs have evolved the structure that we see in terrestrial mammals. The key features of the lungs' passive diffusion system are:

- An adequate diffusion gradient
- A large surface area for contact between air and blood
- A short diffusion distance between air and blood.

It is easy to see how disease can affect all three of these factors, sometimes simultaneously, leading to a reduction in diffusing capacity.

The diffusion gradient is provided by the difference in partial pressure of the gases (P). The partial pressure of a gas is the proportion of the total barometric pressure that the gas contributes. For example, oxygen (O_2) makes up 21% of the atmosphere; if barometric pressure is 760 mmHg ('standard' atmospheric pressure), the partial pressure of oxygen (PO_2) is 20.93% of 760 mmHg, i.e., 159 mmHg. As air enters the alveolus, it is warmed and humidified, and water vapour contributes 47 mmHg pressure. Since total barometric pressure cannot change, the partial pressure of all of the other gases is reduced in proportion to the amount of water added. In the case of PO_2 it is reduced to 149 mmHg:

$$PO_2 = (760 - 47) \times 0.2093 = 149$$

However, the partial pressure of oxygen within the alveoli (P_AO_2) is not 149 mmHg because the inhaled breath is diluted by the air that remained in the lungs at the end of the previous breath (end-expiratory lung volume, EELV). The extent of the dilution depends upon a number of factors, including the EELV and the tidal volume (V_T); typically P_AO_2 will be around 104 mmHg, giving a diffusion gradient of around 65 mmHg. Thus, V_T affects both the flow of gas delivered to the alveoli (via the dead space to V_T ratio; see 'Lung volumes and capacities', below), and the extent to which inspired PO_2 (P_IO_2) is diluted by the EELV (inspired to alveolar gradient). This mixing of old and new gas also affects the diffusion gradient and exchange of CO_2 because it has the effect of raising the partial pressure of CO_2 (PCO_2) in the alveoli (P_ACO_2). Thus, it is easy to see how changes in breathing pattern can influence the driving pressure for gas exchange, leading to hypoxaemia and hypercapnia.

Under normal conditions, the movement of oxygen across the alveolar and capillary membranes is so efficient that the PO_2 of the arterial blood leaving the lungs (P_aO_2) is very close to the P_AO_2. This is known as the a–A gradient, and an increase in this gradient is a sign that all is not well with the process of diffusion. Both the diffusion surface area and the diffusion distance can influence the a–A gradient, as well as how quickly the blood traverses the alveolar capillaries. Despite the diffusion gradient for CO_2 being much smaller than that for O_2 (around 5 mmHg compared with 65 mmHg, respectively), equilibration of pulmonary arterial and alveolar PCO_2 is normally achieved. This is made possible by the fact that the solubility coefficient of CO_2 is 23 times that of O_2.

The reason that solubility affects diffusion efficiency is explained by Fick's law, which describes the rate of movement of gases across a membrane:

$$\text{rate of diffusion} = \frac{A \times S(\Delta C)}{t\sqrt{MW}}$$

where A is the diffusion area, S is the solubility coefficient of the gas, ΔC is concentration gradient for the gas (alveolar to pulmonary arterial), t is the membrane thickness (alveolar plus capillary), and MW is the molecular weight of the gas molecule (its physical size). Although CO_2 is 23 times

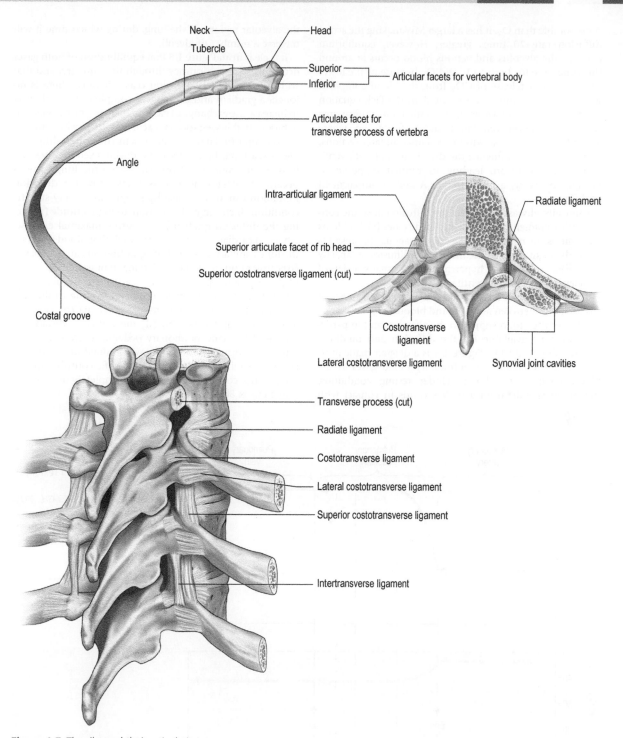

Neck

Tubercle

Head

Superior

Inferior

Articular facets for vertebral body

Articulate facet for
transverse process of vertebra

Angle

Costal groove

Intra-articular ligament

Superior articulate facet of rib head

Superior costotransverse ligament (cut)

Radiate ligament

Costotransverse
ligament

Lateral costotransverse ligament

Synovial joint cavities

Transverse process (cut)

Radiate ligament

Costotransverse ligament

Lateral costotransverse ligament

Superior costotransverse ligament

Intertransverse ligament

Figure 1.7 The ribs and their articulations.

more soluble than O_2, it has a larger MW making the actual diffusion rate 20 times greater. However, equilibrium between the alveolus and venous blood occurs at around the same time for both CO_2 and O_2 because of the lower ΔC and slower release of CO_2 from the blood compared with that of O_2. Importantly, the A in the Fick equation is not the lung surface area, but rather the surface area where there is both ventilation and perfusion, i.e., where air and blood meet. As will be explained in later sections, many factors can influence the distribution of both ventilation and perfusion, leading to ventilation/perfusion ($\dot{V}/\dot{Q}$) inequality, a reduction in A and an impairment of diffusion.

Clinically, disease can affect the diffusion area, the concentration gradient and the diffusion distance (t). Problems with diffusion manifest first as hypoxaemia, because O_2 can be brought closer to the limits of its diffusional capacity by disease. In contrast, hypercapnia is normally a sign of deficiencies of alveolar ventilation.

There is one final factor that influences the efficiency of gas exchange between alveolus and blood, viz., the characteristics of the blood supply to the alveolus, and in particular the time available for the diffusion and binding/release of O_2 and CO_2. Figure 1.8 is a diagrammatic illustration of the change in pulmonary blood gases as the blood traverses the lungs. Under resting conditions, the blood spends around 0.75 seconds in contact with

the alveolar regions of the lung, during which time it will traverse a number of alveoli.

It is clear from Figure 1.8 that equilibration of both gases occurs early in the journey through the capillary, and that within 0.25 seconds diffusion ceases because there is no longer a gradient and exchange is complete. The only way to increase the exchange of gas is to increase the throughput of blood. In this scenario, gas exchange is perfusion limited. Many people find it hard to understand that, in healthy people at sea level, breathing more during exercise does not improve the amount of oxygen leaving the lungs; this is because it's already 'as good as it gets'. However, diffusion limitation can arise in healthy people under very specific conditions including: (1) exposure to high altitude (reducing the diffusion gradient), (2) during maximal exercise, when (a) cardiac output can be so high that blood traverses the lung capillaries before full equilibration can take place, (b) cardiac output can be so high that it outstrips the ability of the respiratory pump to deliver adequate alveolar ventilation (V_A), (c) $\dot{V}/\dot{Q}$ inequality develops due to the mechanical effects of acute pulmonary oedema compressing alveoli and capillaries, and (d) the diffusion distance is increased by acute pulmonary oedema. Exercise-induced arterial hypoxaemia in healthy well-trained individuals at sea level is relatively rare and the specific contributions of the putative contributor remains incompletely understood (Guenette & Sheel, 2007).

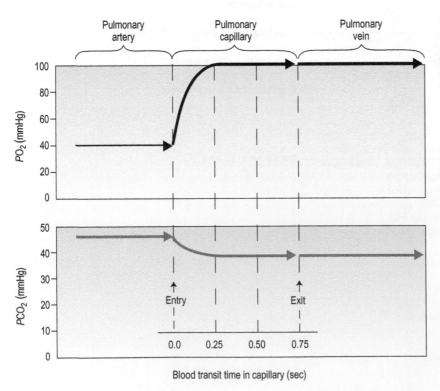

Figure 1.8 Equilibrium time for O_2 and CO_2 as blood traverses the alveolar capillaries under resting conditions.
(With permission from Hicks GH, 2000. Cardiopulmonary anatomy and physiology. WB Saunders, Philadelphia, p. 365, Fig. 12-17.)

In contrast to the rarity of diffusion limitation in healthy people, disease can inflict structural damage and functional changes that render affected individuals diffusion limited. For example:

- Loss of diffusion area due to destruction of lung tissue, and/or lung volume loss
- Alveolar hypoventilation due to mechanical constraints and breathing pattern abnormalities
- $\dot{V}/\dot{Q}$ inequality due to disturbed lung mechanics and breathing pattern abnormalities
- Increased diffusion distance due to fibrosis and oedema.

Perfusion

In the previous section, we touched upon some perfusion-related factors that affected diffusion, e.g., diffusion area. Perfusion is such an important part of the gas exchange process that it merits specific consideration in relation to gas exchange; after all, under normal conditions, gas exchange is perfusion limited.

The pulmonary vasculature is supplied via a separate, low-pressure branch of the cardiovascular system. Deoxygenated blood is returned to the lungs via the right side of the heart and the pulmonary artery. The latter is the only artery in the body to carry deoxygenated blood, which is distributed to a huge capillary network within the lungs (Fig. 1.9).

As well as illustrating the flow of blood through both branches of the circulation, the diagram in Figure 1.9 also illustrates the pressures present within each part. Systolic/diastolic pressure in the pulmonary artery is around only 24/9 mmHg, compared with 120/80 mmHg in the aorta. The pulmonary circuit is at low pressure because of the thin, delicate walls of the capillary network, which minimizes the diffusion distance. Even small increases in pulmonary arterial pressure lead to fluid leakage and pulmonary oedema. Since the pulmonary circulation receives virtually the entire cardiac output, the fact that the pressures

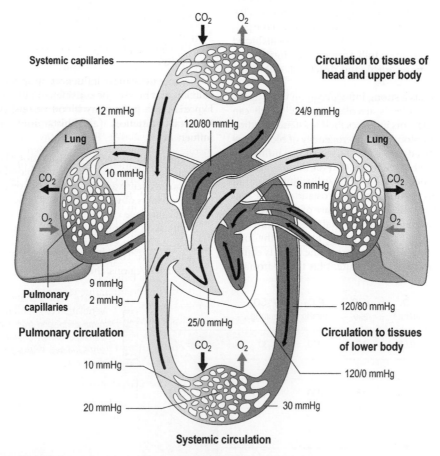

Figure 1.9 Schematic depicting pulmonary and systemic circulations and pressures.
(With permission from Thibodeau GA, Patton KT, 1995. Anatomy and physiology, 3rd edn, Mosby, St Louis.)

within it are low indicates that it has a low resistance. The reason for this low resistance is the extensiveness of its capillary network; as was described above, the capillary network can be thought of as a sheet of blood enveloping the alveoli.

Once gas exchange has taken place, the blood is returned to the left side of the heart to be distributed via the systemic circulation. In this way, the two parts of the circulation function in series, driven by a single pump. The difference in the pressures within the two sides of the circulation has a dramatic influence on the structure of the two sides of the heart: the muscular wall of the right ventricle is much thinner than that of the left, reflecting the lower resistance of the pulmonary circulation.

During exercise, cardiac output may increase from $\sim 5 \, l \cdot min^{-1}$ to $\sim 25 \, l \cdot min^{-1}$. This is accompanied by a small increase in systemic arterial blood pressure, and blood flow increases to exercising muscles because of vasodilatation in their vascular beds. In contrast, the pressure within the pulmonary circulation (receiving the same cardiac output) remains virtually unchanged during exercise. This is because the thin-walled pulmonary blood vessels distend, reducing pulmonary vascular resistance (PVR). In addition, there is recruitment of blood vessels in the pulmonary circulation; under resting conditions, not all blood vessels in the lungs are open fully (patent), but during exercise these vessels are recruited, and distended, stabilizing PVR.

One factor that has a strong influence upon the patency of pulmonary capillaries is alveolar pressure, which can compress the vessels. This increases their resistance, leading to redistribution of blood and heterogeneity of blood flow within the lungs. In addition, gravity, which also influences alveolar pressure (see 'Pressures within the thorax', below), has a potent influence upon blood flow distribution within the lungs. The effect is due to the hydrostatic pressure gradient that exists from the apex to the base of the lungs. It is very potent because pulmonary arterial pressure is so low that it is only just sufficient to pump blood to the lung apices. Perfusion pressure at the base of the lungs is equivalent to pulmonary arterial pressure, plus the hydrostatic

pressure difference between the heart and base of the lungs. At the apex, perfusion pressure is equivalent to pulmonary arterial pressure, minus the hydrostatic pressure difference between the heart and apex of the lungs. This means that blood flow is distributed preferentially to the base of the lungs. As will be described in a later section ('Pressures within the thorax'), ventilation is also distributed preferentially to the base of the lungs. However, the relative distribution of ventilation and perfusion is imperfect; there is around a three- to four-fold difference in ventilation from apex to base, compared with only a 16-fold difference in perfusion. Accordingly, there is a gradient of ventilation perfusion ratios ($\dot{V}/\dot{Q}$), and gas exchange, throughout the lungs. These variations in gas exchange also lead to local variations in the alveolar gas partial pressures. These phenomena are summarized in Figure 1.10.

In summary, the factors influencing blood-flow distribution in the lungs include:

- Gravity (via alveolar pressure and hydrostatic pressure)
- Blood volume
- Cardiac output
- Pulmonary arterial pressure
- Pulmonary arterial resistance
- Lung volume (via alveolar pressure)
- Alveolar gas pressure (influenced by lung volume and gravity).

There are three more influences upon the pulmonary circulation that need to be considered: (1) the direct effect of hypoxia upon pulmonary blood vessels, (2) the effect of humoral substances (e.g., histamine) and (3) neural influences:

- Hypoxic pulmonary vasoconstriction (HPV) is a unique response to hypoxia; in systemic blood vessels, hypoxia elicits vasodilatation. The logic of the differing responses is obvious since there is no point in perfusing areas of the lung that are poorly ventilated. In contrast, in the periphery, hypoxic tissue requires an increase in oxygen delivery and dilatation is the way to achieve this. The effect of HPV is to direct blood to ventilated regions, thereby improving $\dot{V}/\dot{Q}$ for the lung

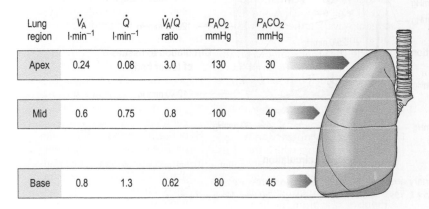

Lung region	$\dot{V}_A$ l·min⁻¹	$\dot{Q}$ l·min⁻¹	$\dot{V}_A/\dot{Q}$ ratio	P_AO_2 mmHg	P_ACO_2 mmHg
Apex	0.24	0.08	3.0	130	30
Mid	0.6	0.75	0.8	100	40
Base	0.8	1.3	0.62	80	45

Figure 1.10 Variations in alveolar ventilation ($\dot{V}_A$) and perfusion ($\dot{Q}$). (With permission from Hicks GH, 2000. Cardiopulmonary anatomy and physiology. WB Saunders, Philadelphia, p. 352, Fig. 12-9.)

as a whole. In patients with conditions such as COPD (chronic obstructive pulmonary disease), in whom alveolar hypoxia is a chronic phenomenon, HPV can result in extensive pulmonary vasoconstriction. This increases PVR and the load placed upon the right side of the heart. As a result, both pulmonary oedema and right heart failure (cor pulmonale) can ensue.

- The pulmonary circulation is also influenced by a number of endogenous substances that induce vasodilatation via nitric oxide (NO) release by pulmonary vessel endothelial cells. These substances include acetylcholine, bradykinin, thrombin, serotonin, adenosine diphosphate and histamine. In addition, mechanical factors such as stretching and vessel wall shear stress may also induce release of NO and vasodilatation.
- The pulmonary vasculature falls under the influence of the autonomic nervous system. Sympathetic stimulation releases norepinephrine (noradrenaline), which stimulates α_1-receptors in the smooth muscle of pulmonary arteries and arterioles, inducing vasoconstriction. The parasympathetic nervous system releases acetylcholine, which induces vasodilatation via the NO system described above. A recent study suggests that sympathoexcitation due to muscle metaboreflex activation induces pulmonary vasoconstriction (Lykidis et al, 2008), which has implications for gas exchange and exercise tolerance.

OXYGEN AND CARBON DIOXIDE TRANSPORT

The primary function of the respiratory system is the delivery of oxygen (O_2) and removal of carbon dioxide (CO_2) from the body. Oxygen is required to liberate energy from food, and CO_2 is a by-product of this chemical process. As we learnt in the previous section, the movement of O_2 and CO_2 occurs via a process of passive diffusion that is driven by the presence of concentration gradients. Oxygen moves down a concentration gradient from the alveoli to the cells, whilst CO_2 moves down a gradient from the cells to the alveoli. The gases are transported between the lungs and tissues via the medium of the blood, which contains specialized cells that have evolved to make this process extremely efficient. The red blood cells (RBCs), or erythrocytes, play an important role in the transport of both O_2 and CO_2, but not before the gases have dissolved briefly in the other important constituent of blood, viz., the plasma. The ability of the plasma to transport O_2 in simple solution is extremely limited (3 ml·l^{-1}), but evolution has provided an answer to this limitation in the form of haemoglobin (Hb). This important molecule is contained within the RBCs, and without it multicellular animals could not have evolved beyond a worm-like collection of cells. Haemoglobin also plays a role in CO_2 transport, but it is only one of a

number of ways in which CO_2 is transported. The addition of CO_2 to the blood must be regulated very carefully because it forms carbonic acid in solution. Hence, the blood contains a number of protein buffers as well as bicarbonate and phosphate that minimize changes in blood pH. As we will see in the section on acid–base balance, breathing has a vital role to play in pH homeostasis.

Oxygen transport

Without haemoglobin, the O_2-carrying capacity of the plasma (3 ml·l^{-1}) would necessitate a blood flow through the lungs of 40 l·min^{-1} in order to meet a typical resting O_2 requirement of ~ 250 ml·min^{-1}. When one considers that the maximal cardiac output of a highly trained young person is only around 30 l·min^{-1}, it is easy to see the need for Hb in an animal the size of a human being.

The molecule Hb allows the blood to carry around 20 ml·l^{-1}, which means that a normal resting cardiac output of 5 l·min^{-1} can deliver the required 250 ml·min^{-1} for resting metabolism. Each Hb molecule consists of a protein (globin) and haem (an iron-containing pigment). Globin consists of four protein chains (two α and two β), each connected to a haem group; thus each Hb contains four protein chains and four haem groups (Fig. 1.11). Each of the four haem groups can bind to one O_2 molecule, so conceptually each Hb molecule has four 'hooks' available to attach to four molecules of O_2.

Oxygen binds to the haem groups of Hb in a reversible reaction, that is driven towards the formation of oxyhaemoglobin (HbO$_2$) by high PO_2, and towards deoxyhaemoglobin (Hb) and O_2 by low PO_2:

$$Hb + O_2 \leftrightarrow HbO_2$$

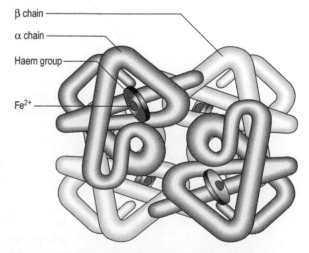

β chain
α chain
Haem group
Fe^{2+}

Figure 1.11 Schematic of the haemoglobin molecule. *(With permission from Davies A, Moores C, 2010. The respiratory system. Churchill Livingstone, London, p. 101, Fig. 8.1, top.)*

Thus, the chemical properties of Hb promote the loading of O_2 (oxygenation) in the high-PO_2 environment of the lungs, and unloading of O_2 by the low-PO_2 environment in the tissues. The binding of O_2 to a haem group changes the shape of its protein chain, making it easier for the next O_2 to bind to an adjacent haem group, and so on. This property is what gives the oxyhaemoglobin dissociation curve its characteristic sigmoid shape (Fig. 1.12).

Healthy men and women have a blood Hb content of $\sim$150 g·l^{-1} and $\sim$130 g·l^{-1} respectively. Each gram of Hb can carry 1.36 ml of O_2. When the blood is 100% saturated with O_2, all of the haem groups are bound to an O_2 molecule. Thus, when fully saturated, each litre of blood contains around 200–175 ml of O_2 (carrying capacity × Hb content). But what determines the degree of saturation?

From Figure 1.12 it is apparent that the partial pressure of oxygen (PO_2) plays a major role in determining Hb saturation (SO_2), i.e., the percentage of haem groups that are bound to O_2. The PO_2 is the partial pressure of dissolved oxygen, and its arterial level is determined by the efficiency of diffusion from alveolus to plasma. i.e., movement of O_2 from an area of high to an area of low PO_2. Although 100% saturation may, on the face of it, indicate efficient O_2 transport, the Hb content needs to be borne in mind when interpreting this (see Fig. 1.12 for details).

Whether O_2 is loaded or unloaded from the Hb is determined by the prevailing PO_2. In Figure 1.12 it is apparent that there is a range over which loading (association) and unloading (dissociation) take place. The difference in the

gradient of the two regions has important functional consequences, since it means that loading takes place over a wide range of PO_2, with the result that over 90% saturation can be achieved from a PO_2 as low as 60 mmHg. Similarly, when the blood reaches the tissues, where unloading is required, relatively small decreases in PO_2 result in a large unloading of O_2. In theory, blood and tissue PO_2 will equilibrate given sufficient time; however, this does not arise under normal circumstances because the blood transits the tissues before equilibration can take place. In anaemia, though, where O_2 content is low, unloading even a small amount of O_2 causes a steep fall in blood PO_2 (because the absolute amount of O_2 is low) reducing the driving pressure for further movement of oxygen to the tissues. Under these conditions, the supply of O_2 to the tissues is impaired, creating tissue hypoxia despite normal arterial PO_2, and saturation levels.

The position of the oxyhaemoglobin dissociation curve on the PO_2 axis undergoes cyclic changes as the blood navigates the body. The curve shifts left or right depending upon the local conditions, and this is another property that has evolved to optimize loading and unloading of O_2. There are four factors that determine the position of the curve on the PO_2 axis (Fig. 1.13):

- *Blood pH:* The hydrogen ion concentration [H^+] influences the affinity of Hb for O_2. Increases in [H^+] (decrease pH) decrease affinity and shift the curve rightwards, a phenomenon known as the Bohr shift.

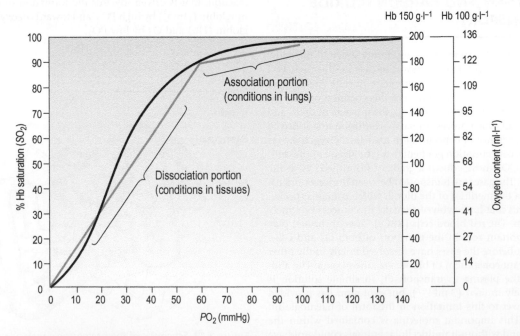

Figure 1.12 Association and dissociation of oxygen from haemoglobin (Hb). Note that the blood of a patient with anaemia, who may have a Hb content of only 100 g·l^{-1}, can carry only 136 ml·l^{-1} of O_2 (O_2 content) when fully saturated, compared to an O_2 content of 175–200 ml·l^{-1} in someone with normal Hb content of 150 g·l^{-1}; but both people may have fully saturated Hb. *(With permission from Beachey W, 1998. Respiratory care anatomy and physiology, 2nd edn. Mosby, St Louis, p. 140, Fig. 8.5.)*

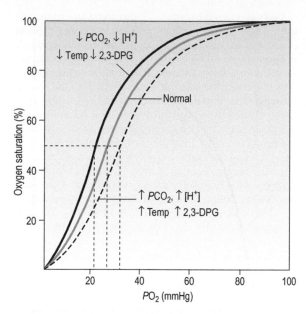

Figure 1.13 Effects of blood pH [H^+], carbon dioxide partial pressure (PCO_2), temperature (Temp), and 2,3-diphosphoglycerate (2,3-DPG) upon the position of the oxyhaemoglobin dissociation curve.
(With permission from Beachey W, 1998. Respiratory care anatomy and physiology, 2nd edn. Mosby, St Louis, p. 143, Fig. 8.10.)

This promotes unloading of O_2, but does not affect loading (because the curve is flat in this region). The conditions under which [H^+] is elevated are the conditions that exist in metabolizing tissues. A decrease of as little as 0.2 pH units can increase the release of O_2 by 25% at tissue levels of PO_2.

- *Carbon dioxide:* As mentioned earlier, CO_2 reacts with Hb (see next section) to form carboxyhaemoglobin. This reaction also shifts the curve rightwards, promoting unloading of O_2 in the tissues, where CO_2 is higher, and vice versa in the lungs.
- *Temperature:* An increase in temperature also shifts the curve to the right. Metabolizing tissues are warmer and have higher O_2 requirements; the shift promotes unloading of O_2 in warm tissues, and vice versa in cold tissues (where metabolism and O_2 requirements are lower).
- *2,3-Diphosphoglycerate (2,3-DPG):* 2,3-DPG is synthesized in RBCs and appears to be an important adaptive mechanism in conditions where tissue oxygen is low (anaemia, high altitude), or tissue O_2 consumption is high (high intensity exercise). Elevation of 2,3-DPG shifts the curve rightwards. The level of 2,3-DPG is also elevated in diseases where there is hypoxaemia, such as COPD.

Thus, under conditions where oxygen demand is high at the tissue level, the associated increases in H^+, CO_2, temperature and 2,3-DPG (e.g., exercise) shift the curve rightwards, promoting the unloading of O_2.

Carbon dioxide transport

The removal of CO_2 from the body is also driven by a concentration gradient from tissue to plasma and RBC. Most of the CO_2 in the blood is transported in the plasma, either in simple solution, as bicarbonate (HCO_3^-), or in combination with proteins (carbamino compounds). The much smaller amount of CO_2 carried in the RBCs belies the huge importance of the RBCs in CO_2 transport; the RBCs are responsible for converting the CO_2 into HCO_3^-, which is then transported in the plasma.

The CO_2 in solution in the plasma undergoes a reversible reaction that produces bicarbonate and hydrogen ions. The latter must be buffered by combining the H^+ with plasma proteins. The direction of the reversible reaction is determined by the concentration of the molecules at each stage, but in plasma, its rate is slow:

$$CO_2 + H_2O \leftrightarrow H_2CO_3 \leftrightarrow HCO_3^- + H^+$$

Plasma proteins also combine with CO_2 directly to form carbamino compounds, a reaction that also liberates H^+, which must be buffered:

$$\text{protein}-NH_2 + CO_2 \leftrightarrow \text{protein}-NHCOO^- + H^+$$

At the tissue level, even small additions of CO_2 to the blood induce a rapid increase in PCO_2, which creates a driving pressure that promotes movement of CO_2 into the RBCs. The combination of CO_2 with water is slow in the plasma, but is catalysed by carbonic anhydrase inside the RBC, driving the production of HCO_3^- and H^+ inside the RBC. The reaction is kept in motion by the removal of H^+ by Hb, and the diffusion of HCO_3^- into the plasma. The loss of the negative HCO_3^- from the RBC would result in a change in the electrical charge of the RBCs, were it not for the movement of chloride ions (Cl^-) into the RBC from the plasma (chloride shift; Fig. 1.14). The chloride shift also ensures the continued production and movement of HCO_3^- out of the RBC.

Inside the RBC, CO_2 combines readily with Hb to form carbamino haemoglobin ($Hb-NHCOO^-$):

$$Hb-NH_2 + CO_2 \leftrightarrow Hb-NHCOO^- + H^+$$

The H^+ produced by this reaction, as well as those produced by the hydration of CO_2 ($CO_2 + H_2O \leftrightarrow H_2CO_3 \leftrightarrow HCO_3^- + H^+$), are also buffered by Hb. It is important to understand that Hb carries O_2 and CO_2 at different sites: O_2 in combination with its haem groups, and CO_2 in combination with its amino groups. The deoxygenation of Hb at the tissue level increases the affinity of Hb for CO_2 (Haldane effect). In contrast, carboxyhaemoglobin has a decreased affinity for O_2 (Bohr effect). Thus, at a given PCO_2, deoxygenated blood carries more CO_2 than oxygenated blood. Deoxyhaemoglobin is also a weaker acid than oxyhaemoglobin and can therefore accept more H^+, increasing the ability of the blood to carry CO_2.

At the lungs, CO_2 is released readily, and the oxygenation of Hb reduces its affinity for CO_2 (see Fig. 1.14). All of the

At the tissues

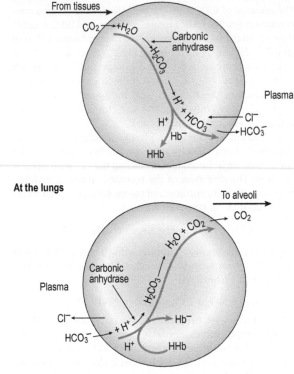

Figure 1.14 Schematic illustrating the formation of bicarbonate within red blood cells.
(With permission from Davies A, Moores C, 2010. The respiratory system. Churchill Livingstone, London, p. 109, Fig. 8.6, top.)

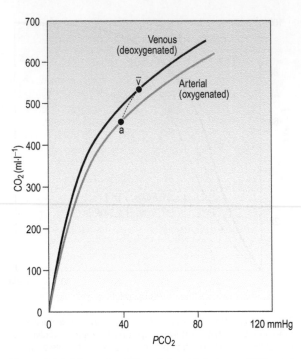

Figure 1.15 Schematic of the relationship between PCO_2 and the CO_2 content of the blood. See text for further explanation.
(With permission from Davies A, Moores C, 2010. The respiratory system. Churchill Livingstone, London, p. 111, Fig. 8.8.)

reactions above move to the left, CO_2 is released from the RBCs, it transits the plasma in solution and is then blown off via the lungs. Of the CO_2 eliminated at the lungs, 8% was transported there in simple solution, 80% as bicarbonate and 12% as carbamino compounds.

Figure 1.15 shows the relationship between PCO_2 and the CO_2 content of the blood. Note two differences compared with the oxygen dissociation curve in Figure 1.13: (1) it is much more linear, and (2) because there is no carrier molecule the *y*-axis is content, not saturation. In addition, because of the Haldane effect described above, the physiological dissociation curve is as indicated by the short dashed line. Consequently, additional CO_2 is loaded and unloaded when O_2 is being unloaded and loaded, respectively.

ACID–BASE BALANCE

Neutral pH is 7.0, but a normal plasma pH is 7.4; a decrease from 7.4 is reflective of acidaemia, whereas an increase reflects alkalaemia. The acid–base balance refers to the regulation of hydrogen ion concentrations [H^+] within the range that is compatible with life (7.0–7.8 pH units). Why are H^+ ions so problematic for biological systems? The most important effect of changes in [H^+] is to alter the ability of proteins to catalyse biochemical reactions. When proteins bind to H^+ the shape of the protein changes; optimal catalytic function is associated with occupancy of a specific number of H^+-binding sites. Accordingly the presence of too many, or too few, H^+ ions affects the efficiency of biochemical processes that are catalysed by enzymes and can stop them altogether, as well as causing irreversible damage to enzymes.

Acids are defined by their ability to donate H^+ ions (protons), whereas bases are defined by their ability to accept H^+. When acids and bases are mixed in aqueous solution, they react with one another to produce a neutral salt and water. For example, when hydrochloric acid (HCl) and sodium hydroxide (NaOH) are mixed in solution, the following reaction takes place:

$$H^+Cl^- + Na^+OH^- \rightarrow Na^+Cl^- + H_2O$$

Metabolism generates H^+ ions constantly, so their continuous regulation is essential for normal physiological function. Cellular proteins play the most important role in this regulation, since their negatively charged regions combine readily with H^+, buffering the H^+. Buffers are chemicals that either take up or release H^+, thereby providing short-term stability of $[H^+]$ and pH. However, the capacity of the protein buffer system is finite and buffers provide only a temporary solution to the H^+ problem, which can only be resolved completely by removal (excretion) of the H^+ ions from the body.

Metabolic acids are of two types: (1) volatile, which are removed from the body in gaseous form (CO_2), and (2) non-volatile, which are excreted in urine (primarily acids of sulphate and phosphate). It will be clear from the preceding section that the respiratory system is able to influence both blood and tissue pH, via control of CO_2; indeed, this is one of its important functions, and around 80% of the body's acid load is removed via the lungs.

Since this book is about the respiratory system, the current section will focus upon the role of breathing in acid–base balance. A more comprehensive description of the broader topic of acid–base balance can be found elsewhere (Davies & Moores, 2010).

The contribution of the respiratory system to acid–base regulation is exerted via its influence upon the volatile carbonic acid (H_2CO_3), which is formed when CO_2 dissolves in water:

$$CO_2 + H_2O \leftrightarrow H_2CO_3 \leftrightarrow HCO_3^- + H^+$$

Carbonic acid is a weak acid, which means that it does not dissociate completely to liberate H^+, i.e., it liberates fewer H^+ ions than a strong acid. Because this reaction is reversible, addition of H^+ or removal of CO_2 drives the equation to the left, effectively mopping up H^+.

Although the system mops up H^+ ions that are added to the blood, its buffering power lies in its ability to get rid of CO_2, and not in the ability of HCO_3^- to combine with H^+. Elevation of both H^+ and CO_2 increases the drive to breathe, thus excreting CO_2 from the lungs. The kidney assists in the buffering process by excreting HCO_3^-, so that the ratio of HCO_3^- to CO_2 remains at 20. The beauty of this respiratory/renal buffering system is that, unlike other buffers such as haemoglobin, it is infinite.

The interrelationship of HCO_3^-, CO_2 and pH is described by the Henderson–Hasselbach equation:

$$pH = pK + \log\frac{[HCO_3^-]}{[CO_2]}$$

where pK is the pH at which the system works best to resist changes in pH; for normal arterial blood, its value is 6.10. By knowing two of the three variables (HCO_3^-, CO_2 or pH), it is possible to calculate the third. Similarly, by knowing pH and pK, the ratio of HCO_3^- to CO_2 can be calculated (normally 20). Thus the equation allows prediction of the consequences of changes to each of the variables, as well as diagnosis of the source of abnormalities. An excellent tool for this purpose is the so-called Davenport diagram (Fig. 1.16), which despite being two dimensional is able to accommodate the three dimensions of HCO_3^-, CO_2 and pH by using isopleths of differing concentrations of CO_2 (PCO_2; the dotted lines on Fig. 1.16).

The Davenport diagram also makes the concepts of respiratory and metabolic acidosis and alkalosis extremely simple to comprehend, as well as illustrating the acute response to changes, and the chronic response after renal compensation (points 1 and 2 on the figure, respectively).

- Respiratory alkalosis results when minute ventilation ($\dot{V}_E$) exceeds that required to remove metabolic CO_2 production leading to loss of CO_2 and an increase in pH (down and to the right).

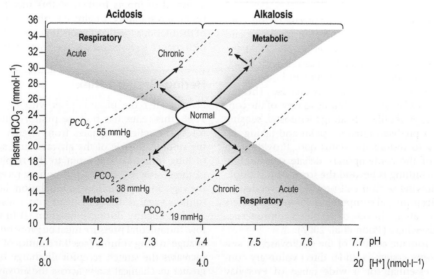

Figure 1.16 The Davenport diagram depicting the interrelationship of HCO_3^-, CO_2 and pH. See text for details. *(With permission from Davies A, Moores C, 2010. The respiratory system. Churchill Livingstone, London, p. 118, Fig. 8.11, top.)*

- Respiratory acidosis results when $\dot{V}_E$ is insufficient to remove metabolic CO_2 production leading to retention of CO_2 and a decrease in pH (up and to the left).
- Metabolic alkalosis results when there is a loss of H^+ (e.g., vomiting) leading to an increase in pH (up and to the right).
- Metabolic acidosis results when there is an excess of H^+ (e.g., exercise) leading to a decrease in pH (down and to the left).

In a clinical context, the $[H^+]$ and PCO_2 of the blood can be assessed readily, and modern equipment calculates a number of associated variables from these. The two most important are:

- Standard bicarbonate is the bicarbonate concentration of the sample if it were exposed to a standard PCO_2 of 5.3 kPa (40 mmHg), at a temperature of 37 degrees centigrade.
- Base excess and base deficit is the quantity of acid or alkali, respectively, required to return the sample (in vitro) to a normal pH at a PCO_2 of 5.3 kPa (40 mmHg), at a temperature of 37 degrees centigrade. It is zero in a normal blood sample, and is represented on Figure 1.16 as the vertical displacement due to movement along the dotted lines.

In deconditioned patients, early metabolic acidosis necessitates ventilatory compensation, which elevates the work of breathing at relatively low intensities of exercise. As a result, $\dot{V}_E$ and dyspnoea tend to be much higher in the presence of deconditioning, contributing to exercise intolerance.

CONTROL OF BREATHING

Despite over a century of research, the precise factors controlling breathing remain one of the great mysteries and controversies of physiology (Forster et al, 2012). At the heart of the mystery is the exquisite precision with which the respiratory controller is able to maintain homeostasis during metabolic disturbances such as exercise. The traditional, some would argue oversimplistic, view of the controller is that it operates like a heating thermostat, sensing departure from a predetermined set point and taking the action necessary to restore the status quo. Providing an understanding of the contemporary debate surrounding the control of breathing is beyond the scope of this book; instead, the following section will provide an overview of the system and its principal components. Interested readers can find out more about the one of the oldest controversies in physiology elsewhere (Poon et al, 2007).

Unlike the automatic control of the cardiovascular system, the respiratory system is under direct voluntary control, which is essential for a wide range of everyday activities, e.g., speaking, blowing, sniffing, straining, lifting, etc. The respiratory control centre resides within the brainstem, receiving a myriad of inputs from somatic receptors, as well as from other parts of the brain. The 'job' of the controller is to deliver a minute ventilation ($\dot{V}_E$) that is appropriate for the prevailing metabolic demand and external environment, thereby minimizing disturbances to internal homeostasis due to states such as exercise and hypoxia. In delivering a given $\dot{V}_E$, the controller must also determine an appropriate breathing pattern, i.e., tidal volume (V_T) and respiratory frequency (f_r). Furthermore, it must have sufficient plasticity that it can adapt to the effects of disease and traumatic injury. This is no mean feat, and it is perhaps unsurprising that a full understanding remains elusive. Figure 1.17 summarizes the principal factors that contribute to the control of breathing.

The rhythm generator

The basic rhythm of breathing originates from a central pattern generator located within the brainstem, which consists of the medulla and pons (Fig. 1.18). The basic pattern is refined by inputs from other regions of the brain and the thorax, producing a smoother, more refined basic pattern of breathing. During resting breathing, which requires only inspiratory muscle activity (see 'Mechanics of breathing'), it is thought that the group of inspiratory neurons in the medulla drives inspiration until a critical level of inhibition from thoracic receptors and higher brainstem centres (pons) switches off their output; this initiates passive exhalation.

Afferent inputs to the respiratory controller

To maintain homeostasis, the respiratory controller requires a myriad of inputs from receptors that monitor both the result of respiratory activity, e.g., the chemical composition of the blood, as well as factors that are linked to impending disturbance to homeostasis, e.g., limb muscle afferents.

Hering–Breuer reflex

Named after the physiologists who first described it in 1868, this reflex has both respiratory and cardiovascular roles. The reflex originates from stretch receptors within the smooth muscle of the airways, and signals the extent of lung inflation. The input to the respiratory controller of these 'slowly adapting pulmonary receptors' occurs via the vagi, and is inhibitory to inhalation, but the signal also inhibits vagal restraint of heart rate, causing heart rate to quicken slightly during inhalation. If lung compliance is low, intrapleural pressure must be more negative for a given change in lung volume (see 'Mechanics of breathing'). This increases the stretch receptor discharge because it creates greater mechanical stress across the airway, thereby terminating inhalation at a lower V_T. This contributes to the rapid shallow breathing that is a feature of conditions that 'stiffen'

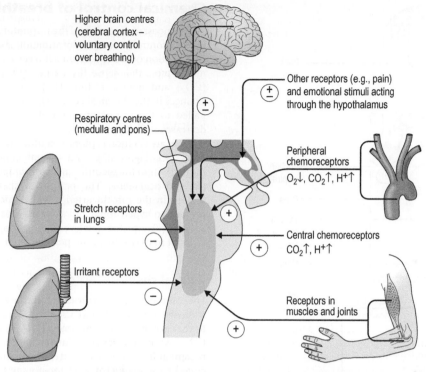

Figure 1.17 The principal afferent inputs to the respiratory control centres of the medulla and pons.

the lungs, e.g., fibrosis, pulmonary hypertension. Another contributor is the sense of effort that arises from the greater contraction force of the inspiratory muscles.

Irritant and other rapidly adapting receptors

Within the larynx and trachea, irritant receptors trigger cough, i.e., a deep inhalation followed by an explosive exhalation; this response overpowers all other inputs to the control of breathing. Within the lung, this group of receptors stimulates a more complex response. The receptors are stimulated by inhalation of irritant gases and vapours, e.g., cigarette smoke. They are also stimulated by distortion of the lung, e.g., during a pneumothorax, initiating what is sometimes referred to as a 'deflation reflex', i.e., an increase in the force and frequency of inspiratory efforts. The receptors themselves are extremely simple, comprising free nerve endings lying close to the airway epithelial surface. These lung receptors trigger either rapid, shallow breathing by curtailment of exhalation, or long, deep inhalations. Its possible that these receptors may contribute to altered breathing patterns in disease conditions such as bronchoconstriction and mucus secretion.

C-fibres (J-receptors)

The endings of these unmyelinated fibres are located close to the pulmonary capillaries (juxtapulmonary, hence

J-receptor), and in the bronchial walls. They are stimulated by increases in interstitial fluid (oedema), pulmonary vascular congestion, and by agents that are released in response to lung damage and inflammation, e.g., histamine, bradykinin and prostaglandins. Stimulation initiates a range of responses that appear appropriate in extreme lung damage, i.e., apnoea, followed by rapid shallow breathing, dyspnoea, hypotension, bradycardia, laryngospasm and skeletal muscle relaxation, but not under normal physiological conditions.

Peripheral proprioceptors and metaboreceptors

The intercostal muscles and diaphragm contain specialized receptors (muscle spindles) that respond to stretch. Muscle contraction stimulates a positive feedback loop via the spinal cord that increases motor drive to the inspiratory muscles. This response ensures that an increase in the resistance to inhalation is met with a compensatory increase in muscle recruitment.

Receptors in the muscles and joints of the locomotor system also provide positive feedback signals to the medullary controller, stimulating hyperpnoea. Some of these receptors are stimulated by passive movement of limbs, and they are thought to play a role in the control of the exercise

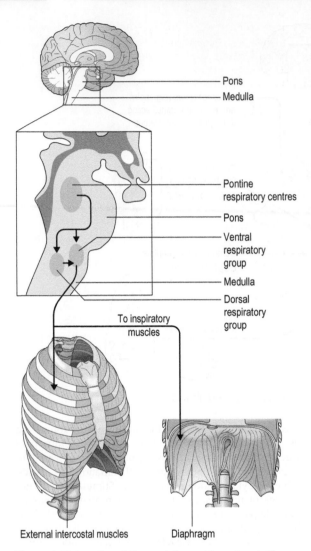

Pons
Medulla

Pontine respiratory centres
Pons
Ventral respiratory group
Medulla
Dorsal respiratory group

To inspiratory muscles

External intercostal muscles   Diaphragm

Figure 1.18 Location of the medullary and pontine rhythm generating neurons of the brainstem, which drive the inspiratory muscles.

hyperpnoea especially at the onset of exercise (phase I of the exercise hyperpnoea).

The respiratory muscles also contain unmyelinated group III and IV afferents that sense the metabolic state of the muscle, specifically the accumulation of metabolites such as lactate. These so-called metaboreceptors are present in all muscles, and although they appear to have no role in the control of breathing they are important in the reflex control of the cardiovascular system. The respiratory muscle metaboreflex has been found to play a very important part in limiting respiratory and limb muscle perfusion during exercise, and will be discussed in more detail in Chapter 3 (Sheel et al, 2001).

Chemical control of breathing

The homeostatic function of the respiratory system requires that the controller receives information about the chemical composition of the blood; thus it receives inputs from chemoreceptors that sense the oxygen (O_2), carbon dioxide (CO_2) and hydrogen ion (H^+) content of the blood. Changes in the chemical composition of the blood are signalled to the respiratory controller, which increases or decreases $\dot{V}_E$ as appropriate.

There are chemoreceptors at central and peripheral locations (see Fig. 1.17). The central chemoreceptors are located within the medulla and are responsive to hypercapnia and acidaemia. The peripheral chemoreceptors are located in the carotid arteries and aortic arch; they also respond to hypercapnia and acidaemia, as well as hypoxia. Around 80% of the total ventilatory response to CO_2 is thought to derive from the peripheral chemoreceptors.

Central chemoreceptors

The central chemoreceptors are located less than 1 mm from the ventral surface of the medulla, and respond only to changes in H^+ concentration ($[H^+]$). Their response to CO_2 is indirect, occurring via changes in $[H^+]$ in the cerebrospinal fluid (CSF). The arterial blood and CSF are separated by a semipermeable membrane that is porous to CO_2, but not to H^+ ions. Elevation of the partial pressure of CO_2 (PCO_2) of arterial blood causes diffusion of CO_2 molecules into the CSF, where they react with water to form carbonic acid (H_2CO_3). The H^+ part of H_2CO_3 stimulates the medullary chemoreceptors to increase $\dot{V}_E$. The CSF contains no protein buffers, so changes in PCO_2 stimulate breathing very quickly, but not as quickly as the peripheral chemoreceptors; thus the central chemoreceptors are thought to act primarily as monitors of steady-state PCO_2 and brain perfusion. There is no medullary sensitivity to O_2, and there is no response to changes in PCO_2 below about 35 mmHg, or above about 70 mmHg.

Peripheral chemoreceptors

The peripheral chemoreceptors are located within the carotid bodies and aortic arch, the latter making the least important input to the respiratory controller (Fig. 1.19). The receptors in these locations respond extremely quickly to changes in CO_2 by stimulating $\dot{V}_E$, and they are regarded as being the main sensing mechanisms for rapid changes in PCO_2. The peripheral chemoreceptors also provide the only means of sensing hypoxaemia and acidaemia (H^+ cannot cross the blood–brain barrier to stimulate the central chemoreceptors). The structures in which the chemoreceptors are located are highly vascular, and have an extremely high blood flow – so high that their own metabolic requirements make virtually no impact on the composition of the blood flowing through them.

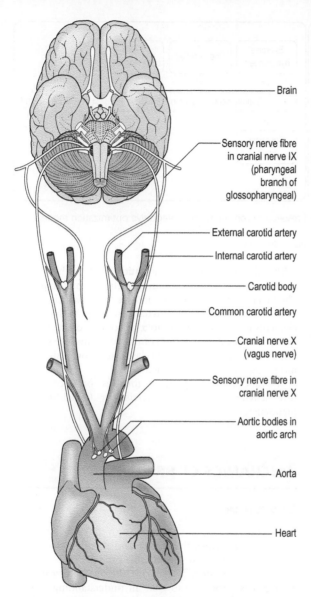

Brain

Sensory nerve fibre in cranial nerve IX (pharyngeal branch of glossopharyngeal)

External carotid artery

Internal carotid artery

Carotid body

Common carotid artery

Cranial nerve X (vagus nerve)

Sensory nerve fibre in cranial nerve X

Aortic bodies in aortic arch

Aorta

Heart

Figure 1.19 The peripheral chemoreceptors of the carotid bodies and aortic arch communicate with the respiratory controller via cranial nerves IX and X (glossopharyngeal and vagus, respectively).

At normal arterial PCO_2 and $[H^+]$, the partial pressure of oxygen (PO_2) in arterial blood must fall below around 60 mmHg before an increase in $\dot{V}_E$ is stimulated. This is because of the sigmoid shape of the oxygen dissociation curve (see 'Oxygen and carbon dioxide transport'), which dictates that haemoglobin saturation is relatively unaffected by changes in PO_2 until the 60 mmHg threshold is exceeded. Accordingly, O_2 plays no role in the control of breathing in healthy people at sea level. However, hypercapnia and acidaemia increase the sensitivity of the peripheral

chemoreceptors, so in disease states where hypoxaemia and hypercapnia coexist breathing can be stimulated very strongly, especially during exercise. In contrast hypocapnia, which arises during acute exposure to hypoxia, depresses the ventilatory response to hypoxia. The peripheral chemoreceptors are also sensitive to a reduction in their perfusion.

Control of exercise hyperpnoea

Exercise hyperpnoea has been perhaps the greatest source of controversy within respiratory physiology. One of the problems that exists in gaining an understanding of the control mechanisms is the difficulty of isolating specific inputs to the controller; there appears to be a huge amount of redundancy within the system, i.e., if one input is removed experimentally the responses appear to remain normal because another input is able to compensate for its loss. This has led to individual inputs being ruled in, or ruled out, of the control of the exercise hyperpnoea according to the specific research paradigms utilized. This is one reason why these reductionist approaches to understanding complex control systems have proved inadequate.

Traditionally, the exercise hyperpnoea was suggested to be the result of an integrated response to a range of inputs that included: (1) feedforward signals that were activated simultaneously with locomotor drive, (2) feedback signals from limb mechano- and metabo-receptors, and (3) chemical signals from the arterial blood. Unfortunately, this so-called neurohumoral theory of control has proved inadequate; it does not satisfactorily explain the ability of a system that is able to adapt to the challenges of exercise in different environments, and disease states.

Most recently, a new model has emerged, one that has its origin in the 1960s (Priban & Fincham, 1965), and has the process of optimization at its heart (Poon, 1983). The model proposes that the respiratory controller regulates $\dot{V}_E$ and breathing pattern in such a way as to 'keep the operating point of the blood at the optimum while using a minimum of energy' (Priban & Fincham, 1965). This model is attractive for a number of reasons, but primarily because it recognizes the importance of respiratory sensation in the breathing strategy that is adopted. In addition, the model predicts not only the exercise hyperpnoea, but also respiratory system responses to a range of other challenges including chemoreceptor stimulation and loaded breathing, as well as respiratory muscle fatigue and weakness. Hitherto, the ventilatory response, and the breathing pattern used to deliver it, were thought to be regulated independently via a hierarchy of discrete feedbacks (Poon et al, 1992); the optimization model incorporates control of both $\dot{V}_E$ and breathing pattern into a single, unifying paradigm. Figure 1.20 contrasts the optimization model with the traditional, reductionist approach.

Numerous studies have shown that the ventilatory response to feedback stimuli, and to integrated responses such as exercise, is modulated by the work of breathing,

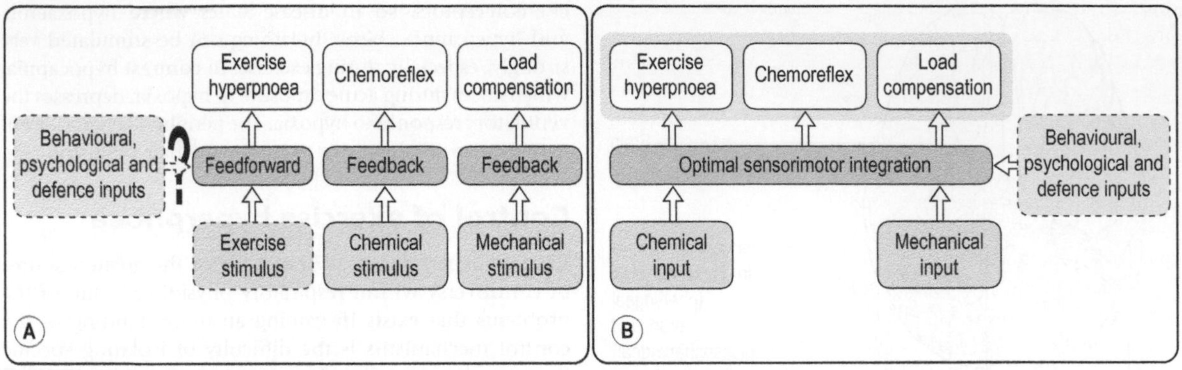

Figure 1.20 (A) The traditional hierarchical reductionist model of respiratory control, (B) the integrative optimization model of respiratory control.
(With permission from Poon CS, Tin C, Yu Y, 2007. Respir. Physiol. Neurobiol. 159, 1–13.)

suggesting that the final $\dot{V}_E$ and breathing pattern are a 'negotiated' response by the controller to a range of feedback signals (Poon et al, 2007). Importantly, the optimization model of control also predicts correctly the behaviour of breathing pattern after a period of inspiratory muscle training, since an important facet of the model is the capacity of the respiratory pump to deliver a given ventilatory response; this capacity is related directly to the condition of the inspiratory muscles, entering the model via the 'Mechanical input' and modulated via the 'Behavioural, physiological and defence inputs' in Figure 1.20B.

Respiratory muscle control

The nerves supplying the diaphragm are probably the most well known of the nervous system, but the phrenic nerves are unusual in that they are controlled almost entirely by direct innervation from the cervical region (C3–5). Furthermore, the phrenic alpha (α) motor neurons are also unusual in: (1) lacking a feedback mechanism that is responsible for terminating neural 'after-discharge' (Renshaw cells), and (2) the 'cycling' behaviour of motor unit activation; phrenic motor neurons take turns during successive inspirations, thereby recruiting different populations of fibres within the diaphragm with each contraction. This adaptation may enhance fatigue resistance.

The inspiratory and expiratory motor neurons within the spinal cord operate under a system of reciprocal inhibition such that inspiration is inhibited during expiration, and vice versa. In contrast to other skeletal muscles, this inhibition does not originate from muscle spindles within the diaphragm, but rather it occurs within the medulla.

The transition between breathing phases is smoothed by a continuation of inspiratory activity into early expiration, but also by the actions of the larynx (adduction), both of which have a braking influence on expiratory air flow. As was described above, the laryngeal abductors are activated by the respiratory controller just prior to the initiation of inspiratory air flow.

The rib cage possesses innervation from both α motor neurons, and γ (gamma) motor neurons (fusimotor nerves). The latter innervate intrafusal muscle fibres, which possess muscle spindles that sense stretch. Stretching of the spindle elements feeds back directly to α motor neurons within the spinal cord producing reflex contraction; thus, the spindles respond to increased loading (elastic and flow resistive) by increasing the force of contraction.

The abdominal expiratory muscles produce expiratory activity only during exercise or forced-breathing manoeuvres.

MECHANICS OF BREATHING

Overview

This section will explain how air is moved in and out of the lungs, and describes the elastic and flow-resistive forces that must be overcome during this process. These properties of the respiratory system are affected by disease and ageing; it is important to gain an understanding of how the work of breathing is affected by normal physiology, so that the impact of pathophysiological changes can be comprehended.

The mechanical actions of breathing are extremely familiar to everyone. These actions involve a rhythmic pumping of the chest 'bellows' that sucks air in and blows air out of the lungs. Conceptually, the breathing apparatus can be thought of as a pump consisting of an elastic balloon (lungs) inside an expandable and compressible cavity (thorax). The expansion and compression of the thoracic cavity are brought about by the actions of the complex group of muscles that surround the lungs (i.e., the respiratory muscles). These muscles bring about movements of the cavity that surrounds the lungs; changes in the volume of this cavity produce changes in the pressure within it, and this creates the gradient for movement of air in and out of the cavity.

In high-school biology classes, a simple model is often used to explain how changes in volume and pressure bring about the movement of air. The model consists of a glass bell jar (rib cage) containing a balloon (lungs); the jar is sealed at its open base by an elastic membrane (diaphragm). The model is imperfect because the walls of the bell jar, which represent the rib cage, do not expand; however, the elastic membrane provides a perfect illustration of what happens in response to movements of the major inspiratory muscle, the diaphragm. It is not difficult to see how moving the walls of the bell jar (expanding the rib cage) would bring about precisely the same changes as moving the diaphragm, i.e., an increase in volume and a fall in pressure (analogous to intrapleural pressure), which creates movement of air because of the effects of Boyle's law (see below).

The balloon in the bell jar model also illustrates another important feature of the lungs: they are elastic. In fact, both the lungs and the rib cage are elastic structures that naturally spring back to their resting positions once the forces acting on them are removed. You can experience this yourself by taking a deep breath and then relaxing; the air 'falls' out of your lungs under the pressure generated by the recoil of the lungs and rib cage (recoil pressure). During inhalation, the inspiratory muscles expand the thoracic compartment and stretch the lungs and rib cage. This stores some elastic energy within these tissues in the same way that inflating a party balloon stores elastic energy within the wall of the balloon. At the start of an inhalation, the inspiratory muscles are relaxed, and any elastic energy stored within the lungs and chest wall has been dissipated during the preceding exhalation. Thus, in healthy lungs, each intake of breath is initiated from a point where all of the forces acting on the lungs are in a state of balance. This is not the case in obstructive lung diseases such as chronic obstructive pulmonary disease, where there is premature airway closure trapping air in the lungs, thereby maintaining a positive intrapulmonary pressure. This pressure is known as intrinsic positive end-expiratory pressure ($PEEP_i$), and will be described in more detail later in the context of its effect upon inspiratory muscle loading.

The balloon analogy has another important principle to convey about the lungs and rib cage: because they are elastic, the more inflated they are the greater is the force required to change their volume. In other words, in the case of the balloon, the balloon is relatively easy to inflate at first, but greater effort is required to inflate it as it becomes larger. This property has important implications for how people breathe during exercise, especially those with airway obstruction, who are forced to breathe at higher lung volumes where the elastic load is greater. The latter phenomenon in known as 'hyperinflation' and will be described in more detail later in the context of its effect upon inspiratory muscle loading.

Turning to the balloon analogy once more, it is possible to illustrate the final principle that affects the work of breathing, i.e., the inherent air-flow resistance of the lungs. The size of the force (pressure) required to draw air into the balloons is influenced by the diameter of the tube connecting them to the outside world. If this tube is narrow, it requires a greater force to overcome the inherent air-flow resistance of the tube. The diameter of the tube is analogous to airway diameter, and airway resistance is affected by disease acutely (e.g., asthma) and chronically (e.g., bronchitis).

Pressures within the thorax

In the simple 'balloon in jar' model of the thorax described above, changes in the volume of the thorax induced changes in pressure that caused the movement of air into and out of the lungs. The drop in pressure inside the thorax when its volume is expanded is a manifestation of Boyle's law, which dictates that pressure multiplied by volume is a constant. Or, to look at it another way, if pressure decreases then volume must increase proportionately in order to maintain constancy of their interrelationship:

$$P \times V = \text{constant}$$
$$\text{therefore } P_1 \times V_1 = P_2 \times V_2 \text{ (Boyle's law)}$$

where P_1 and V_1 are the original pressure and volume, and P_2 and V_2 are the new pressure and volume.

There are a number of different pressures within the thorax, each created by the physical properties of the surrounding tissues and their movements. Furthermore, some of these pressures also differ because of the effects of gravity upon the thoracic structures. The pressure that provides the primary driving force that links respiratory muscle actions to movement of air is intrapleural pressure, which is the pressure surrounding the lungs. Even when the respiratory muscles are relaxed, intrapleural pressure (P_{pl}) remains slightly negative relative to the inside of the alveoli (alveolar pressure, P_{alv}) and to atmospheric pressure. The P_{pl} is created by a balance of two forces: the elasticity of the lungs pulling inwards and the chest wall pulling outwards (Fig. 1.21); the result is a slight vacuum of the intrapleural space (P_{pl}). Any connection between either the alveoli, or the atmosphere (through the chest wall), will

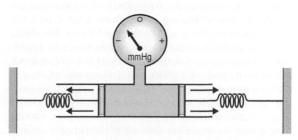

Figure 1.21 A simple model illustrating how intrapleural pressure is generated by the opposing forces of lung and chest wall elasticity.
(With permission from Davies A, Moores C, 2010. The respiratory system. Churchill Livingstone, London, p. 30, Fig. 3.2.)

cause P_{pl} to increase and the lung to collapse, as occurs in a pneumothorax.

As mentioned previously, gravity influences thoracic pressures, resulting in gradients between the uppermost point and the lowermost point within the thorax. The gradients are largest in the upright position, and are the result of the fluid behaviour of the lung parenchyma (tissue). The lungs literally hang inside the thoracic cavity, and the effect of this mass upon P_{pl} can be measured as a slightly more negative pressure at the apex of the lung than at the base. This occurs because the elastic force pulling inwards is supplemented at the top of the lungs by the force of gravity pulling the lungs downwards and away from the inside of the upper thoracic cavity. In contrast, at the base of the thorax the lungs are pressing outwards slightly against the lower thoracic cavity. This is also the reason why the basal regions of the lung are better ventilated. This may appear counterintuitive, but the more negative apical P_{pl} means that the apical alveoli are more distended, have a higher recoil pressure and are therefore less compliant (less easy to expand; see 'Lung compliance'). Accordingly, air will flow preferentially to the more compliant, basal alveoli.

Lung and thoracic cage compliance

Recalling the earlier 'balloon in jar' model of the thorax can also assist in understanding another important property of the lungs, viz., compliance. Compliance is the reciprocal of elastance, representing the ease with which a material can be stretched; the lung behaves to a certain extent according to Hooke's law, which states that an elastic structure changes dimensions in proportion to the force applied to it. In the case of the lungs, the force is pressure and the dimension is volume. The interrelationship of pressure and volume of the lungs is more complex than Hooke's law implies, because the proportionality (linearity) of the relationship is limited. Indeed, the pressure and volume relationship of the lungs is sigmoid, and also shows a property called hysteresis, i.e., it is different during inflation and deflation (Fig. 1.22).

The sigmoid shape of the pressure and volume relationship is the result of the combined effects of inherent elastic properties of the lungs and their liquid lining. The elastic and collagen fibres within the lung parenchyma are responsible for its inherent elasticity (elastance). Whilst collagen is not of itself elastic, the fibres interact with one another in such a way that the resulting structure is elastic. In diseases such as COPD there is a loss of elastin, which reduces recoil pressure and increases compliance. In contrast, fibrotic lung disease increases the amount of both elastin and collagen, increasing recoil pressure and reducing compliance.

Around half of the total elastance of the lungs derives from its millions of bubble-like alveoli, and their liquid lining. The liquid lining of the lungs processes a property

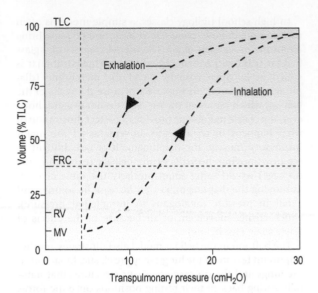

Figure 1.22 Diagram illustrating the pressure–volume relationship of the lungs during inhalation and exhalation. The differing characteristics during inflation and deflation are called hysteresis (see text for details). TLC, total lung capacity; FRC, functional residual volume; RV, residual volume; MV, minimal volume.
(With permission from Berne RM, Levy MN, 1993. Physiology, 3rd edn, Mosby, St Louis.)

called surface tension (as do all air–liquid interfaces), which acts almost like a surface skin. The tension created at the surface is the manifestation of a fundamental property of liquid surfaces, i.e., the molecules are drawn closer together to minimize the surface area of the liquid, creating surface tension. This is seen clearly in the behaviours of water droplets, which form spheres. The liquid lining of the alveoli creates a force that tends to collapse the alveoli, contributing to recoil pressure. The alveoli are prevented from collapsing by two forces: the pressure inside the alveoli and the recoil force from adjacent alveoli pulling on each other's walls. Laplace's law dictates interrelationships of the radius of curvature of a sphere (or partial sphere), the tension in its wall, and the pressure inside it:

$$P = \frac{4T}{r} \text{ (Laplace's law)}$$

where P is pressure inside the sphere, T is wall tension and r is radius of curvature. Because the alveoli have only one surface exposed to the air, $4T$ becomes $2T$ for the alveoli.

Somewhat counterintuitively, Laplace's law predicts that small spheres have a greater recoil pressure than larger spheres. In a structure like the lungs, with alveoli of differing sizes, small alveoli might be expected to empty into larger ones. However, the presence of lung surfactant in the alveolar lining fluid prevents this from happening, because surfactant lowers liquid surface tension. The net effect upon total alveolar recoil pressure is for the Laplace effect and the surface tension effects to cancel one another out, resulting in stability. It is easy to see how the destruction of alveoli by diseases such as emphysema reduce recoil pressure and increase compliance; in the next section we will see how this impacts upon airway resistance.

The compliance of the thoracic cage is the sum of chest wall compliance and compliance of the diaphragm, which transmits pressure from the abdominal compartment. The latter makes an important contribution to thoracic cage compliance (usually called chest wall compliance) in conditions where abdominal pressure is elevated, e.g., obesity, pregnancy, venous congestion. Compliance of the chest wall is affected by conditions that reduce the mobility of the rib cage, as well as factors that impede outward expansion of the surface of the skin, such as extensive burns, or tight clothing.

The individual compliances of the respiratory system behave as parallel elements, rather than series elements. Accordingly, total respiratory system compliance is given by the following equation:

$$\frac{1}{C_{Tot}} = \frac{1}{C_L} + \frac{1}{C_T}$$

where C_{Tot} is total compliance, C_L is lung compliance and C_T is thoracic compliance. Note that the combined compliance in parallel is always smaller than any of the individual compliances, whereas the opposite is true for compliances in series.

Airway resistance

Recalling the earlier 'balloon in jar' model once more, the rate of air flow into the balloon is determined by two factors: the pressure gradient (driving pressure) between atmosphere and alveolus, and the diameter of the airway. In fact, the system behaves in a similar manner to an electric circuit and follows the principle of Ohm's law, where driving pressure (voltage) equals the product of flow (current) and resistance. Accordingly, airway resistance is given by:

$$R = \frac{P_1 - P_2}{\dot{V}}$$

where R is resistance, $P_1 - P_2$ is driving pressure, and $\dot{V}$ is air flow.

The resistance to air flow through a tube is produced by friction between the gas molecules themselves, as well as friction between the gas molecules and the wall of the tube. Accordingly, resistance is greater when gas density or viscosity is higher, and tube diameter is narrower. The resistance of the respiratory system is a dynamic property that is determined by both anatomy and physiology. The anatomy of the airways is such that their branching structure results in an increase in the total cross-sectional area of the airways, which expands exponentially after the 10th generation (Fig. 1.23).

Accompanying the increase in total surface area is a decrease in the individual surface area of each airway generation. As can be seen from Figure 1.23, the rapid increase in the number of airways more than offsets the effect of their decreasing diameter upon total airway resistance. Accordingly, of the airway resistance emanating below the larynx, 80% derives from the trachea and bronchi.

Total airway resistance decreases during lung inflation, and increases during deflation. This effect is due primarily to the effect of 'parenchymal pull', also known as 'radial traction', which tethers the airways holding them open. The lung parenchyma forms a supportive structure around the airways, which upon lung inflation pulls them open, increasing their diameter and reducing their resistance to air flow. The influence of this phenomenon is especially important at low lung volumes, where resistance increases rapidly during deflation, resulting in airway closure. In young healthy individuals, radial traction ensures that airway collapse (closing capacity) occurs below functional residual capacity (FRC), but senescent degeneration of connective tissue, as well as destruction by diseases such as emphysema, elevates the closing capacity so that it occurs at or above FRC. This increases the physiological dead space, which increases the risk of hypoxaemia due to mismatch between ventilation and perfusion.

Another important factor that influences airway resistance is bronchial smooth muscle tone, which exerts an extremely powerful influence upon airway resistance. This site of variable airway resistance is in a part of the bronchial tree (generations 7–14) where the beneficial effects of airway proliferation upon total cross-sectional area are relatively modest. Accordingly, any reduction in their diameter exerts a potent influence upon resistance in this part of the bronchial tree. Conditions such as asthma influence bronchial smooth muscle tone. Readers are referred elsewhere for further information about the pathophysiology of asthma (Murphy & O'Byrne, 2010).

Exhalation mechanics

The mechanical properties of the lung determine its function, which can be assessed by measuring flow and volume-generating capacity, especially during exhalation. Before considering lung volumes and their measurement, it is helpful to gain an understanding of the mechanical factors that influence the behaviour of the airways and determine the characteristics of the expiratory flow profile.

During passive exhalation, which occurs through elastic recoil, intrapleural pressure remains negative and the pressure across the intrathoracic airways tends to keep the airways open. However, during exercise hyperpnoea and forced exhalation, the intrapleural pressure becomes positive and mechanical factors that were holding the airways open, such as radial traction, are reduced. As a result, airway diameter reduces, leading to dynamic airway collapse and attendant expiratory flow limitation (Fig. 1.24). The small airways are most vulnerable to collapse as they depend entirely upon factors such as radial traction for their patency.

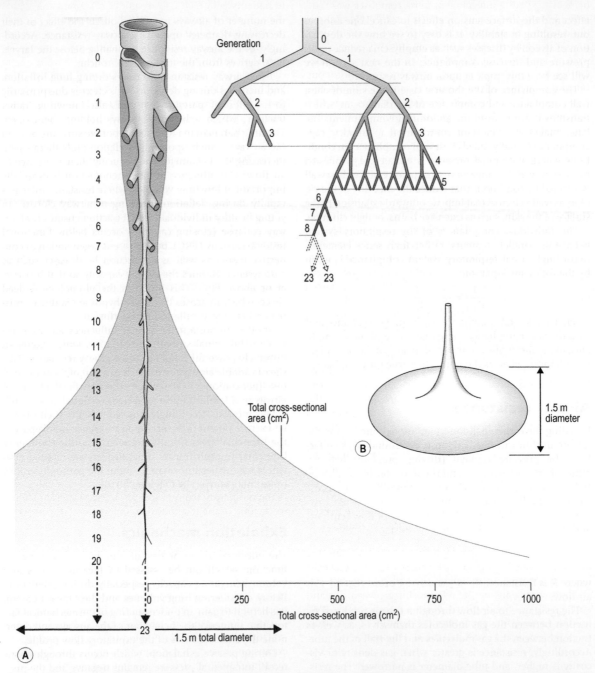

Figure 1.23 Schematic illustrating changes in airway diameter and total cross-sectional area with successive airway generation in two (A) and three dimensions (B).
(With permission from Davies A, Moores C, 2010. The respiratory system. Churchill Livingstone, London, p. 47, Fig. 4.9.)

As can be seen in Figure 1.24, during forced exhalation there is a pressure gradient inside the airways (most positive at the alveolar end, decreasing to atmospheric pressure at the mouth); there is a point along the airway tree where intrapleural pressure equals the pressure inside the airway.

This point is known as the equal pressure point (EPP), which moves progressively towards the smaller airways as lung volume decreases. This migration occurs because the contribution of the elastic recoil of the lung to the production of a positive pressure inside the airway diminishes as

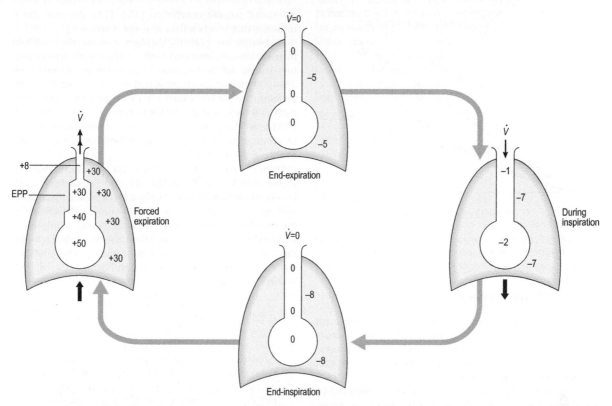

Figure 1.24 Schematic illustrating pressure changes (in cmH$_2$O) across intrathoracic airways during different phases of respiration. See text for details. EPP, equal pressure point.
(With permission from Davies A, Moores C, 2010. The respiratory system. Churchill Livingstone, London, p. 55, Fig. 4.18.)

lung volume diminishes. Air is trapped behind the collapsed airways, but exerting more expiratory force simply tightens the collapse. In healthy lungs, the EPP does not arise above FRC, but where airway walls and/or alveoli have been damaged by disease the lungs' elastic recoil and radial traction are reduced and the EPP arises above FRC. Dynamic airway collapse underlies the characteristic triangular shape of the expiratory limb of a flow volume loop in healthy lungs, as well as its scooped appearance in obstructive lung disease (see 'Lung volumes and capacities').

Effects of lung properties upon breathing

The lungs have a heterogeneous distribution of compliance, resistance and intrapleural pressure, which affect the dynamics of inflation, the distribution of air flow and the work of breathing. This arises because the system connects to the atmosphere via a single conduit (trachea), and all parts must respond within the same duration of inspiratory and expiratory time. Thus, the parts of the lung with high resistance and/or low compliance fill more slowly and/or less completely. During exercise, the time available for filling and emptying the lungs is reduced, exacerbating heterogeneity. In addition, expiratory flow limitation may slow exhalation to the extent that inhalation may commence whilst the pressure inside some airways is still positive, creating an intrinsic (i.e., auto) positive end-inspiratory pressure (PEEP$_i$). These phenomena induce a process known as hyperinflation, which maintains expiratory air flow but at a cost. Hyperinflation forces tidal volume (V_T) towards total lung capacity (TLC), where the elastic load to breathing is higher. Thus, somewhat counter-intuitively, the work of the inspiratory muscles is increased by expiratory flow limitation (see also Fig. 3.1). The heterogeneity of air distribution in the lungs also affects gas exchange via its effect upon ventilation/perfusion inequalities, i.e., parts of the lung may be perfused, but not ventilated, and vice versa, reducing the area available for gas exchange (see 'Gas exchange', above). Areas of the lung where ventilation and perfusion are mismatched, and do not contribute effectively to gas exchange, are known as alveolar dead space.

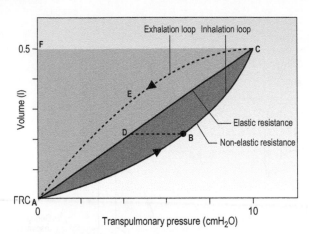

Figure 1.25 Schematic representation of the pressure–volume relationship of the lungs, illustrating the elastic and resistive work of breathing. See text for details.

Work of breathing

The elastic and flow-resistive forces described above must be overcome in order to create inspiratory air flow. Under resting conditions, exhalation is normally a passive process that recovers stored potential energy (elastic energy) that has been generated by the inspiratory muscles.

Respiratory work is done when pressure (generated by respiratory muscles) moves air into or out of the lungs. Figure 1.25 is a schematic pressure–volume relationship, illustrating the elastic and resistive work of breathing (WOB) for a 0.5-litre tidal inhalation above FRC. The inspiratory work done in overcoming elastic opposition to lung inflation is given by the area ADCFA, whilst the work done to overcome the flow-resistive (frictional) forces is given by ABCDA. The total WOB is therefore given by the area ABCFA. If inspiratory effort is halted mid-inhalation, and the airway is occluded, pressure falls to point D. Slightly more than half ($\sim$65%) of the WOB at rest overcomes elastic forces, with the remainder overcoming airway resistance. Exercise and disease alter this ratio; for example, increasing V_T elevates elastic work, whereas higher flow rates increase the flow-resistive component of the WOB. By mechanisms that are not fully understood, the respiratory control system selects a balance of V_T and breathing frequency that tends to minimize the WOB for a given situation.

Lung volumes and capacities

The mechanical changes described above bring about a process that ventilates the lungs. Typically, this is expressed globally as a flow in litres per minute ($l \cdot min^{-1}$), measured at the mouth, and is the product of tidal volume (V_T) and breathing frequency (f_r). The V_T can be either inspired or expired, but conventionally the expired volume is reported

as expired minute ventilation ($\dot{V}_E$). (The dot over the V indicates that this is a flow and not a volume.)

In healthy people, $\dot{V}_E$ displays a more than 10-fold increase between rest and peak exercise, with typical resting values of 8–$10\,l \cdot min^{-1}$ and values approaching 150–$200\,l \cdot min^{-1}$ during maximal exercise in highly trained athletes. The highest values for $\dot{V}_E$ are recorded in athletes such as rowers, where it is not uncommon for $\dot{V}_E$ to reach $250\,l \cdot min^{-1}$ at peak exercise in elite, open-class oarsmen. In contrast, peak $\dot{V}_E$ in a patient with moderate COPD may be only $40\,l \cdot min^{-1}$.

During exercise $\dot{V}_E$ increases via a combination of increases in V_T and f_r (see Ch. 2), and the increase in V_T occurs by utilizing reserve lung capacities for inspiration and expiration. All but one of the volume subdivisions of the total lung capacity can be measured using a simple spirometer (residual volume, and thus also functional residual capacity, requires specialized equipment). The so-called static lung volumes are illustrated in Figure 1.26 and definitions are provided below:

- *Total lung capacity (TLC):* The volume of air in the lungs at full inspiration. This cannot be measured without access to specialized equipment.
- *Vital capacity (VC):* The maximum volume that can be exhaled/inhaled between the lungs being completely inflated and the end of a full expiration. VC can be measured during either a 'forced' (with maximal effort; FVC) or relaxed manoeuvre (VC). The relaxed manoeuvre is more appropriate for patients with lung disease whose airways tend to collapse during a forced manoeuvre.
- *Residual volume (RV):* The volume of air remaining in the lungs at the end of a full expiration. This cannot be measured without access to specialized equipment.
- *Functional residual capacity (FRC):* The volume of air remaining in the lungs after a resting tidal breath. This changes during exercise, when it becomes known as end-expiratory lung volume (EELV).
- *Expiratory and inspiratory reserve volumes (ERV/IRV):* The volumes available between the beginning or end of tidal breath and TLC and RV, respectively.

Lung function is influenced by a number of physiological and demographic factors, as well as by the presence of disease. For example, there is a strong influence of body size, gender and age, as well as ethnicity. For this reason, there are population-specific prediction equations that assist in the interpretation of measured values. Generally, lung volumes are greater in larger individuals, are lower in women, and decrease with age. A component of the effect of gender appears to be independent of the effect of body size (Becklake, 1986).

A description of the methods used to assess lung volumes is beyond the scope of this book, and the reader is referred to the joint American Thoracic Society and European Respiratory Society guidelines for further information on

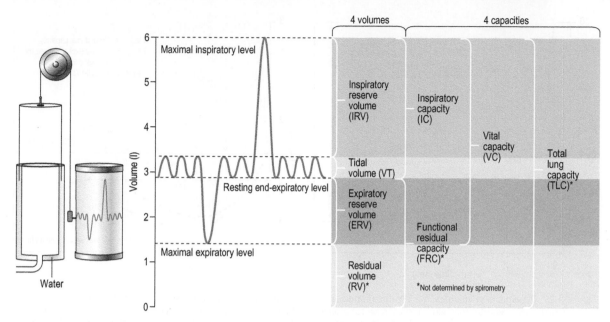

Figure 1.26 Static lung volumes and capacities on a volume–time spirogram, with typical healthy adult values shown.

assessment (Wanger et al, 2005) and interpretation (Pellegrino et al, 2005).

The condition of the airways (as distinct from the measurement of lung volumes) can be assessed by referencing changes in volume to time, thereby deriving flow (dynamic lung function). Obstructive lung diseases such as asthma are diagnosed by measuring the rate of expiratory air flow during forced expiratory manoeuvres. By plotting either volume against time (Fig. 1.27A) or flow against volume (by integration of the flow signal) (Fig. 1.27B), a 'spirogram' is constructed. Figure 1.27A and B illustrate each of these approaches and identify a number of parameters that provide information about airway function (see figure legend for details). The most commonly used index of airway calibre is the forced expiratory volume in 1 second (FEV_1), which can be assessed using either a bellows (wedge) spirometer, or using electronic spirometry. Because FEV_1 is influenced by vital capacity, it is expressed as a fraction of vital capacity (FEV%).

Electronic spirometers allow the construction of so-called flow–volume loops (Fig. 1.27B). A description of the methods used to undertake spirometry is beyond the scope of this book, and the reader is referred to the joint American Thoracic Society and European Respiratory Society guidelines for further information on assessment (Miller et al, 2005) and interpretation (Pellegrino et al, 2005).

Finally, consideration of the effect of the dead-space volume is required, since this becomes more important functionally in older people and those with lung and/or heart disease. Gas exchange takes place only in areas of the lung that have alveoli, and within these regions it takes place only in those units where there is adequate ventilation and perfusion. Accordingly, there are two types of dead space in the lung: (1) the conducting airways, and (2) alveolar dead space; their sum is known as physiological dead space. Only that part of V_T entering perfused alveoli contributes to gas exchange; the remainder ventilates the dead space and is 'wasted'. The proportion of wasted total ventilation is determined by the ratio of dead space volume to tidal volume (V_D/V_T). It therefore depends not only upon the influence of anatomy and physiology, but also upon breathing pattern. If V_T is low then a greater proportion of the breath is wasted in the dead space. As a consequence, in order to deliver the required level of alveolar air flow ($\dot{V}_A$), breathing frequency and total $\dot{V}_E$ must increase, raising the work of breathing. For instance, consider an example in which the gas exchange requirement of running on level ground corresponds to an alveolar ventilation of $54 \, l \cdot min^{-1}$. Table 1.1 illustrates the repercussions of two different breathing strategies that will both deliver this $\dot{V}_A$.

Mechanical properties of respiratory pump muscles

To generate a breath, the respiratory pump muscles must produce a pressure differential between the atmosphere outside the body and the inside of the lungs. Broadly speaking, the inspiratory muscles pull outward to expand the thorax, and the expiratory muscles pull inward to compress the thorax. The size and speed of the pressure differential that the muscle contractions generate determine how large the

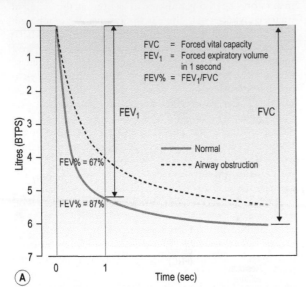
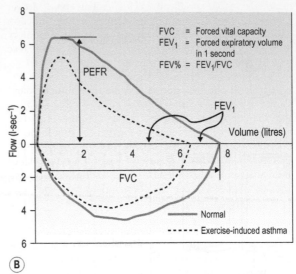

Figure 1.27 Dynamic lung volumes. (A) Volume plotted against time, (B) flow plotted against volume, with values shown before (solid lines) and after (dashed lines) exercise for a patient with exercise-induced asthma. In (B) the volume corresponding to FEV_1 under the normal and obstructed conditions is identified. BTPS, body temperature and pressure saturated; PEFR, peak expiratory flow rate.

Table 1.1 Influence of V_T upon the $\dot{V}_E$ requirement of exercise	
Deep breathing	**Shallow breathing**
Alveolar ventilation = 54 l·min^{-1}	Alveolar ventilation = 54 l·min^{-1}
Dead-space ventilation = 4.3 l·min^{-1}	Dead-space ventilation = 9.5 l·min^{-1}
Minute ventilation = 58.3 l·min^{-1}	Minute ventilation = 63.5 l·min^{-1}
Physiological dead space = 0.15 l	Physiological dead space = 0.15 l
Tidal volume = 2.0 l	Tidal volume = 1.0 l
Dead space/tidal volume = 0.15/2 = 7.5%	Dead space/tidal volume = 0.15/1 = 15%
Breathing frequency = 29.2 breaths·min^{-1}	Breathing frequency = 63.5 breaths·min^{-1}

breath is and how fast the air moves into (or out of) the lungs, respectively. During exercise, air must flow in and out of the lungs more quickly than at rest, and the respiratory pump muscles must contract more quickly and forcefully to generate the required increase in volume and air-flow rate. Like other muscles, the respiratory pump muscles have a finite ability to generate force (which results in the generation of pressures within the thorax), and this finite ability is one of the limiting factors to breathing during exercise.

The ability of the respiratory muscles to generate the pressure differentials that bring about lung ventilation is influenced by the act of breathing itself. Breathing results in changes in the length (lung volume) and the speed (air-flow rate) of muscle shortening, both of which change the ability of the respiratory muscles to generate pressure (Leblanc et al, 1988). The implications of these interactions are important, especially in patients where disease exacerbates the detrimental influence of changing volume and flow.

The length–tension (volume–pressure) relationship of the respiratory pump muscles is illustrated in Figure 1.28.

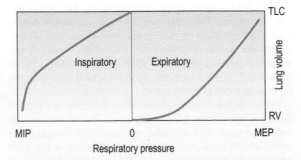

Figure 1.28 Schematic illustrating the effect of lung volume on the static pressure generating capacity of the respiratory muscles. Note that MIP is maximized at RV, whereas MEP is maximized at TLC. The pressure lines do not intersect at TLC and RV because of the effects of gas compression and decompression upon lung volume, respectively. RV = residual volume; TLC = total lung capacity; MIP = maximal inspiratory pressure; MEP = maximal expiratory pressure.

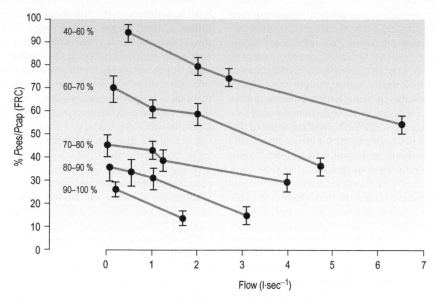

Figure 1.29 Maximum inspiratory oesophageal pressure (*Poes*). *Pcap*, maximal pressure generating capacity. *(Reproduced from Leblanc P, Summers E, Inman MD, et al, 1988. J. Appl. Physiol. 64, 2482–2489 with permission of JAP.)*

The capacity to generate inspiratory pressure is greatest when the lungs are empty and smallest when they are full (Rahn et al, 1946). Conversely, the capacity to generate expiratory pressure is greatest when the lungs are full and smallest when they are empty. Thus, inhalation and exhalation commence at the lung volumes where the respective muscles are strongest. This relationship has functional implications because, as V_T increases with increasing exercise intensity, it expands into the inspiratory reserve volume. Thus, the end of inhalation (end-inspiratory lung volume, EILV) occurs closer to TLC, which is also the region where the inspiratory muscles are weakest (see also Ch. 2, Fig. 2.1). This so-called functional weakening of the inspiratory muscles during lung inflation increases susceptibility to fatigue, for two reasons: (1) the muscles are weaker, and (2) they must overcome a higher elastic load (see 'Mechanics of breathing', below). Functional weakening also has implications for the perception of dyspnoea (see 'Dyspnoea and breathing effort', below), as well as how the respiratory muscles can be overloaded during resistance training, which will be considered in Chapter 6.

The force–velocity (pressure–flow) relationship of the respiratory pump muscles also has important repercussions. Unfortunately, this relationship is impossible to study in isolation from the volume–pressure relationship since the velocity component is the velocity of shortening, which implies a change in length. In the only study of its kind to date (Leblanc et al, 1988), the effects of both the volume–pressure and pressure–flow relationships of the inspiratory muscles were characterized and their influence upon pressure generating capacity quantified; the capacity of the inspiratory muscles to generate dynamic pressure was predicted to decrease by 17% for each 10% of the total lung capacity that is accounted for by an increased V_T above functional residual capacity, and by 5% for each $l·s^{-1}$ increase in inspiratory flow (Fig. 1.29).

Thus, as V_T and inspiratory flow increase with exercise, a given level of tension represents a relatively greater percentage of the maximum tension that can be developed, and requires a greater inspiratory motor drive. In moderately fit, healthy individuals, the peak dynamic pressure generated by the inspiratory muscles, expressed relative to the ability to generate pressure at the lung volumes and flows adopted during maximal exercise, is only 40–60% (Leblanc et al, 1988). However, in circumstances where muscle-operating length is reduced (e.g., hyperinflated patients with COPD), or where the velocity of shortening must increase to meet elevated flow requirements (e.g., tachypnoeic patients with heart failure), this percentage may increase considerably. Such conditions arise in a number of disease states, and they render the inspiratory muscles, in particular, vulnerable to fatigue.

The non-respiratory roles of the respiratory muscles are described in Chapter 3, and the assessment of respiratory muscle function is described in Chapter 6 ('Assessment of respiratory muscle function').

DYSPNOEA AND BREATHING EFFORT

Dyspnoea, or breathlessness, is defined as an 'uncomfortable sensation of breathing', or 'the consciousness of the necessity for increased respiratory effort' (Meakins, 1923).

By definition then, dyspnoea is a subjective experience, and one that is therefore influenced by a combination of physiological and psychological factors (Williams et al, 2010). Patients with conditions as wide ranging as cancer and neurological disorders experience disabling bouts of dyspnoea, but the clinical groups that most commonly present with disabling dyspnoea as their primary symptom are those with asthma, COPD and heart failure. A comprehensive review of the pathophysiology of dyspnoea is beyond the scope of this book, but what follows is an overview of the subject, with particular emphasis upon the role of breathing mechanics and the respiratory muscles in its genesis.

Dyspnoea is essentially an increased sense of effort associated with breathing and/or a sense that breathing is inadequate. Whilst some degree of dyspnoea is a very normal part of exercise for everyone (even athletes get out of breath), there comes a point where the intensity becomes disabling. If intolerable dyspnoea is experienced during an activity as modest as carrying one's shopping home on level ground at walking pace, then dyspnoea is arguably disabling.

The conscious awareness of dyspnoea is a distillation of the somatic feedback arising from numerous chemical and mechanical receptors, modulated by psychological factors related to the affective state of the individual (Williams et al, 2010). There are three principal dimensions of dyspnoea: (1) 'air hunger', (2) work/effort and (3) chest tightness.

In healthy people, 'air hunger', is perceived as being more unpleasant than work/effort, and its unpleasantness varies independently of its intensity (Banzett et al, 2008). The relative importance of different descriptors of dyspnoea has also been explored by applying a technique called principal component analysis (Smith et al, 2009). Descriptors were compared in patients with asthma, COPD, interstitial lung disease and idiopathic hyperventilation and in healthy people. Interestingly, air hunger was found to be the dominant quality of dyspnoea during exercise, irrespective of the pathophysiological differences between the individuals reporting it. The authors suggest that the attainment of a mechanical limit to breathing at the end of exercise may provide a unifying explanation for their observations. Of course, the attainment of this limit is influenced to some extent by the ability of the inspiratory muscles to utilize the available inspiratory reserve volume to expand tidal volume. Thus, the mechanical work of the inspiratory muscles may also contribute to the sensation of air hunger during exercise. This is consistent with the notion that dyspnoea can be explained by a single model that is applicable to a wide range of clinical conditions (Moxham & Jolley, 2009). This model is based upon the balance, or lack of it, between the demand for inspiratory muscle work and the capacity of the muscles to meet this demand.

The closest functional correlates of dyspnoea are not indices of airway obstruction or gas exchange impairment, but inspiratory muscle function (O'Donnell et al, 1987; Killian & Jones, 1988) and the degree of lung hyperinflation (O'Donnell et al, 1998; Marin et al, 2001) – in other words, the relative load upon the inspiratory muscles. The sense of effort associated with any muscular act is the result of a balance between the force that is being demanded and the muscle's capacity to supply force (its strength), i.e., the demand/capacity relationship. A helpful analogy is to consider the sensations associated with lifting an object. If the object is heavy, the sense of effort associated with lifting it is high compared with lifting a light object. However, if we increase the strength of the muscles (give them greater capacity) then the effort of lifting a given object is reduced because the muscles' capacity to supply force has been increased. These principles apply equally well to the muscles employed during breathing.

Central to this demand/capacity model of dyspnoea are the neurophysiological mechanisms responsible for sensing the breathing effort or, as Meakins (1923) put it, 'the consciousness of the necessity for increased respiratory effort'. Meakins' definition of dyspnoea was the first to provide a unifying theory to explain the presence of dyspnoea in both patients and healthy people, and was developed further in the 1960s, when the term 'length–tension inappropriateness' (LTI) was created to explain how the sensation of dyspnoea might be transduced to consciousness (Campbell, 1966). Campbell argued that human beings have a quantitative, conscious appreciation of the degree of effort associated with breathing and that dissociation, or a mismatch, between the central respiratory motor activity (efferent output) and the mechanical response of the respiratory system (afferent feedback) produces a sensation of respiratory discomfort, or dyspnoea. More recently, the LTI paradigm has been 'rebranded' as neuromechanical uncoupling, and generalized to include not only afferent sensory inputs from respiratory muscles but also information emanating from receptors throughout the respiratory system (ATS, 1999). When viewed in the context of neuromechanical uncoupling, the role of respiratory muscle function in the perception of dyspnoea becomes intuitively predictable. Thus the intensity of dyspnoea is increased when changes in respiratory muscle length (i.e., volume) or tension (i.e., pressure) are inappropriate for the outgoing motor command. In turn, changes in capacity of the muscles to deliver ventilation, or in the mechanical loads that they must overcome in doing so, contribute to the perceived appropriateness of the ventilatory response, relative to the motor command. Furthermore, the size of the motor command itself is influenced by the contractile properties of the inspiratory muscles and the loads they overcome during breathing. The greater the magnitude of the discrepancy between efferent drive and afferent feedback, the greater is the intensity of dyspnoea.

Disease affects both sides of the demand/capacity relationship, weakening respiratory muscles and increasing the mechanical loads that they must overcome in order to sustain breathing (see Ch. 3, 'Changes in breathing mechanics and respiratory muscle function'). Acting via neuromechanical uncoupling, this imbalance is perceived as dyspnoea. Thus, dyspnoea is the inevitable consequence of inspiratory muscle weakness combined with an increase in the elastic and/or resistive work of breathing. In the early and mild stages of disease, this imbalance may manifest itself only during exercise, but as the severity of the impairments increases then dyspnoea occurs also at rest.

The assessment of dyspnoea and breathing effort is described in Chapter 7 ('Assessing patient needs').

REFERENCES

ATS, 1999. Dyspnea: Mechanisms, assessment, and management: A consensus statement. Am. J. Respir. Crit. Care Med. 159, 321–340.

Banzett, R.B., Pedersen, S.H., Schwartzstein, R.M., et al., 2008. The affective dimension of laboratory dyspnea: air hunger is more unpleasant than work/effort. Am. J. Respir. Crit. Care Med. 177, 1384–1390.

Beachey, W., 1998. Respiratory care anatomy and physiology, second ed. Mosby, St Louis.

Becklake, M.R., 1986. Concepts of normality applied to the measurement of lung function. Am. J. Med. 80, 1158–1164.

Berne, R.M., Levy, M.N., 1993. Physiology, third ed. Mosby, St Louis.

Boucher, V.J., Ahmarani, C., Ayad, T., 2006. Physiologic features of vocal fatigue: electromyographic spectral-compression in laryngeal muscles. Laryngoscope 116, 959–965.

Brancatisano, T.P., Dodd, D.S., Engel, L.A., 1984. Respiratory activity of posterior cricoarytenoid muscle and vocal cords in humans. J. Appl. Physiol. 57, 1143–1149.

Buchler, B., Magder, S., Katsardis, H., et al., 1985. Effects of pleural pressure and abdominal pressure on diaphragmatic blood flow. J. Appl. Physiol. 58, 691–697.

Campbell, E.J.M., 1966. The relationship of the sensation of breathlessness to the act of breathing. In: Howell, J.B.L. (Ed.), Breathlessness. Blackwell Scientific, London, pp. 55–64.

Davies, A., Moores, C., 2010. The respiratory system: basic science and clinical conditions. Churchill Livingstone Elsevier, London.

Forster, H.V., Haouzi, P., Dempsey, J.A., 2012. Control of breathing during exercise. Comp. Physiol. 2 (1), 743–777.

Gollnick, P.D., Armstrong, R.B., Saubert, C.W., et al., 1972. Enzyme activity and fiber composition in skeletal muscle of untrained and trained men. J. Appl. Physiol. 33, 312–319.

Guenette, J.A., Sheel, A.W., 2007. Exercise-induced arterial hypoxaemia in active young women. Appl. Physiol. Nutr. Metab. 32, 1263–1273.

Hicks, G.H., 2000. Cardiopulmonary anatomy and physiology. WB Saunders, Philadelphia.

Hoh, J.F., 2005. Laryngeal muscle fibre types. Acta Physiol. Scand. 183, 133–149.

Hussain, S.N., 1996. Regulation of ventilatory muscle blood flow. J. Appl. Physiol. 81, 1455–1468.

Killian, K.J., Jones, N.L., 1988. Respiratory muscles and dyspnea. Clin. Chest Med. 9, 237–248.

Leblanc, P., Summers, E., Inman, M.D., et al., 1988. Inspiratory muscles during exercise: a problem of supply and demand. J. Appl. Physiol. 64, 2482–2489.

Li, Z.B., Lehar, M., Nakagawa, H., et al., 2004. Differential expression of myosin heavy chain isoforms between abductor and adductor muscles in the human larynx. Otolaryngol. Head Neck Surg. 130, 217–222.

Lumb, A.B., 2010. Nunn's applied respiratory physiology. Churchill Livingstone Elsevier.

Lykidis, C.K., White, M.J., Balanos, G.M., 2008. The pulmonary vascular response to the sustained activation of the muscle metaboreflex in man. Exp. Physiol. 93, 247–253.

Marin, J.M., Carrizo, S.J., Gascon, M., et al., 2001. Inspiratory capacity, dynamic hyperinflation, breathlessness, and exercise performance during the 6-minute-walk test in chronic obstructive pulmonary disease. Am. J. Respir. Crit. Care Med. 163, 1395–1399.

Meakins, J., 1923. The cause and treatment of dyspnea in cardiovascular disease. Br. Med. J. 1, 1043–1045.

Miller, M.R., Hankinson, J., Brusasco, V., et al., 2005. Standardisation of spirometry. Eur. Respir. J. 26, 319–338.

Moxham, J., Jolley, C., 2009. Breathlessness, fatigue and the respiratory muscles. Clin. Med. 9, 448–452.

Murakami, Y., Kirchner, J.A., 1972. Mechanical and physiological properties of reflex laryngeal closure. Ann. Otol. Rhinol. Laryngol. 81, 59–71.

Murphy, D.M., O'Byrne, P.M., 2010. Recent advances in the pathophysiology of asthma. Chest 137, 1417–1426.

O'Donnell, D.E., Sanii, R., Anthonisen, N.R., et al., 1987. Effect of dynamic airway compression on breathing pattern and respiratory sensation in severe chronic obstructive pulmonary disease. Am. Rev. Respir. Dis. 135, 912–918.

O'Donnell, D.E., Lam, M., Webb, K.A., 1998. Measurement of symptoms, lung hyperinflation, and endurance during exercise in chronic obstructive pulmonary disease. Am. J. Respir. Crit. Care Med. 158, 1557–1565.

Pellegrino, R., Viegi, G., Brusasco, V., et al., 2005. Interpretative strategies for lung function tests. Eur. Respir. J. 26, 948–968.

Polla, B., D'Antona, G., Bottinelli, R., et al., 2004. Respiratory muscle fibres: specialisation and plasticity. Thorax 59, 808–817.

Poon, C.S., 1983. Optimal control of ventilation in hypoxia, hypercapnia and exercise. Elsevier, New York.

Poon, C.S., Lin, S.L., Knudson, O.B., 1992. Optimization character of inspiratory neural drive. J. Appl. Physiol. 72, 2005–2017.

Poon, C.S., Tin, C., Yu, Y., 2007. Homeostasis of exercise hyperpnea and optimal sensorimotor integration: the internal model paradigm. Respir. Physiol. Neurobiol. 159, 1–13; discussion 14–20.

Priban, I.P., Fincham, W.F., 1965. Self-adaptive control and respiratory system. Nature 208, 339–343.

Rahn, H., Otis, A.B., Chadwick, L.E., et al., 1946. The pressure–volume diagram of the thorax and lung. Am. J. Physiol. 146, 161–178.

Sheel, A.W., Derchak, P.A., Morgan, B.J., et al., 2001. Fatiguing inspiratory muscle work causes reflex reduction in resting leg blood flow in humans. J. Physiol. 537, 277–289.

Smith, J., Albert, P., Bertella, E., et al., 2009. Qualitative aspects of breathlessness in health and disease. Thorax 64, 713–718.

Suzuki, M., Kirchner, J., 1969. The posterior cricoarytenoid as an inspiratory muscle. Ann. Otol. Rhinol. Laryngol. 78, 849–863.

Thibodeau, G.A., Patton, K.T., 1996. Anatomy and physiology, third ed. Mosby, St Louis.

Wanger, J., Clausen, J.L., Coates, A., et al., 2005. Standardisation of the measurement of lung volumes. Eur. Respir. J. 26, 511–522.

Williams, M., Cafarella, P., Olds, T., et al., 2010. Affective descriptors of the sensation of breathlessness are more highly associated with severity of impairment than physical descriptors in people with chronic obstructive pulmonary disease. Chest 138 (2), 315–322.

Chapter | 2 |

Exercise physiology and training principles

In Chapter 1, we learned of the close anatomical and functional relationships between the respiratory and cardiovascular systems; indeed, they are so integrated that we often refer to the 'cardiorespiratory' system. This intimacy is essential for the efficient transport of respired gases to and from the metabolizing tissues of the body. Whilst the cardiorespiratory system operates comfortably within its capacity under resting conditions, during exercise the system imposes a limit upon oxygen delivery, and thence exercise tolerance. In order to understand how the respiratory system contributes to exercise limitation, it is necessary to understand a little of the integrated response of the healthy cardiorespiratory system to exercise, as well as how the individual systems respond to training. This chapter will describe the responses of the cardiorespiratory system to exercise, the limitations it imposes upon exercise tolerance, the concept of cardiorespiratory fitness, and the responses of the cardiorespiratory system to different types of training.

CARDIORESPIRATORY RESPONSES TO EXERCISE

During exercise the cardiovascular and respiratory systems must operate as an integrated 'machine' for the transport of respired gases. In this section, we will consider the responses of each system to exercise.

Respiratory

Introduction

At rest, the average adult takes 10 to 15 breaths per minute, with a volume of about 0.5 litres, producing a 'minute ventilation' ($\dot{V}_E$) of 7.5 l·min^{-1} (15 × 0.5). The volume of each breath (tidal volume: V_T) depends on body size and metabolic rate. Larger people have larger lungs and take larger breaths; they also require more energy and oxygen (O_2) to support their metabolism; accordingly, they require a larger $\dot{V}_E$.

During heavy exercise, breathing frequency (f_r) rises to around 40 to 50 breaths per minute. In a physically active young male, V_T rises to around 3 to 4 litres, generating a $\dot{V}_E$ of 120 to 160 l·min^{-1}. However, in Olympic-class male endurance athletes, V_T can be over 5 litres, resulting in a $\dot{V}_E$ of 250 to 300 l·min^{-1}.

Kilogram for kilogram, Olympic oarsmen can achieve a $\dot{V}_E$ that is equivalent to that seen in thoroughbred racehorses! Take the rower Sir Matthew Pinsent as an example. In his 20s, this four-time Olympic gold medalist (1992, 1996, 2000, 2004) and 13-time senior world champion possessed the largest lungs of any British athlete; his forced vital capacity (FVC) was 8.25 litres. Sir Matthew stood just under 2 m (6 feet 5 inches) tall and weighed around 108 kg (240 pounds); a man of his size would normally have a FVC of about 6 litres, whilst the average man has a FVC closer to 5 litres. During a 2000-meter rowing race, Sir Matthew would generate a massive 460 watts of propulsive power for around 6 minutes, requiring a peak oxygen uptake ($\dot{V}O_{2peak}$) of around 8 l·min^{-1} and a $\dot{V}_E$ of close to 300 l·min^{-1}. The total volume of air that was moved into and out of his lungs during a race would have been close to 1700 litres, requiring a power output by his respiratory muscles of around 85 watts. These are truly staggering statistics, and they give some insight into what the human cardiorespiratory system is capable of achieving.

The respiratory pump during exercise

During exercise, the rate and depth of breathing are increased in order to deliver a higher $\dot{V}_E$ and oxygen uptake ($\dot{V}O_2$); this response is known as the exercise hyperpnoea, and requires the respiratory muscles to contract more forcefully and to shorten more quickly. At rest, expiratory muscles make very little contribution to breathing, but during exercise they contribute to raising V_T and expiratory airflow rate. However, at all intensities of exercise the majority of the work of breathing is undertaken by the inspiratory muscles; expiration is always assisted to some extent by the elastic energy that is stored in the expanded lungs and rib cage from the preceding inhalation. This elastic energy is 'donated' by the contraction of the inspiratory muscles as they stretched and expanded the chest during inhalation. Recent studies have estimated that, during maximal exercise, the work of the inspiratory respiratory muscles demands approximately 16% of the available oxygen (Harms & Dempsey, 1999), which puts into perspective how strenuous breathing can be in healthy young people.

The strategy that the respiratory controller adopts in order to deliver a given $\dot{V}_E$ depends upon a number of factors, especially in the presence of disease. Chapter 1 described how the respiratory controller most likely regulates ventilation and breathing pattern so as to 'keep the operating point of the blood at the optimum while using a minimum of energy' (Priban & Fincham, 1965). Figure 2.1 illustrates how tidal volume changes as exercise intensity increases, placing it within the subdivisions of the lung volumes that are illustrated in Figure 2.1. Initially, during light exercise, V_T increases by the person exhaling more deeply, and utilizing the expiratory reserve volume,

but this increase is quickly supplemented as a result of the deeper inhalation and utilization of the inspiratory reserve volume.

Eventually, V_T reaches a point where it does not increase any further, despite a continuing need to increase $\dot{V}_E$. This can be seen more clearly in Figure 2.2, which shows how $\dot{V}_E$, V_T, f_r and $\dot{V}O_2$ change during incremental cycling to the limit of tolerance in a well-trained athlete. Each point on the plot represents an individual breath, and there are two key features to note. Firstly, unlike the linear response of $\dot{V}O_2$ to incremental exercise, $\dot{V}_E$ is non-linear, rising steeply at about 70% of maximal intensity. As a result, the $\dot{V}_E$ required at 80% of maximum capacity is not twice the amount required at 40%; rather, it is more like four or five times greater. Secondly, as V_T levels off, f_r rises steeply to meet the need for an escalating $\dot{V}_E$.

The non-linear increase of $\dot{V}_E$ results from the role that breathing plays in compensating for the escalating metabolic acidosis. Chapter 1 described how breathing plays an important role in regulating blood and tissue pH by manipulating the excretion of CO_2 at the lungs. At the lactate threshold (LaT), lactic acid (also known as lactate) production exceeds its degradation leading to accumulation of lactic acid in the muscles and blood (see 'Cardiorespiratory fitness, Lactate threshold' below). Above the LaT, $\dot{V}_E$ exceeds that required to deliver O_2, and the primary role of the respiratory system is stabilizing pH by removal of CO_2 via the lungs. This process is known as a ventilatory compensation for a metabolic acidosis (see

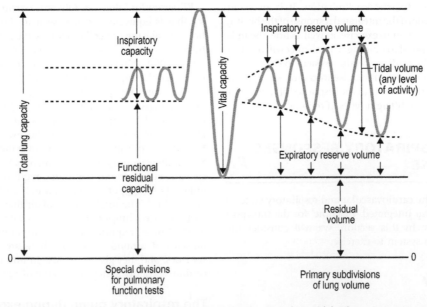

Figure 2.1 Changes in tidal volume during exercise of increasing intensity. Note how tidal volume increases as exercise intensity increases. This increase in tidal volume results from utilization of both the inspiratory and expiratory reserve volumes.
(From Astrand P-O, Rodahl K, Stromme S, 2003. Textbook of work physiology: physiological bases of exercise, 4th edn. Human Kinetics, Champaign, IL, p. 185, with permission.)

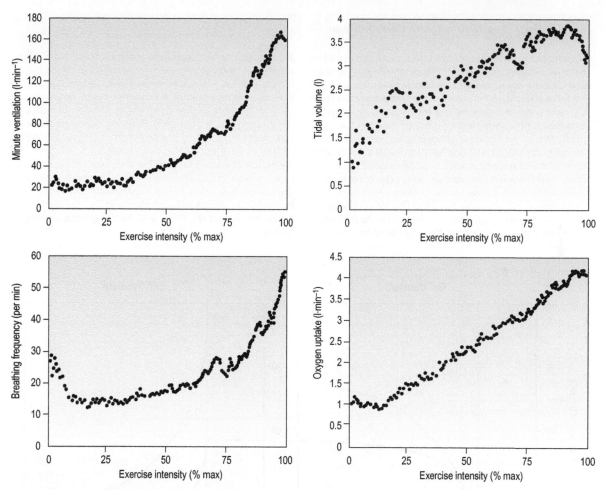

Figure 2.2 Changes in breathing during incremental cycling in a well-trained triathlete. Each dot corresponds to 1 breath. *(Adapted from McConnell AK, 2011. Breathe strong, perform better. Human Kinetics, Champaign, IL, with permission.)*

Ch. 1, 'Acid–base balance'). The steep increase in $\dot{V}_E$ at the LaT is a response to stimulation of the peripheral chemoreceptors by the hydrogen ion component of lactic acid (see Ch. 1, 'Chemical control of breathing'). This ventilatory response is central to the system that minimizes the acidification of the body and the negative influence of this upon muscle function and fatigue (Box 2.1). As will be described in the section 'Lactate threshold' below, the inflection of the response of $\dot{V}_E$ can be used to estimate the exercise intensity at which blood lactate accumulation commences, i.e., the so-called ventilatory threshold. The LaT and ventilatory threshold are related to the same physiological phenomenon, and are often used synonymously. However, they are not identical: the ventilatory threshold lags behind the LaT slightly because it is a response to the elevated hydrogen ion concentration in the blood.

The increasing reliance upon f_r to raise $\dot{V}_E$ at high intensities of exercise arises because it becomes too uncomfortable to continue to increase V_T; typically, this occurs when V_T is around 60% of FVC. As V_T increases, progressively greater inspiratory muscle force is required to overcome the elastance of the respiratory system. Higher inspiratory muscle force output increases effort and breathing discomfort (see Ch. 1, 'Dyspnoea and breathing effort'). Eventually, the sensory feedback from the inspiratory muscles signals the respiratory centre to change the pattern of breathing, and to increase f_r more steeply instead of V_T. The respiratory centre has an exquisite system for minimizing breathing discomfort, which also optimizes efficiency. This drive to optimize is also observed in the breathing pattern derangements that are seen in the presence of disease (see Ch. 3).

The influence of the LaT upon the exercise hyperpnoea can also be observed during constant intensity exercise. Figure 2.3 illustrates the typical ventilatory responses to two intensities of exercise, one below and one above the LaT. In both intensity domains, the 'on' transient response

Box 2.1 **How breathing helps to delay fatigue**

Muscles can liberate energy from stored substrates using two types of metabolic pathways: (1) those requiring O_2 (aerobic), and (2) those not requiring O_2 (anaerobic). Aerobic pathways are more efficient and terminate in the production of harmless CO_2 and water, but they liberate energy slowly. In contrast, anaerobic pathways are less efficient, terminate in the production of lactic acid (also known as lactate), and liberate energy much faster. Lactic acid has been linked to the onset of muscle fatigue because it leads to acidification of the muscle fibres, which interferes with the normal process of contraction.

Muscles are able to use aerobic pathways for low- to moderate-intensity exercise, but these liberate energy too slowly to meet the requirements of high-intensity exercise, so anaerobic pathways supplement energy liberation. The

accumulation of lactic acid from anaerobic metabolism is the reason that high-intensity exercise cannot be sustained for more than a few minutes. However, the ability to sustain high-intensity exercise would be even shorter were it not for the ability of the body to slow down the acidification of muscles using a process called buffering. Buffering neutralizes the acid component of lactic acid (the hydrogen ion: H^+) by pairing it with an alkali, a process that slows down the acidification of the muscle and delays fatigue. The buffering is made possible by the removal of CO_2 from the blood by hyperventilation (see Ch. 1, 'Acid–base balance'). The need to buffer lactic acid is the reason that breathing increases steeply at the 'so-called' lactate threshold (LaT). This is how breathing helps to delay fatigue.

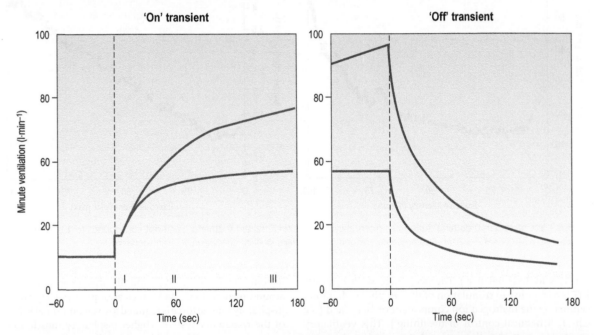

Figure 2.3 Diagram of the three-phase 'on' transient response of 'minute ventilation' to fixed-intensity exercise during moderate (bottom line) and heavy (top line) exercise.
(Copyright AKM.)

of $\dot{V}_E$ has three phases: phase I is an almost instantaneous increase, which is followed by the monoexponential increase of phase II, and finally phase III, which is either a plateau or a continued, slow increase. During light and moderate-intensity exercise, phase III is a plateau (steady state); in contrast, during heavy exercise phase III continues to show a gradual increase throughout exercise, never achieving a steady state. The absence of a steady state in phase III is due to the presence of a ventilatory

compensation for the metabolic acidosis. Unfortunately, this compensation is imperfect, and does not offset the fall in pH completely; accordingly, exercise above the LaT is non-sustainable. At exercise cessation, the 'off' transient also displays an abrupt fall in $\dot{V}_E$, followed by exponential decline; the recovery of $\dot{V}_E$ following heavy exercise takes much longer than that following light and moderate exercise because of a continued drive to breathe originating from the metabolic acidosis.

Cardiovascular

A detailed description of the cardiovascular system is beyond the scope of this book, and readers are referred to the numerous excellent textbooks on cardiovascular physiology for a comprehensive description of cardiovascular structure and function (e.g., Levick, 2009). The following section provides an overview of the integrated response of the cardiovascular system to exercise.

Introduction

At rest, the average adult heart beats at a frequency of around 65 beats per minute. With each beat, around 75 ml of blood are ejected from the heart (stroke volume: SV), providing a cardiac output ($\dot{Q}$) of around 5 l·min^{-1} (65×0.075 l). The SV depends upon body size, training status and metabolic rate. Larger and fitter people both have larger hearts, which eject a larger SV. In the case of fitter people, this may be around 100 ml, and the increase results in a lower resting heart rate (f_c) since resting $\dot{Q}$ is unchanged. In contrast, the larger SV of larger individuals is supporting a higher energy and oxygen (O_2) demand, which requires a higher $\dot{Q}$; thus their resting f_c is unchanged.

During maximal exercise, f_c rises to over 200 beats per minute in a healthy young person. Accompanying this increase in f_c is a rise in SV, to around 110 ml, such that $\dot{Q}$ reaches around 22 l·min^{-1} at maximal exercise. In Olympic-class endurance athletes, $\dot{Q}$ has been measured at 40 l·min^{-1}, thanks to a SV that can be as high as 210 ml.

In contrast to the 'trainability' of stroke volume, maximal f_c tends to remain the same in a given individual, but does decline with advancing age. Accordingly, an approximate estimate of a maximal f_c (f_{cMax}) can be obtained by using equations such as:

$$f_{cMax} = 220 - \text{age}$$

In the previous section, Sir Matthew Pinsent's phenomenal lung capacity and respiratory power output were described. Along with his extraordinary ability to deliver fresh air to his alveoli, was an equally astonishing ability of his cardiovascular system to collect oxygen from the lungs, and deliver it to the exercising muscles. Sir Matthew's $\dot{V}O_{2peak}$ of around 8 l·min^{-1} would have required a maximal cardiac output of around 40 l·min^{-1}.

The cardiovascular system during exercise

During exercise, both f_c and SV increase progressively in order to deliver an appropriate $\dot{Q}$ to the pulmonary and peripheral circulations. As is the case with the increase in respiratory V_T during exercise, SV also displays a non-linear response, showing a plateau at around 40–50% of maximal exercise capacity. The reasons for this are complex, but include a number of mechanical limitations that arise from both the filling of the ventricle during diastole and the

ability of the heart to eject blood during systole (Gonzalez-Alonso, 2012).

Commensurate with this plateau in SV is a plateau in $\dot{Q}$. As was mentioned above, SV is very amenable to training, and provides the only mechanism by which maximal $\dot{Q}$ can be increased; this will be described in the section 'Principles of cardiorespiratory training, Training adaptations' (below).

In the acute response to exercise, SV is enhanced by two main mechanisms: (1) an intrinsic mechanism whereby an elevation in the volume of blood returning to the heart (venous return) stimulates a more forceful ventricular contraction, and (2) an increase in the force of ventricular contraction due to neurohumoral influences (sympathetic drive to the heart and circulating catecholamine levels). Venous return is enhanced by both the pumping action of the exercising muscles (see below) and the more negative intrathoracic pressure swings that arise from increased V_T and inspiratory flow rate. The muscle pump 'pushes' blood towards the heart, whilst the thoracic pump 'sucks' it towards the heart. The result is an increased pre-load during diastole, which stretches the myocardial wall stimulating it to contract more forcefully. This response is possible because stretching of the myocardial muscle fibres leads to a pre-stretch that stores elastic energy within the fibres. This energy is released during contraction, leading to an increase in the force of myocardial contraction. The increase in force expels a greater proportion of the ventricular end-diastolic volume, as well as the additional blood that had caused the myocardial stretch. The result is an increase in SV, a reduction in the end-diastolic volume (EDV; akin to RV of the lungs) and an increase in the ejection fraction (proportion of EDV that is ejected). This mechanical response of the heart was first described in the early 1900s by Otto Frank and Ernst Starling, and is known as the Frank–Starling law of the heart. This intrinsic mechanism for enhancing SV is enhanced by the effects of the sympathetic neural and hormonal influences upon the myocardium, which also enhance the contractility of the myocardial wall.

As well as increasing $\dot{Q}$ during exercise, the integrated response of the cardiovascular system must also distribute blood to the parts of the body where it is needed most. So far as exercising muscle blood flow is concerned, this regulation takes place with exquisite precision such that muscle O_2 demand and supply are regulated tightly. However, if this increase were to take place without a compensatory restriction of blood flow elsewhere in the peripheral circulation, arterial blood pressure would be in jeopardy. Accordingly, the integrated response of the cardiovascular system during exercise includes redistribution of blood flow such that it is directed to areas of urgent O_2 demand, at the expense of areas such as the splanchnic circulations. For example, renal blood flow falls by about 75% during maximal exercise.

The control of exercising muscle blood flow is complex, and the factors responsible change as exercise progresses

(Hussain & Comtois, 2005). At the immediate onset of exercise, rhythmic contraction of exercising muscles facilitates unidirectional ejection of blood through the venules and deep veins (backflow is prevented by venous valves); during relaxation, venous pressure drops, facilitating the inflow of blood via the arterial circulation. This pumping action also stimulates an increase in muscle blood flow via the release of local vessel endothelial factors that respond to 'shear stress' inside the arterioles; in other words, the physical stress exerted on the vessel endothelium by flowing blood stimulates the vessel to relax and dilate. As exercise progresses, muscle metabolism leads to an increase in local metabolites such as CO_2, lactic acid, adenosine, potassium ions and osmolarity, as well as a decline in O_2. This vasodilator stimulus supplements that from endothelial factors to produce a full-blown exercise hyperaemia (Hussain & Comtois, 2005).

The maximal capacity of the exercising muscles to accommodate blood flow far exceeds the ability of the $\dot{Q}$ to supply it. Accordingly, blood flow to exercising muscles, as well as non-exercising tissues, must be regulated by the sympathetic nervous system, whose job it is to defend arterial blood pressure (ABP). Without this regulatory restraint by the sympathetic nervous system, ABP would fall precipitously. One important component of the mechanism(s) contributing to this restraint is feedback from muscle metaboreceptors (Sinoway & Prophet, 1990). The afferent arm of the resulting reflex response (metaboreflex) is mediated by simple group III and IV afferents residing within skeletal muscles. These afferents sense both mechanical and metabolic stimuli during exercise, and, amongst other things, induce sympathetically mediated, active vasoconstriction in all tissues, including exercising muscles. In tissues with low metabolism this output stimulates powerful vasoconstriction, whist in exercising muscles the resultant vasoconstriction is a balance between the local vasodilatory influence and the neural vasoconstrictor influence.

In Chapter 3 (section 'Respiratory muscle involvement in exercise limitation, Healthy people') we will consider the ramifications of activation of the metaboreflex originating from exercising respiratory muscles.

MECHANISMS OF FATIGUE

Fatigue is a complex phenomenon that has been studied extensively for over a century. Fatigue and exercise are linked inextricably, and it is impossible to consider exercise without also considering fatigue. But precisely what factors lead human beings to slow down and/or stop exercising, or muscles to cease to generate the force they once could? Despite the extensive literature addressing the phenomenon of fatigue, our understanding remains incomplete. This section is intended to provide a 'working knowledge' of fatigue mechanisms for the purposes of understanding

the factors that contribute to exercise intolerance in patients, and of specific respiratory muscle fatigue. For a more comprehensive review of fatigue the reader is referred to the excellent overview of skeletal muscle physiology by David Jones and colleagues (Jones et al, 2004), and to the comprehensive guide to muscle fatigue edited by Williams & Ratel (2009).

Fatigue means very different things to different people, encompassing everything from the condition associated with general tiredness, to failure of muscle contraction at the level of the contractile machinery. For the purposes of this section, the focus will be on factors that limit the tolerability of physical activity. Ultimately, whether one is a frail elderly person or an aspiring Olympian, exercise is limited by tolerance to the unpleasant sensations it provokes. The extent to which those unpleasant sensations are also associated with failure of function at a physiological level is a moot point, but one that should not place limits on the definition of fatigue. In other words, long-lasting contractile dysfunction of locomotor muscles at the cessation of exercise is not a prerequisite that distinguishes fatiguing exercise from malingering. As this section will demonstrate, the complex, integrative nature of fatigue makes such reductionist definitions wholly inadequate.

Definition of fatigue

Even agreeing upon a definition of fatigue has proved elusive – not least because its presence, or otherwise, can be specific to the test, timing and conditions used to detect it. For example, changes in muscle responses to electrical stimulation can differ at different stimulation frequencies such that 'fatigue' is revealed only at the 'right' frequency. Similarly, any definition of fatigue must recognize that force-generating capacity is not the only muscle property that is affected by the process of fatigue; reductions in muscle power and speed are also indicators of fatigue (see below). Early definitions were oversimplistic, relying upon measurement of isometric force, e.g., 'the inability to maintain the required or expected force' (Bigland-Ritchie, 1981). This is not to imply that such definitions are invalid; indeed, this definition is used extensively in the literature as a method to identify respiratory muscle fatigue and to test its relationship to exercise tolerance (Romer & Polkey, 2008). However, this definition is limited and, in 1992, Enoka & Stuart proposed the following definition of fatigue, which encapsulates a number of important characteristics of fatigue that previous definitions had neglected: 'an acute impairment of performance that includes both an increase in the perceived effort necessary to exert a desired force and an eventual inability to produce this force' (Enoka & Stuart, 1992). Although Enoka & Stuart's 1992 definition still focuses upon force as the outcome measure of function, it acknowledges a number of important features of fatigue: (1) the transiency of fatigue,

(2) that fatigue can be manifested during movements (not just isometric contractions), (3) that fatigue is associated with sensations, and (4) that fatigue is a process (not an end point). However, although this definition hints at the fact that fatigue can be present before performance declines, and/or task failure occurs, it is not explicit. This important concept is explored in the section 'Task failure and task dependency'

Indicators of fatigue

For reasons of technical expediency, laboratory studies of fatigue have tended to focus upon measurement of isometric force in the identification of fatigue. These contractions are used to both induce and to measure a decline in function. When asked to maintain a maximal isometric contraction of a limb muscle, with biofeedback of force and encouragement, people can typically sustain the contraction for around a minute. Over the course of the minute, force declines progressively and muscle discomfort rises. Eventually there is an almost complete loss of force, which is followed swiftly by intolerance and cessation of contraction. The difficulty with tests such as this is two-fold: (1) they are not physiological, and (2) it is impossible to distinguish loss of force due to declining effort from loss due to declining function. One way to overcome the second issue is to stimulate the muscle briefly with an electrical stimulus to assess the contractile state of the muscle *per se*. However, this process is not without its own limitations (see above), and also does not distinguish between decline in effort and decline in the motor drive to the muscle from the spinal cord and brain. Notwithstanding this, electrical stimulation experiments have revealed that fatigue at the level of the contractile machinery is not only associated with a decline in maximal force, it is also associated with slowing of the rate of force development and the rate of relaxation (Cady et al, 1989). Since muscle power is the product of force and speed of contraction, it is obvious that fatigue is associated with a loss of muscle power output.

As should be apparent from the preceding paragraph, exercise-induced decline in muscle functional properties (fatigue) can be due to failure at the level of the contractile machinery, or to failure of nervous system activation of muscle contraction. Inevitably, this influences the techniques used to identify the presence of fatigue and their limitations. The following section considers the potential sites of fatigue, before moving on to consider some of the underlying mechanisms.

Potential sites and causes of fatigue

In 1981, Brenda Bigland-Ritchie published a model that identified a number of potential sites/factors influencing fatigue, extending from the motor cortex to the muscle contractile machinery; it also included the influence of the

supply the energy for interaction between the contractile proteins (Bigland-Ritchie, 1981). In sequence, these sites/factors were:

1. Excitatory input to the motor cortex
2. Excitatory drive to lower motoneurons
3. Motorneuron excitability
4. Neuromuscular transmission
5. Sarcolemma excitability
6. Excitation–contraction coupling
7. Contractile machinery
8. Metabolic energy supply.

Traditional models of fatigue have separated the sites/factors numbered 1 to 6, and classified these as being 'central', whilst those numbered 4 to 8 have been classified as being 'peripheral'. Thus, some locations are involved in both central and peripheral fatigue. Moreover, central fatigue can be located within both the central and peripheral nervous systems, being characterized by a decrease in the neural drive to the muscle. To a large extent, these early classifications of fatigue were made artificially on the basis of the experimental techniques available to study changes in muscle functional properties. In particular, the so-called twitch interpolation technique was used as a method of distinguishing fatigue originating upstream and downstream of the site of electrical stimulation (motor nerve or muscle) (Merton, 1954). The technique was first described by Denny-Brown (1928) and involves the electrical (or latterly, magnetic) stimulation of the muscle of interest, or its motor nerve. The stimulus is delivered during a voluntary contraction of the muscle, and the resulting total force depends upon the extent to which the pool of motor units accessed by the external stimulus has been activated by the voluntary effort. For example, if 100% of motor units accessible to the stimulus are activated by the voluntary drive, no additional force will be evoked by the external stimulation. In contrast, if the voluntary drive has activated only a proportion of this motor unit pool, more motor units will be recruited by the stimulation, and a 'twitch' of additional force will be measureable. The latter is indicative of a failure of voluntary neural drive, or 'central fatigue'. Thus, as Merton (1954) put it, 'If the equality [between voluntary and electrically evoked forces] still holds, then the site of fatigue must be peripheral to the point [of stimulation] of the nerve; otherwise it is central, wholly or partly'. Using electrical stimulation techniques, it has also been possible to demonstrate that well-motivated people are capable of activating muscles maximally, such that no additional force is generated electrically, compared with voluntary muscle contraction (Merton, 1954), including the respiratory muscles (Similowski et al, 1996).

Most recently, a new technique has emerged for evaluating the role of the brain in fatigue – that of transcranial magnetic stimulation. The technique involves placing a magnetic coil over the motor cortex. By harnessing electromagnetic induction, an electric current passing through a coil excites adjacent nervous tissue, generating an action potential. This method can also be used to stimulate motorneurons in the spine, as well as peripheral nerves. By careful positioning of the coil, different parts of the motor cortex can be stimulated, evoking brief contractions of specific muscles. Using these muscle activation techniques, it has become clear that feedback from contracting muscles influences the neural drive to the muscles at a number of sites; this will be considered in more detail in the section below 'Afferent feedback and fatigue'.

Early research on fatigue mechanisms tended to focus upon the sites located at the muscle level. This was partly for pragmatic reasons, but also because Merton's muscle stimulation studies (Merton, 1954) had shown that, during maximal isometric contractions of the adductor pollicis, force could not be restored by strenuous stimulation of the muscles. Because the muscle action potential remained unchanged, the finding indicated the decline in force was due to failure within the muscle and not to failure of neuromuscular transmission. Consequently the neuromuscular junction, the influence of fuel availability and the role of accumulated metabolic 'waste products' became a focus of research. At one time, prolonged exercise was understood to be limited by running out of fuel, whereas high-intensity exercise was limited by running out of fuel and/or accumulation of lactic acid (McKenna & Hargreaves, 2008). In other words, fatigue was considered to be a sign of a system in crisis. However, contemporary research on fatigue recognizes not only the important contribution of the brain, but also the fact that fatigue is not a sign of catastrophic failure, but of a system making an integrated response that conserves and optimizes function. For these reasons, and for those explored below in the section 'Afferent feedback and fatigue', classification of fatigue as either 'central' or 'peripheral' has become increasing irrelevant.

Before considering the role of feedback from exercising muscles in fatigue processes, the potential causes of fatigue at the level of the muscle will be discussed briefly (sites 4 to 8; Bigland-Ritchie, 1981). In theory, the neuromuscular junction could present a limit to muscle activation by 'running out' of the neurotransmitter acetylcholine. However, there appears to be little evidence to support a role for the neuromuscular junction in fatigue (Bigland-Ritchie et al, 1982). In contrast, a reduction in sarcolemmal excitability is a potential contributor to fatigue. Failure of action potential propagation can arise for a number of reasons. For example, changes in the concentrations of sodium and potassium ions around the muscles fibres can reduce the excitability of those fibres, with a result that force is reduced (Jones et al, 2004). The next step in the process of muscle contraction is excitation–contraction coupling, which involves the release of calcium from the sarcoplasmic reticulum (SR). Calcium release, its interaction with troponin, and reuptake into the SR, are fundamental to the contraction and relaxation of muscle fibres. Hence, if release or binding of calcium to troponin

is impaired, force can be reduced. Similarly, if reuptake is impaired, relaxation could be slowed. Experiments using single fibres of mouse muscle indicate that repeated bouts of high-intensity exercise can lead to a reduction in calcium release, which is associated with a loss of force (Westerblad et al, 1993). The intramuscular factors implicated in impairing calcium release are ATP, magnesium ions and inorganic phosphate, either separately or in combination; studies in patients with McArdle's syndrome suggest that pH does not contribute to impaired release of calcium (Jones et al, 2004). However, pH does influence the interaction between calcium and troponin, as do phosphate ions. Although both pH and the concentration of phosphate ions change during fatiguing exercise, the interaction between calcium and troponin is not thought to play an important role in human muscle fatigue (Jones et al, 2004). Finally, calcium removal has for many years been considered responsible for the slowing of muscle relaxation in fatigued muscle. However, there is no evidence for this association in human muscle (Jones et al, 2004).

The final stage of muscle contraction is the interaction between the contractile proteins actin and myosin, which generates muscle shortening. Studies on single fibres of fatigued mouse muscle indicate that, even when the fibres are saturated with calcium, the force generated is around 20% lower than that of the unfatigued muscle (Westerblad et al, 1993). This suggests that failure of cross-bridge function contributes to fatigue-related force deficits. Cross-bridge kinetics also influence rates of muscle shortening and relaxation and, since changes in maximum shortening velocity can be accounted for only by slowing of cross-bridge kinetics, this is a key index of cross-bridge dysfunction (Jones et al, 2004). But what factors induce such dysfunction? Because of the reversible nature of the reactions that liberate energy from ATP, it is theoretically possible that accumulation of inorganic phosphate and ADP, or depletion of ATP are responsible. However, there is currently no evidence that accumulation of inorganic phosphate and ADP, or depletion of ATP, lead to cross-bridge dysfunction (Jones et al, 2004), so other candidates must be sought. The 'usual suspect' is pH, but substantial detrimental effects of increases in hydrogen ion concentration ($[H^+]$) appear to be limited to unphysiological ranges of muscle temperature (Jones et al, 2004). To date, there is no consensus regarding the specific metabolites that are responsible for cross-bridge dysfunction. Experiments have typically manipulated one metabolite at a time, and it is conceivable that when changes in metabolites are combined their effects become far more potent (Jones et al, 2004), but for now this remains speculation.

In summary, there appears to be no single weak link in the chain of events that produce muscle contraction, thereby triggering fatigue. In much the same way that efforts to identify a single control factor for the exercise hyperpnoea have resulted in failure, so too has the quest to find a single cause of fatigue. For such a thing to exist, it is implicit that the other links are 'overbuilt', which does not tend to be how evolution operates. Instead, it is more likely that all links approach 'failure' together, and thus all have the potential to be 'the weakest link'. In this scheme, variations in the exercise conditions are what determine the weakest link for any given situation. This is yet another reason why reductionist models of fatigue have, and will continue to be, inadequate.

Afferent feedback, fatigue and perception of effort

Latterly, feedback signals from exercising muscles have been recognized as making an important contribution to central fatigue mechanisms, as well as to perception of effort. These afferents, their sites of action, and influences upon muscle activation are complex, and beyond the scope of this section (see Gandevia, 1998). However, one group of afferents has particular relevance in the context of respiratory muscle training, viz., group III and IV non-myelinated fibres (see Chs 3 and 4). Virtually silent at rest, these small-diameter afferents increase their discharge during muscle contraction in response to stimuli from changes in the temperature, chemical and mechanical properties of the muscle milieu. For this reason, they are often referred to as 'metaboreceptors', and they project to a number of sites within the central nervous system. This means they have many roles, including cardiovascular and respiratory system regulation, and effort perception (Amann et al, 2010), as well as fatigue.

Feedback from group III and IV afferents has been implicated in central fatigue mechanisms via inhibition of central motor output (Gandevia, 2001). It has been suggested (Gandevia, 2001) that afferent feedback from exercising muscles protects locomotor and respiratory muscles from catastrophic fatigue, indeed: 'An extreme example [of central fatigue] occurs with exercise of the inspiratory muscles in which task failure can occur with minimal peripheral fatigue' (Gandevia, 2001). Observations such as this, and more recent studies on leg muscles, have led to the hypothesis that, 'feedback from fatiguing muscle plays an important role in the determination of central motor drive and force output, so that the development of peripheral muscle fatigue is confined to a certain level' (Amann & Dempsey, 2008b) – in other words, that the magnitude of exercise-induced muscle fatigue is a regulated variable (Amann & Dempsey, 2008a).

The importance of group III and IV afferent feedback in regulating integrated exercise responses was illustrated recently by an elegant study in which a cycle time trial was undertaken with and without the selective μ-opioid receptor agonist fentanyl, an agent affecting only afferent fibres (Amann et al, 2009). During a self-paced 5 km (5000 m) time trial, intrathecal fentanyl was associated with greater quadriceps fatigue, a higher central motor output and greater perceived exertion compared with placebo.

A higher power output in the first half of the fentanyl time trial was offset by a lower power output in the second, resulting in no change in performance time. However, compared with placebo the decline in quadriceps twitch force was greater with fentanyl (45.6% vs 33.1%) and was associated with ambulatory problems post-exercise. The authors suggest their data 'emphasize the critical role of locomotor muscle afferents in determining the subject's choice of the "optimal" exercise intensity that will allow for maximal performance while preserving a certain level of locomotor muscle "functional reserve" at end-exercise' (Amann et al, 2009). The specific contribution of respiratory muscle groups III and IV afferents to central fatigue during whole-body exercise awaits investigation. Given the importance of protecting diaphragm function, it is reasonable to speculate that the inhibitory feedback from inspiratory muscle afferents during exercise influences both respiratory and locomotor central motor output. As we will discover in Chapters 3 and 4, feedback from inspiratory muscle metaboreceptors makes an important contribution to cardiovascular control, regulation of limb blood flow and hence to factors that affect development of muscle fatigue (McConnell & Lomax, 2006; Romer et al, 2006).

Task failure and task dependency

An important distinction that has been made within the past two decades is between the concepts of fatigue and task failure (Barry & Enoka, 2007; Astrand et al, 2003). Typical experimental designs used to elucidate fatigue are to quantify: (1) the decline in maximum contraction force (voluntary or evoked electrically) during a bout of fatiguing contractions, and (2) the decline in force or power immediately after the fatiguing contractions (Enoka & Duchateau, 2008). These experiments reveal that fatigue is an evolving process that may or may not lead to task failure and cessation of exercise (Bigland-Ritchie & Woods, 1984). In their 2007 update of Enoka & Stuart's 1992 review, Barry & Enoka (2007) acknowledge that 'The most common definition of fatigue in the past decade is that it corresponds to an exercise-induced reduction in the ability of the muscle to produce force or power, whether or not the task can be sustained'. For this reason, the notion of *fatiguing contractions* is an important one, since is describes an intensity domain in which fatigue begins early in the task, but does not necessarily lead to an inability to sustain the task, or indeed to any measurable failure in, say, maximum voluntary contraction force at its cessation. This is an important concept, since the lack of residual respiratory muscle fatigue post-exercise (e.g., an impairment of diaphragm function) is often cited as an argument for the futility of inspiratory muscle training (Polkey & Moxham, 2004). As has been explained above, failure of muscle activation can occur at any number of sites, not just the contractile machinery.

Furthermore, just as any *definition* of fatigue must accommodate multiple factors, the *process* of fatigue itself is multifactorial and, ultimately, task dependent. Research has now shown that the factors precipitating fatigue are specific to the task, and include participant motivation, pattern of muscle activation, intensity and duration of activity, and continuous or intermittent activity (Barry & Enoka, 2007). For example, studies comparing the responses of older and younger men to two types of muscle contractions showed that older men were more fatigable during dynamic contractions, whilst younger men were more fatigable during isometric contractions (Barry & Enoka, 2007). The explanation for these differences resides in an understanding that there is no single cause of fatigue. As was described above, several linked processes contribute to muscle contraction, and impairment of any one process, or any combination of processes, can result in fatigue. Different tasks impair different physiological processes, thereby determining the task specificity of fatigue. For maximal-intensity tasks, the development of fatigue is linked closely to the decline in performance, and task failure. In contrast, for submaximal intensity tasks, fatigue may develop but might not lead to task failure. Because an activity such as breathing generally requires sub-maximal intensity work by the respiratory pump muscles, contractile fatigue of these muscles may not be the cause of task failure, even when the task involves breathing against a load.

Indeed, task failure may not be the result of fatigue of the principal muscles involved in the task (Enoka & Duchateau, 2008). For example, when human beings inhale against inspiratory loads ranging between 75% and 90% of the maximal strength of their inspiratory muscles, all reach task failure within 20 minutes (McKenzie et al, 1997). However, none exhibited inspiratory muscle fatigue; instead, task failure was associated with hypercapnia and dyspnoea. Even in similar studies, where the work history of the inspiratory muscles has been manipulated to induce prior fatigue, task failure was not related to the severity of inspiratory muscle fatigue (Rohrbach et al, 2003). Rather, task failure appeared to be related to hypercapnia and/or arterial oxygen desaturation.

Because of the seeming futility of identifying any unifying cause(s) of fatigue, research has shifted to focus upon task failure, i.e., the duration for which a task can be sustained. This is not only pragmatic scientifically, but also in terms of the relevance of the findings to everyday life, since it is the failure to sustain the task that impacts upon the individual, not the mechanism(s) of fatigue; individuals can seemingly continue to function in the presence of fatigue, and it may only be when the point of task failure is approached that performance of the task is impaired.

An enlightening model used to elucidate the mechanisms contributing to task failure of limb muscles has been to compare the responses to two tasks of differing difficulty (Hunter et al, 2004). In one task the limb is fixed, and a predetermined isometric force must be sustained for as long as possible. In the second task, an inertial load (requiring the same muscle force as the first task) must be maintained in a specified position for as long as possible. The latter is the

more difficult task, which is reflected in the shorter time to task failure (Hunter et al, 2004). By comparing performance of these two tasks it is possible to identify the adjustments that limit the duration of the more difficult task. These studies have revealed that the neural strategies utilized to deliver the two tasks differ. In the more difficult task, heightened activation of the muscle stretch reflex from the unsupported limb appears to lead to earlier recruitment of the motor unit pool and more rapid termination of the task (Maluf & Enoka, 2005). The additional challenge generated by postural control of the limb has also been studied in the context of the role of synergistic and accessory muscle contributions to the task (Rudroff et al, 2007). Unsurprisingly, tasks that required an accessory muscle contribution were briefer than those that did not.

These data provide empirical confirmation of the anecdotal observation that lifting free weights is more challenging than lifting 'machine' weights (where there is typically only one plane of movement). Confirmation of the highly task-dependent nature of fatigue supports an argument for the development of 'functional' tests of muscle fatigue, as well as for the application of functional principles to muscle training, especially where the objective is to improve performance in activities of daily living (Maluf & Enoka, 2005).

As will be described in Chapter 3, the respiratory muscles are engaged in a number of non-respiratory tasks related to postural control and stabilization of the trunk. Based upon knowledge gained from limb muscles (Maluf & Enoka, 2005), it is reasonable to postulate that a respiratory task such as sustaining exercise hyperpnoea will be more challenging, and potentially limiting, under conditions where these muscles are also engaged in non-respiratory tasks.

Summary

The preceding section might seem to create more questions than answers, but fatigue is an extremely complex phenomenon that contributes to exercise limitation. Fatigue is a process with no single cause, and which may or may not result in task failure. Fatigue also displays plasticity, being influenced by changes in an individual's characteristics, such as the presence of disease or improvements in the neuromuscular system brought about by training. This plasticity may create weak links in the 'fatigue chain', just as it may strengthen them, thereby changing the balance of factors contributing to exercise limitation.

CARDIORESPIRATORY LIMITATION OF EXERCISE TOLERANCE

Whether one is an Olympic athlete or a patient with cardiorespiratory disease, exercise is limited by the unpleasant sensations that it precipitates; even athletes cannot ignore the discomforts of exercise. Principally, these sensations originate from the work of the muscles involved, i.e., the locomotor and respiratory muscles. When overloaded, the former provoke feelings of local discomfort and 'fatigue', whereas the latter stimulate the central sensation of dyspnoea and 'fatigue'. When the contributions of leg effort and dyspnoea to exercise limitation are assessed, over 60% of healthy people cease exercise because of the combined contribution of the two symptoms (Hamilton et al, 1996). Interestingly, the Borg CR-10 rating of dyspnoea at exercise cessation in healthy people can be higher (6 units) than the rating in a similar group of patients with respiratory disease (5 units) (Hamilton et al, 1996). These data indicate that, even in healthy people, dyspnoea is a troubling symptom that makes an important contribution to the decision to stop exercising.

In the absence of disease, the sensations of leg discomfort and dyspnoea originate from an inability of the cardiorespiratory system to deliver adequate O_2 to support the current metabolic requirements of the muscles involved. Failure to meet this demand contributes to muscle fatigue and discomfort (locomotor and respiratory), muscle metaboreflex activation, as well as considerable dyspnoea.

The transport of O_2 to the working muscles involves five stages:

1. *Alveolar ventilation:* Delivery of atmospheric air to the alveoli (breathing)
2. *Pulmonary diffusion:* Transfer of O_2 from the alveoli to the capillary blood
3. *Transport by the blood I:* Loading of O_2 at the lungs
4. *Transport by the blood II:* Delivery of O_2 to the muscle cells via the circulation
5. *Tissue diffusion:* Transfer of O_2 from the muscle capillary blood to the muscle cells.

In Chapter 1 we learned that, in healthy people, the ability of the lungs to oxygenate the pulmonary arterial blood (stages 1 and 2) is not a limiting factor in the supply of O_2 to the tissues, and that, at sea level, most human beings are 'perfusion limited'. In other words, the amount of blood flowing through the pulmonary capillaries limits the amount of O_2 that can be delivered to the periphery (stages 3 and 4). As is the case with stage 1, stage 5 is not a limiting factor at sea level.

To understand the influence of the factors that contribute to stage 3, let's consider the amount of O_2 in $l \cdot min^{-1}$ that can be delivered to the working muscles under two conditions that increase the ability of the blood to transport O_2: (1) if the concentration of haemoglobin [Hb] in the blood is increased, and (2) if the $\dot{Q}$ is increased (Table 2.1).

Thus, increasing [Hb] and/or $\dot{Q}$ can increase the amount of O_2 delivered to the exercising muscles by more than 20%. In practice, athletes can increase [Hb] legally by only one means, i.e., acclimatization to high altitude. However, the capacity to increase [Hb] by this method is very limited, and not all individuals respond to altitude exposure by increasing [Hb] – hence the temptation to partake in the illegal practice of 'blood doping'. In contrast to difficulties in manipulating [Hb], SV is very amenable to training, and can be elevated by around 30% (see 'Training adaptations, Cardiovascular', below).

There are two final stages in the process of transporting the O_2 to the metabolizing muscle cells, i.e., delivery of O_2 to the tissues and tissue diffusion (stages 4 and 5). In common with the loading of O_2 at the lungs, the unloading at the tissues is not diffusion limited, but perfusion limited. In other words, stage 4 is also limited by the amount of blood available to perfuse the muscles, as well as the proximity of the capillaries to the muscle fibres.

Table 2.1 The factors contributing to the loading of O_2 at the lungs

	Control	Increased [Hb]	Increased $\dot{Q}$
O_2 saturation (%)	97	97	97
[Hb] $(g \cdot l^{-1})$	140	170	140
O_2 content per litre of blood (ml)	*$1.36 \times 140 =$ 190	*$1.36 \times 170 =$ 231	*$1.36 \times 140 =$ 190
Stroke volume (l)	0.100	0.100	0.125
f_{cMax} (beats·min^{-1})	200	200	200
$\dot{Q}$ $(l \cdot min^{-1})$	20	20	25
O_2 content per beat (ml)	$0.100 \times 190 =$ 19.00	$0.100 \times 231 =$ 23.10	$0.125 \times 190 =$ 23.75
O_2 delivery $(l \cdot min^{-1})$	**$19.00 \times 200 =$ 3.80**	**$23.10 \times 200 =$ 4.62**	**$23.75 \times 200 =$ 4.75**

* Each gram of Hb can carry 1.36 ml of O_2.

A helpful analogy for this transport process (stages 1 to 5) is to conceptualize it as a haulage business, supplying goods (O_2) to individual stores (muscle cells). The goods are loaded onto trucks in series, at a central depot (the lungs), where there is no limit to the quantity of goods available for transport. However, there are only a finite number of trucks available to be loaded (Hb), and their throughput is also finite ($\dot{Q}$), which determines the carrying capacity of the entire system. For example, if another truck is added to the fleet ([Hb] is increased), or the throughput of trucks can be increased ($\dot{Q}$), then the quantity of goods departing the depot can also be increased. Now consider what happens at the delivery end of the process. With a finite number of trucks, and many stores to supply, the trucks must have access to a network of roads (blood vessels) that allow them to take their goods as close to the stores as possible. If the road network is plentiful and the fleet has lots of trucks, then it is possible to deliver the goods to the doorstep of every store; delivery is fast and efficient, and the stores do not run out of goods. However, if there aren't enough trucks to go around, then the trucks must prioritize the stores they deliver to, and not all stores are supplied promptly; consequently, the delivery service fails to keep pace with customer demand, with the result that the stores run out of goods before the next truck arrives. The limiting factor at both ends of the delivery process is the throughput of trucks; similarly, the rate-limiting step in the oxygen transport system is therefore $\dot{Q}$.

There is one more stage in the process of O_2 *usage*, as compared with O_2 *transport*, to be considered, i.e., the ability of the muscles to consume the O_2 that is supplied. In our analogy above, this is akin to the customer demand for the goods in the stores. Demand generally exceeds the ability to supply, and muscles could do more work if they were supplied with more O_2. This is known because in studies comparing one-legged and two-legged cycling at the same power output the oxygen consumption of two-legged cycling is lower than twice that of one-legged cycling (Davies & Sargeant, 1974). In other words, when one leg has exclusive access to the entire $\dot{Q}$, it is capable of consuming more oxygen, and doing more work, than when the work and $\dot{Q}$ are shared by two legs. The concept of O_2 usage will be considered in the section 'Maximal oxygen uptake and oxygen uptake kinetics' (below).

Before closing this section on cardiorespiratory limitations, we need to consider a breathing-related limitation that has an impact upon O_2 transport. This may appear to be a contradictory statement, because earlier in this section it was stated that breathing does not limit stages 1 and 2, above. However, this is not the site at which breathing influences O_2 transport. The mechanical and metabolic work of breathing has been shown to affect the delivery of O_2 to exercising muscles (Harms et al, 1998). Breathing influences the share of $\dot{Q}$ that the locomotor muscles receive, such that an increase in the work of breathing reduces locomotor muscle blood flow, thereby reducing exercise tolerance (Harms et al, 2000). This influence is exerted via a respiratory muscle metaboreflex (see above), which is discussed in more detail in Chapter 3 (section 'Respiratory muscle involvement in exercise limitation, Healthy people').

CARDIORESPIRATORY FITNESS

Maximal oxygen uptake

In the previous section we considered how $\dot{Q}$ is the rate-limiting step in the transport of O_2 to exercising muscles. In this section the ability of the body to utilize O_2 to undertake external work will be discussed.

In the previous section the analogy of a haulage company supplying goods to stores was used to illustrate the role of $\dot{Q}$ in O_2 transport. In an extension to that analogy, we can think of O_2 uptake ($\dot{V}O_2$) by the muscles as being akin to the sales of the goods, which are a function of the rate of delivery and the customer demand; both are required in order to achieve sales. In the same way, muscle $\dot{V}O_2$ is a function of blood flow and O_2 utilization. The utilization of O_2 is the amount of O_2 extracted from the blood as it passes through the tissue, i.e., the arterial to mixed venous O_2 difference (a–$\bar{v}O_2$). Thus, the $\dot{V}O_2$ of a muscle is given by the equation:

$$\dot{V}O_2 = \dot{Q} \times \text{a–}\bar{v}O_2$$

During exercise, not only does blood flow to a muscle increase, but the extraction of oxygen from the blood is also enhanced, widening the a–$\bar{v}O_2$.

The $\dot{V}O_2$ of the entire body can be measured by using the a–$\bar{v}O_2$ difference measured at the lungs. Typically, this gradient is around 5 ml at rest, but can be three times this value during heavy exercise. The change is generated by an increased extraction of O_2 by the muscles, which produces a reduction in mixed venous O_2 content and a wider a–$\bar{v}O_2$ difference. However, measuring $\dot{Q}$ and pulmonary a–$\bar{v}$ O_2 difference is a highly invasive method of assessing total body $\dot{V}O_2$; fortunately, it can also be estimated by subtracting the amount of oxygen exhaled from the amount inhaled at the mouth.

The maximal oxygen uptake ($\dot{V}O_{2max}$; also called maximal oxygen consumption or aerobic capacity) is an index that combines both the maximal ability to transport and to utilize O_2. It can be defined for an exercising muscle group, but is more frequently defined for the whole body during exercise by measuring $\dot{V}O_2$ at the mouth. During exercise at sea level requiring the involvement of >30% of the total muscle mass, $\dot{V}O_{2max}$ is limited by $\dot{Q}$, and not by the ability of the muscles to consume O_2 (Gonzalez-Alonso & Calbet, 2003). For this reason, $\dot{V}O_{2max}$ is used as an index of cardiovascular function, as well as of 'aerobic fitness'.

Typically, $\dot{V}O_{2max}$ is estimated by undertaking an incremental exercise test to the limit of tolerance. An example of the $\dot{V}O_2$ response to such a test is provided in the bottom right panel of Figure 2.2. The gold standard criterion for a test that is limited by physiological factors is a plateau of $\dot{V}O_2$, despite an increase in the external work done. If this plateau is not observable, a number of secondary criteria can be used to imply maximality. These include, either individually or in combination, the following (Poole et al, 2008):

- Respiratory exchange ratio ≥ 1.00, 1.10, or 1.15
- Peak heart rate within 10 beats·min^{-1}, or 5% of age-predicted maximum
- Blood lactic acid concentration of 8–10 mmol·l^{-1}.

However, use of these indirect criteria has been shown to underestimate $\dot{V}O_{2max}$ by as much as 27% (Poole et al, 2008). Accordingly, prudence is advised, and the term $\dot{V}O_2$ peak ($\dot{V}O_{2peak}$) should be used in order to distinguish the value from a true $\dot{V}O_{2max}$ that was limited by central cardiovascular function ($\dot{Q}$). The term $\dot{V}O_{2peak}$ is also used in situations where none of these criteria have been met, as will be the case in many patients who are symptom limited by factors such as dyspnoea.

The ability to sustain high levels of external work without becoming fatigued is very closely related to one's $\dot{V}O_{2max}$. Hence, endurance athletes tend to have high values, but so too do very large people with a large muscle mass. Accordingly, $\dot{V}O_{2max}$ is often expressed as a relative value by dividing the value expressed in ml·min^{-1} by body mass in kilograms to give relative $\dot{V}O_{2max}$ in ml·min^{-1}.kg^{-1}. Body mass also needs to be borne in mind when considering weight-bearing and non-weight-bearing exercise. For example, being heavy is no disadvantage when cycling a stationary ergometer, but is a considerable disadvantage during walking and running. Accordingly, compared with an overweight individual with a low relative $\dot{V}O_{2max}$, a slight individual with a high relative $\dot{V}O_{2max}$ may have a lower ability to sustain a moderate power output on a cycle ergometer, but a much greater ability to sustain ambulation at a moderate speed.

Furthermore, for athletes, having a high relative $\dot{V}O_{2max}$ does not necessarily imply that they will be a good marathon runner. Although, as a population, marathon runners all have a high relative $\dot{V}O_{2max}$, within this population, performance is not predicted by $\dot{V}O_{2max}$. In other words, two athletes with the same relative $\dot{V}O_{2max}$ can have very different marathon running times. This is because of the influence of two other factors upon performance: (1) the lactate threshold (LaT) and (2) exercise economy. Each will be considered below.

The response of $\dot{V}O_{2max}$ to training will be considered in the section 'Training adaptations', below.

Lactate threshold

The term lactate threshold (LaT) is slightly misleading, because it implies that it corresponds to an exercise intensity at which anaerobic metabolism is switched on abruptly. This is not the case, because anaerobic metabolism takes place constantly. Even at very low intensities of exercise, inhomogeneity of blood flow distribution within muscles means that some muscle fibres and groups of fibres receive inadequate blood flow, resulting in reliance upon anaerobic metabolic pathways. The production of lactic acid (La; also known as lactate) therefore takes place constantly, but La is also metabolized constantly, in a continuous cycle of production and breakdown. So long as there is sufficient spare aerobic capacity to metabolize La, the concentration in the blood may be elevated slightly, but there is no accumulation of La. However, when the intensity of exercise exceeds the capacity to break down La, it will continue to accumulate in the tissues and blood until exercise is terminated. Because of the detrimental influence of La upon pH and muscle function, exercise above the LaT is non-sustainable and the inevitable end point is exercise intolerance. The LaT should be thought of as an intensity domain during exercise that results in an elevated concentration of La in the blood ([La]); further increases in exercise intensity above this level result in a progressive increase in the [La] and eventual exercise intolerance.

The impact of the LaT upon exercise tolerance is therefore to determine the maximum exercise intensity at which exercise is sustainable for prolonged periods of time. Typically, the LaT occurs at around 50–60% of $\dot{V}O_{2max}$. However, in highly trained endurance athletes it may be as high at 90% $\dot{V}O_{2max}$. This is why athletes with the same $\dot{V}O_{2max}$ can have very different marathon performances; the athlete whose LaT occurs at the highest percentage of his or her $\dot{V}O_{2max}$ can sustain a higher running speed over the course of the marathon.

The LaT is highly responsive to training, which will be considered in 'Training adaptations' (below).

Exercise economy

The final piece in the performance jigsaw is exercise economy, i.e., the oxygen cost of exercise. At the very top of elite sport, where $\dot{V}O_{2max}$ and LaT have been optimized, economy appears to be the factor that differentiates world champions from 'also rans' (Foster & Lucia, 2007).

As well as being determined by external factors such as the effects of aerodynamic drag, movement economy is determined by a number of intrinsic factors (Saunders et al, 2004):

1. Motor skills (e.g., pedalling efficiently in cycling)
2. Biomechanical factors (e.g., the return of elastic energy during running)
3. Anthropometry (e.g., small, light limbs)
4. Metabolic adaptations within muscles that enhance the amount of energy liberated per unit of oxygen utilized.

Exercise economy is responsive to training, but improvements are difficult to obtain, and scientific evidence to support particular training interventions is limited (Midgley et al, 2007). Accordingly, this aspect of performance will not be considered any further. However, it should be clear that, in patients with obvious difficulties with ambulation, interventions that improve exercise economy also improve exercise tolerance.

PRINCIPLES OF CARDIORESPIRATORY TRAINING

In the preceding section, a number of factors were identified as contributing to exercise tolerance/performance. For the average person, the greatest gains in exercise tolerance can be made from improving $\dot{V}O_{2max}$ and LaT, and these factors will be the focus of this section.

The principles of training specificity are discussed in detail in relation to muscle training in Chapter 5, 'General training principles'. Suffice to say for the purposes of the following section, the principles of overload, specificity and reversibility also apply to whole-body training. In short, muscles and systems need to be *overloaded* in order to elicit adaptation, these adaptations are *specific* to the training stimulus that is applied, and they *reverse* if the overload is removed.

In the following sections, the respective adaptations of the cardiovascular and respiratory systems to training are described.

Cardiovascular training adaptations

Oxygen delivery to the exercising muscles can be increased by improving the function of both the heart and the circulatory system. From the preceding sections it will be apparent that the limitations imposed by $\dot{Q}$ upon O_2 transport make the pumping capacity of the heart a prime candidate for improvement. Since the heart's main function is as a pump, the specificity principle dictates that overload must tax the heart's ability to eject a bolus of blood into the circulation, i.e., improving SV. The determinants of SV are the volume of blood returning to the heart (venous return), the ability of the left ventricle to accommodate blood and the efficiency with which the ventricle is able to eject the blood it contains. In practice this means undertaking whole-body activities that elevate heart rate; however, just as the resistance training of skeletal muscles requires the right combination of load and duration (repetitions), so too does training the myocardium. Typically, for very-high-intensity exercise, the duration of the training stimulus should be ≥90 seconds, whilst for sub-maximal exercise it should be ≥10 minutes (Jones & Poole, 2009). These types of 'aerobic' activities also deliver a training stimulus to the rest of the circulatory system, and to the exercising muscles. Improving circulatory and muscle function will improve $\dot{V}O_{2max}$ and LaT, with $\dot{V}O_{2max}$ typically having the potential to increase by around 20% in a previously sedentary individual. However, the magnitude of this increase can be greater in people with extremely low baseline function, and also depends upon the intensity and duration of the training stimulus, as well as the frequency and duration of the training programme. Responsiveness to training also varies enormously between individuals owing to genetic predisposition. Just as training can 'give' $\dot{V}O_{2max}$, inactivity can 'taketh away', with a loss of $\dot{V}O_{2max}$ at the rate of around 1% per day over a period of up to 30 days of bed rest (Convertino, 1997).

The specific adaptations that result in the functional outcome of an improvement in $\dot{V}O_{2max}$ and LaT fall into three main categories: myocardial, circulatory and muscle adaptations.

Myocardial adaptations

The intrinsic efficiency of the heart improves such that myocardial oxygen cost at a given metabolic rate is lower. The lower f_c (bradycardia) at any given metabolic rate is a manifestation of the increase in SV that follows aerobic training (Wilmore et al, 2001a). This increase is made possible by both an increase in the volume of blood returning to the heart (venous return or pre-load) and an increase in left and right ventricular volumes (Scharhag et al, 2002), which is required to accommodate a larger volume of blood at the end of diastole (end-diastolic volume, EDV). Another critical feature of the myocardial response to training is an improvement in the efficiency with which blood is ejected from the ventricles. The resulting reduction in end-systolic volume (ESV) (Scharhag et al, 2002) is due to hypertrophy of the muscle cells, as well as the potentiating influence of pre-load stretch upon the Frank–Starling mechanism (see above). Many of the changes to myocardial function are mutually reinforcing; for example, the increased SV results in a bradycardia, which improves ventricular filling (pre-load) by lengthening diastole. The bradycardia also contributes to lowering myocardial work and thus O_2 cost.

Circulatory adaptations

Exercise requires vasodilatation in muscle vascular beds, and vasoconstriction in regions with low metabolic requirements, the latter being a compensatory measure to defend ABP. The volume of fluid within a closed, pump-driven system represents an obvious limitation to the ability to accommodate large changes in the volume of the system (active muscle vasodilatation), without jeopardizing its driving pressure (ABP). Aerobic training stimulates an immediate expansion of the plasma volume, which results from fluid shifts that are secondary to an increased blood albumin concentration (Gillen et al, 1991). A week or so after the increase in plasma volume is an increase in the number of red blood cells (RBCs); however, plasma volume expands relatively more than the number of RBCs, with the result that [Hb] is lower in the trained state. The increase in the number of RBCs increases O_2-carrying capacity, whilst the decrease in [Hb] improves flow, thanks to a decrease in viscosity (El-Sayed et al, 2005). Accompanying these improvements in the properties of the blood are enhancements to the structure and function of the vasculature that improve its blood-flow capacity (Laughlin & Roseguini, 2008). Larger blood vessels undergo arteriogenesis, increasing their diameter, whilst the capillary network is expanded through angiogenesis. The former increases the capacitance of the peripheral vasculature, whilst the latter slows capillary transit time and brings blood closer to the muscle cells, increasing oxygen extraction (Wilmore et al, 2001a). There is also an improvement in the functional properties of the vasculature, which increase exercise blood-flow capacity; these are underpinned by changes to vessel endothelial and smooth muscle properties (Laughlin & Roseguini, 2008). These vascular changes appear to show a high degree of heterogeneity and are specific to the type of training (e.g., high vs moderate intensity). Finally, training induces a lower sympathetic nervous system activity, resulting in an attenuated ABP response to exercise, and a slight (<3 mmHg) reduction in resting ABP (Wilmore et al, 2001b).

Muscle adaptations

The enhancement is the efficiency of the O_2 delivery system are accompanied by an enhanced ability of the muscle cells to utilize O_2 to liberate energy for work. Oxygen is utilized within the cells' mitochondria to liberate energy from pyruvate, in the form of ATP, to fuel muscle contraction. Endurance training induces an increase in the size and number of muscle cell mitochondria, which results in an increase in overall mitochondrial enzyme activity (Holloszy & Booth, 1976). Amongst other metabolic changes elicited by the enhanced enzyme activity is a reduction in lactic acid production (Stallknecht et al, 1998), which is the alternative destination for pyruvate when the oxidative capacity of the cells is limited.

Respiratory training adaptations

In light of the huge capacity of the cardiovascular system to adapt to training, one might expect the lungs to exhibit a similar degree of plasticity. To most people's surprise, the lungs show no training response. Unlikely though it seems, training does not increase lung volumes, improve lung function, or enhance the ability of the lungs to transfer oxygen to the blood, even in athletes who have trained for many years (Wagner, 2005).

Notwithstanding this inability to adapt to training, the observation that the lung function of athletes such as swimmers and rowers is superior to that of their non-athletic contemporaries has led to speculation that physical training, especially during childhood and adolescence, may enhance the development of the lungs (Armour et al, 1993). However, one cannot exclude the possibility that, for some sports, having large lungs may provide an advantage that leads to success. Hence only competitors with larger than normal lungs succeed and remain to compete in their chosen sport as adults.

Notwithstanding the intransigence of the lungs *per se* to adapt to training, the musculature of the respiratory pump (Powers & Criswell, 1996) and upper airway (Vincent et al, 2002) has been shown to respond to endurance training. There is also evidence that endurance training raises the intensity of inspiratory muscle work required to activate the inspiratory muscle metaboreflex (Callegaro et al, 2011). This reflex is know to impair O_2 delivery to exercising locomotor muscles (Harms et al, 1997) and to exacerbate fatigue (Romer et al, 2006).

Whole-body exercise training also results in higher peak $\dot{V}_E$ during exercise, as well as a lower ventilatory equivalent for oxygen ($\dot{V}_E / \dot{V}O_2$), i.e., a reduced breathing requirement for exercise. The latter results from an increase in V_T, and a corresponding improvement in the dead space to tidal volume ratio (V_D / V_T), which increases alveolar ventilation (V_A), lessening the $\dot{V}_E$ requirement. As was discussed above (see 'Cardiorespiratory limitation of exercise tolerance'), an improved respiratory-pumping capacity does not enhance blood oxygenation, but it does enhance the ability to make a respiratory compensation for a metabolic acidosis.

The response of the respiratory musculature to specific resistance training and the associated functional benefits are described in detail in Chapter 4.

METHODS OF CARDIORESPIRATORY TRAINING

The physiological changes that underpin a training-induced increase in aerobic exercise performance/tolerance involve the integrated overload of the cardiovascular, respiratory and neuromuscular systems. The optimal training stimulus is therefore any exercise that overloads the entire aerobic energy transfer system, from lungs to mitochondria. The activities that facilitate this type of overload involve repeated, rhythmic contractions of large muscle groups at intensities that can be sustained for ≥10 minutes (see 'Exercise modality', below).

The two physiological indices of function normally associated with an improvement in the ability to undertake aerobic exercise are $\dot{V}O_{2max}$ and the LaT. As we learned above, these two parameters normally increase in concert with one another, but it is also possible to tailor training to emphasize the overloading stimulus to one or other parameter. In the following sections, the characteristics of training programmes to increase in $\dot{V}O_{2max}$ and LaT are described.

Exercise modality

Overload of the cardiorespiratory system can be achieved using a wide variety of exercise modalities. Traditional activities include, brisk walking, running, cycling, swimming, rowing, cross-country skiing, and even dancing. In a health-club setting, machines have been created that provide the involvement of large muscles mass, with some of the discomforts and injury risks of traditional activities, including stair climbers, elliptical walkers, arm crank ergometers, etc. When selecting an exercise modality for training, a large number of highly personal factors come into play, e.g., personal preference, orthopaedic limitation, skill, personal finances, etc. In practical terms, the optimal training mode is the one that the individual is most likely to engage with in accordance with the requirements of the training regimen.

However, the specificity principle limits the extent to which cardiorespiratory improvements transfer between different exercise modalities (Millet et al, 2009). In other words, a 15% increase in $\dot{V}O_{2max}$ achieved through cycle training will not necessarily result in the same improvement in $\dot{V}O_{2max}$ during running. The reasons for this are not fully understood, but probably arise because of the specificity of the peripheral adaptations to muscle structure and function, as well as biomechanics. Notwithstanding these limitations, many athletes uses a range of exercise modalities, so-called 'cross training', as a means of lessening boredom, and of reducing the risk of overuse injuries. Cross training can also enhance adherence to training, especially at a recreational level.

With the specificity principle in mind, it is also important to consider how exercise modality impacts upon the broad range of training benefits. Whilst $\dot{V}O_{2max}$ might be one of the main physiological outcomes that a particular training programme targets, maximizing $\dot{V}O_{2max}$ is unlikely to be the goal from the perspective of the individual undertaking the training. For example, an amateur competitive runner is more likely to be focussed on, say improving their 10 km time. Although $\dot{V}O_{2max}$ improvement may contribute to the achievement of personal goals, it is not an end in itself particularly, as the limitation to the 10 km performance may not reside in $\dot{V}O_{2max}$ but in the running speed corresponding to the LaT. With goals and specificity in mind, if one is training to increase 10 km running performance then this is best achieved through the practice of running, and using a training regimen that overloads both $\dot{V}O_{2max}$ and LaT.

Before closing this section, there is one final aspect of specificity to consider, i.e., the role of the trunk musculature in specific exercise modalities (see also Ch. 3, 'Non-respiratory functions of the respiratory muscles'). A striking phenomenon, particularly in non-athletes, is the greater intensity of dyspnoea at equivalent $\dot{V}O_2$ during walking/running than during cycling. The mechanism underpinning this is the involvement of the respiratory musculature in postural control during running – a challenge that is not present during cycling, especially on a stationary ergometer. In other words, the respiratory muscles are required to multi-task during running, which increases respiratory muscle work and exacerbates dyspnoea. The implications of this are three-fold: (1) if training overload is limited by dyspnoea during walking/running, then an alternative modality (e.g., cycling) might enhance the overall aerobic training response, (2) if reducing dyspnoea during activities of daily living is a goal, then using cycling as a means of training does not deliver a sufficiently specific training overload, because it does not address the postural role of the trunk muscles during exercise, and (3) supplementing or preceding the aerobic training with specific respiratory muscle and postural training may enhance the final training outcome by reducing limitations arising from dyspnoea.

Aerobic capacity ($\dot{V}O_{2max}$)

The ability of the cardiovascular system to deliver oxygenated blood to the exercising muscles is the weakest link in the O_2 delivery system determining aerobic capacity, i.e., $\dot{V}O_{2max}$. Improvement of $\dot{V}O_{2max}$ is therefore underpinned principally by the improvement of O_2 delivery by the cardiovascular system. Accordingly, training interventions that are intended to increase $\dot{V}O_{2max}$ must overload the cardiovascular contribution to O_2 delivery. Improvement in $\dot{V}O_{2max}$ has become synonymous with the concept of 'endurance' training, i.e., undertaking prolonged, moderate-intensity exercise. However, this traditional view is changing and there is evidence supporting alternative training to enhance $\dot{V}O_{2max}$.

In common with many interventions that influence biological processes, exercise possesses a dose–response relationship. Accordingly, when devising a training regimen there are a number of key factors that make up the exercise 'prescription', and the thresholds for each differ according to the starting level of $\dot{V}O_{2max}$:

- *Intensity:* The percentage of $\dot{V}O_{2max}$ of the training. This can be expressed in range of ways, including the percentage of: (1) total $\dot{V}O_{2max}$, (2) $\dot{V}O_2$ reserve ($\dot{V}O_{2maxR}$), (3) maximal f_c, (4) f_c reserve and (5) metabolic equivalent of the task (MET). Irrespective of baseline function, the improvements in $\dot{V}O_{2max}$ are greater with exercise of vigorous intensity than with moderate intensity (Swain, 2005) (Table 2.2).
- *Duration:* The duration of each individual bout of exercise has received much attention, and current recommendations advise a minimum daily goal of $\geq$ 30 minutes per day (5 days per week), which can be accumulated in individual bouts of $\geq$10 minutes (Garber et al, 2011). Because the duration of exercise required to elicit a training effect is inversely related to duration, higher-intensity exercise requires a daily accumulation of only 20 minutes (Table 2.2).
- *Frequency:* The weekly frequency of training has also received specific attention, and current recommendations advise a minimum daily goal of 5 days per week ($\geq$30 minutes per day) (Garber et al,

Table 2.2 Minimum intensity and effective intensity ranges, duration and frequency of training required to increase $\dot{V}O_{2max}$ in individuals with low, moderate and high baseline $\dot{V}O_{2max}$[1]

	Low $\dot{V}O_{2max}$	Moderate $\dot{V}O_{2max}$	High $\dot{V}O_{2max}$
Intensity	[1]40–50% $\dot{V}O_{2max}$	[2]65–80% $\dot{V}O_{2max}$	[2]95–100% $\dot{V}O_{2max}$
Duration	[1]30 min·day^{-1} (low) [3]20 min·day^{-1} (moderate)	30 to 90 min·day^{-1}	Interval training
Frequency	[4]2–5 days·week^{-1}	[3]5 days·week^{-1}	5–7 days·week^{-1}

[1] Garber et al, 2011; [2] Midgley et al, 2006; [3] Haskell et al, 2007; [4] Meyer et al, 2006.

2011). However, in previously untrained individuals, accumulating the same total duration (150 minutes per week) in as little as 2 days per week can yield the same increase in $\dot{V}O_{2max}$ (Meyer et al, 2006) (Table 2.2).

There is no 'magic bullet' training regimen for increasing $\dot{V}O_{2max}$, but Table 2.2 attempts to provide some approximate, evidence-based guidance. As well as bearing in mind the enormous heterogeneity of responsiveness to training, the necessity to vary and progress the stimulus must also be borne in mind. In addition, the table provides *minimum* thresholds; optimized benefits are achieved by *maximizing* training intensity. For example, in previously sedentary men, training at 80% $\dot{V}O_{2max}$ three times per week elicited a greater increase in $\dot{V}O_{2max}$ than training at 60% $\dot{V}O_{2max}$, at equivalent caloric expenditure per training session (400 kcal).

The progression of training is essential, as improvements in absolute $\dot{V}O_{2max}$ will render a given percentage of $\dot{V}O_{2max}$ relatively less intense. Any of the three aforementioned components of the training prescription can be varied in order to maintain overload. Current guidelines make no specific recommendations, but common sense suggests that a combination of all three components is required (Garber et al, 2011).

Lactate threshold

The intensity of exercise corresponding to the LaT is determined primarily by the oxidative capacity of the active muscle mass (Ivy et al, 1980). As was discussed above, the LaT represents the intensity at which the production of lactic acid exceeds its breakdown. Endurance training appears to increase the intensity of exercise corresponding to the LaT by enhancing the ability to break down lactic acid (Donovan & Brooks, 1983). Thus exercise regimens that overload the lactate clearance mechanisms are required in order to elicit improvement in LaT. A typical training session to achieve this goal will be $\sim$20 minutes in duration at an intensity of $\sim$90% $\dot{V}O_{2max}$. However, there are a variety of methods that can be used to enhance LaT, including interval training at maximal (100% $\dot{V}O_{2max}$) and supramaximal (130% $\dot{V}O_{2max}$) intensities, in bouts that are sustained for $\sim$3 minutes and 30 seconds, respectively (Esfarjani & Laursen, 2007). These training regimens also improve $\dot{V}O_{2max}$, with the largest increase in both parameters ($\sim$10%) observed after interval training at 100% $\dot{V}O_{2max}$ for $\sim$3 minutes (8 bouts per session, two times per week) (Esfarjani & Laursen, 2007).

High-intensity interval training is not only a very time-efficient method of enhancing both LaT and $\dot{V}O_{2max}$, it may also be better tolerated in individuals in whom the escalating intensity of exercise-related symptoms can limit the ability to undertake continuous exercise, e.g., dyspnoeic patients. Notwithstanding this, high-intensity training may also be contraindicated for certain individuals, especially those with cardiovascular disease. Accordingly, the design of a training regimen needs to be made on the basis of the clinical profile of the individual involved.

REFERENCES

Amann, M., Dempsey, J.A., 2008a. The concept of peripheral locomotor muscle fatigue as a regulated variable. J. Physiol. 586, 2029–2030.

Amann, M., Dempsey, J.A., 2008b. Locomotor muscle fatigue modifies central motor drive in healthy humans and imposes a limitation to exercise performance. J. Physiol. 586, 161–173.

Amann, M., Proctor, L.T., Sebranek, J.J., et al., 2009. Opioid-mediated muscle afferents inhibit central motor drive and limit peripheral muscle fatigue development in humans. J. Physiol. 587, 271–283.

Amann, M., Blain, G.M., Proctor, L.T., et al., 2010. Group III and IV muscle afferents contribute to ventilatory and cardiovascular response to rhythmic exercise in humans. J. Appl. Physiol. 109, 966–976.

Armour, J., Donnelly, P.M., Bye, P.T., 1993. The large lungs of elite swimmers: an increased alveolar number? Eur. Respir. J. 6 (2), 237–247.

Astrand, P.O., Rodahl, K., Stromme, S., 2003. Textbook of work physiology: Physiological bases of exercise, fourth ed. Human Kinetics, Champaign, IL, p. 185.

Barry, B.K., Enoka, R.M., 2007. The neurobiology of muscle fatigue: 15 years later. Integrative and Comparative Biology 47, 465–473.

Bigland-Ritchie, B., 1981. EMG and fatigue of human voluntary and stimulated contractions. In: Porter, R., Whelan, J. (Eds.), Human muscle fatigue: physiological mechanisms. Pitman Medical, London, pp. 130–156.

Bigland-Ritchie, B., Woods, J.J., 1984. Changes in muscle contractile properties and neural control during human muscular fatigue. Muscle Nerve 7, 691–699.

Bigland-Ritchie, B., Kukulka, C.G., Lippold, O.C., et al., 1982. The absence of neuromuscular transmission failure in sustained maximal voluntary contractions. J. Physiol. 330, 265–278.

Cady, E.B., Elshove, H., Jones, D.A., et al., 1989. The metabolic causes of slow relaxation in fatigued human skeletal muscle. J. Physiol. 418, 327–337.

Callegaro, C.C., Ribeiro, J.P., Tan, C.O., et al., 2011. Attenuated inspiratory muscle metaboreflex in endurance-trained individuals. Respir. Physiol. Neurobiol. 177, 24–29.

Convertino, V.A., 1997. Cardiovascular consequences of bed rest: effect on maximal oxygen uptake. Med. Sci. Sports Exerc. 29, 191–196.

Davies, C.T., Sargeant, A.J., 1974. Physiological responses to one- and two-leg exercise breathing air and 45 percent oxygen. J. Appl. Physiol. 36, 142–148.

Denny-Brown, D.E., 1928. On inhibition as a reflex accompaniment of the tendon jerk and of other forms of active muscular response. Proc. R. Soc. Lond. B Biol. Sci. 103, 321–326.

Donovan, C.M., Brooks, G.A., 1983. Endurance training affects lactate clearance, not lactate production. Am. J. Physiol. 244, E83–E92.

El-Sayed, M.S., Ali, N., El-Sayed Ali, Z., 2005. Haemorheology in exercise and training. Sports Med. 35, 649–670.

Enoka, R.M., Duchateau, J., 2008. Muscle fatigue: what, why and how it influences muscle function. J. Physiol. 586, 11–23.

Enoka, R.M., Stuart, D.G., 1992. Neurobiology of muscle fatigue. J. Appl. Physiol. 72, 1631–1648.

Esfarjani, F., Laursen, P.B., 2007. Manipulating high-intensity interval training: effects on VO2max, the lactate threshold and 3000 m running performance in moderately trained males. J. Sci. Med. Sport 10, 27–35.

Foster, C., Lucia, A., 2007. Running economy: the forgotten factor in elite performance. Sports Med. 37, 316–319.

Gandevia, S.C., 1998. Neural control in human muscle fatigue: changes in muscle afferents, motoneurones and motor cortical drive [corrected]. Acta Physiol. Scand. 162, 275–283.

Gandevia, S.C., 2001. Spinal and supraspinal factors in human muscle fatigue. Physiol. Rev. 81, 1725–1789.

Garber, C.E., Blissmer, B., Deschenes, M.R., et al., 2011. American College of Sports Medicine position stand. Quantity and quality of exercise for developing and maintaining cardiorespiratory, musculoskeletal, and neuromotor fitness in apparently healthy adults: guidance for prescribing exercise. Med. Sci. Sports Exerc. 43, 1334–1359.

Gillen, C.M., Lee, R., Mack, G.W., et al., 1991. Plasma volume expansion in humans after a single intense exercise protocol. J. Appl. Physiol. 71, 1914–1920.

Gonzalez-Alonso, J., 2012. Human thermoregulation and the cardiovascular system. Exp. Physiol. 97, 340–346.

Gonzalez-Alonso, J., Calbet, J.A., 2003. Reductions in systemic and skeletal muscle blood flow and oxygen delivery limit maximal aerobic capacity in humans. Circulation 107, 824–830.

Hamilton, A.L., Killian, K.J., Summers, E., et al., 1996. Quantification of intensity of sensations during muscular work by normal subjects. J. Appl. Physiol. 81, 1156–1161.

Harms, C.A., Dempsey, J.A., 1999. Cardiovascular consequences of exercise hyperpnea. Exerc. Sport Sci. Rev. 27, 37–62.

Harms, C.A., Babcock, M.A., McClaran, S.R., et al., 1997. Respiratory muscle work compromises leg blood flow during maximal exercise. J. Appl. Physiol. 82, 1573–1583.

Harms, C.A., Wetter, T.J., McClaran, S.R., et al., 1998. Effects of respiratory muscle work on cardiac output and its distribution during maximal exercise. J. Appl. Physiol. 85, 609–618.

Harms, C.A., Wetter, T.J., St Croix, C.M., et al., 2000. Effects of respiratory muscle work on exercise performance. J. Appl. Physiol. 89, 131–138.

Haskell, W.L., Lee, I.M., Pate, R.R., et al., 2007. Physical activity and public health: updated recommendation for adults from the American College of Sports Medicine and the American Heart Association. Med. Sci. Sports Exerc. 39, 1423–1434.

Holloszy, J.O., Booth, F.W., 1976. Biochemical adaptations to endurance exercise in muscle. Annu. Rev. Physiol. 38, 273–291.

Hunter, S.K., Duchateau, J., Enoka, R.M., 2004. Muscle fatigue and the mechanisms of task failure. Exerc. Sport Sci. Rev. 32, 44–49.

Hussain, S.N.A., Comtois, A.S., 2005. Regulation of skeletal muscle blood flow during exercise. In: Hamid, Q., Shannon, J., Martin, J. (Eds.), Physiologic basis of respiratory disease. Decker, Hamilton, ONT, pp. 555–566.

Ivy, J.L., Withers, R.T., Van Handel, P.J., et al., 1980. Muscle respiratory capacity and fiber type as determinants of the lactate threshold. J. Appl. Physiol. 48, 523–527.

Jones, A.M., Poole, D.C., 2009. Physiological demands of endurance exercise. In: Maughan, R.J. (Ed.), Olympic textbook of science in sport. Blackwell, Oxford, pp. 43–55.

Jones, D.A., de Haan, A., Round, J.M., 2004. Skeletal muscle: from molecules to muscles. Churchill Livingstone, London.

Laughlin, M.H., Roseguini, B., 2008. Mechanisms for exercise training-induced increases in skeletal muscle blood flow capacity: differences with interval sprint training versus aerobic endurance training. J. Physiol. Pharmacol. 59 (Suppl. 7), 71–88.

Levick, R.J., 2009. An introduction to cardiovascular physiology. Hodder Arnold, London.

Maluf, K.S., Enoka, R.M., 2005. Task failure during fatiguing contractions performed by humans. J. Appl. Physiol. 99, 389–396.

McConnell, A.K., 2011. Breathe strong, perform better. Human Kinetics Publishers, Champaign, IL.

McConnell, A.K., Lomax, M., 2006. The influence of inspiratory muscle work history and specific inspiratory muscle training upon human limb muscle fatigue. J. Physiol. 577, 445–457.

McKenna, M.J., Hargreaves, M., 2008. Resolving fatigue mechanisms determining exercise performance: integrative physiology at its finest! J. Appl. Physiol. 104, 286–287.

McKenzie, D.K., Allen, G.M., Butler, J.E., et al., 1997. Task failure with lack of diaphragm fatigue during inspiratory resistive loading in human subjects. J. Appl. Physiol. 82, 2011–2019.

Merton, P.A., 1954. Voluntary strength and fatigue. J. Physiol. 123, 553–564.

Meyer, T., Auracher, M., Heeg, K., et al., 2006. Does cumulating endurance training at the weekends impair training effectiveness? Eur. J. Cardiovasc. Prev. Rehabil. 13, 578–584.

Midgley, A.W., McNaughton, L.R., Wilkinson, M., 2006. Is there an optimal training intensity for enhancing the maximal oxygen uptake of distance runners? Empirical research findings, current opinions, physiological rationale and practical recommendations. Sports Med. 36, 117–132.

Midgley, A.W., McNaughton, L.R., Jones, A.M., 2007. Training to enhance the physiological determinants of long-distance running performance: can valid recommendations be given to runners and coaches based on current scientific knowledge? Sports Med. 37, 857–880.

Millet, G.P., Vleck, V.E., Bentley, D.J., 2009. Physiological differences between cycling and running: lessons from triathletes. Sports Med. 39, 179–206.

Polkey, M.I., Moxham, J., 2004. Improvement in volitional tests of muscle function alone may not be adequate evidence that inspiratory muscle training is effective. Eur. Respir. J. 23, 5–6.

Poole, D.C., Wilkerson, D.P., Jones, A.M., 2008. Validity of criteria for establishing maximal O2 uptake during ramp exercise tests. Eur. J. Appl. Physiol. 102, 403–410.

Powers, S.K., Criswell, D., 1996. Adaptive strategies of respiratory muscles in response to endurance exercise. Med. Sci. Sports Exerc. 28, 1115–1122.

Priban, I.P., Fincham, W.F., 1965. Self-adaptive control and respiratory system. Nature 208, 339–343.

Rohrbach, M., Perret, C., Kayser, B., et al., 2003. Task failure from inspiratory resistive loaded breathing: a role for inspiratory muscle fatigue? Eur. J. Appl. Physiol. 90, 405–410.

Romer, L.M., Polkey, M.I., 2008. Exercise-induced respiratory muscle fatigue: implications for performance. J. Appl. Physiol. 104, 879–888.

Romer, L.M., Lovering, A.T., Haverkamp, H.C., et al., 2006. Effect of inspiratory muscle work on peripheral fatigue of locomotor muscles in healthy humans. J. Physiol. 571, 425–439.

Rudroff, T., Barry, B.K., Stone, A.L., et al., 2007. Accessory muscle activity contributes to the variation in time to task failure for different arm postures and loads. J. Appl. Physiol. 102, 1000–1006.

Saunders, P.U., Pyne, D.B., Telford, R.D., et al., 2004. Factors affecting running economy in trained distance runners. Sports Med. 34, 465–485.

Scharhag, J., Schneider, G., Urhausen, A., et al., 2002. Athlete's heart: right and left ventricular mass and function in male endurance athletes and untrained individuals determined by magnetic resonance imaging. J. Am. Coll. Cardiol. 40, 1856–1863.

Similowski, T., Duguet, A., Straus, C., et al., 1996. Assessment of the voluntary activation of the diaphragm using cervical and cortical magnetic stimulation. Eur. Respir. J. 9, 1224–1231.

Sinoway, L., Prophet, S., 1990. Skeletal muscle metaboreceptor stimulation opposes peak metabolic vasodilation in humans. Circ. Res. 66, 1576–1584.

Stallknecht, B., Vissing, J., Galbo, H., 1998. Lactate production and clearance in exercise. Effects of training. A mini-review. Scand. J. Med. Sci. Sports 8, 127–131.

Swain, D.P., 2005. Moderate or vigorous intensity exercise: which is better for improving aerobic fitness? Prev. Cardiol. 8, 55–58.

Vincent, H.K., Shanely, R.A., Stewart, D.J., et al., 2002. Adaptation of upper airway muscles to chronic endurance exercise. Am. J. Respir. Crit. Care Med. 166, 287–293.

Wagner, P.D., 2005. Why doesn't exercise grow the lungs when other factors do? Exerc. Sport Sci. Rev. 33 (1), 3–8.

Westerblad, H., Duty, S., Allen, D.G., 1993. Intracellular calcium concentration during low-frequency fatigue in isolated single fibers of mouse skeletal muscle. J. Appl. Physiol. 75, 382–388.

Williams, C., Ratel, S. (Eds.), 2009. Human muscle fatigue. Routledge, London.

Wilmore, J.H., Stanforth, P.R., Gagnon, J., et al., 2001a. Cardiac output and stroke volume changes with endurance training: the HERITAGE Family Study. Med. Sci. Sports Exerc. 33, 99–106.

Wilmore, J.H., Stanforth, P.R., Gagnon, J., et al., 2001b. Heart rate and blood pressure changes with endurance training: the HERITAGE Family Study. Med. Sci. Sports Exerc. 33, 107–116.

Chapter 3

The respiratory muscles

An important concept that will be explored in this chapter is that of imbalance in the demand/capacity relationship of the respiratory muscles, and, in particular, the inspiratory muscles. Evaluating function in the context of relative demand is a pragmatic method of defining 'weakness', since it incorporates context. A muscle might not be considered 'weak' in absolute terms, but if the demands that are placed upon a 'normal muscle' are excessive then it is rendered 'weak' functionally. For example, morbidly obese people with normal quadriceps muscle strength have functional weakness by virtue of their greater body mass. The same principle applies to the respiratory muscles: patients with lung fibrosis may have normal inspiratory muscle strength, but the elevated intrinsic inspiratory load generates functional weakness that manifests as reduced inspiratory muscle endurance (Hart et al, 2002). Traditionally, weakness has been defined by reference to measures of strength, but it is important to appreciate that strength is a one-dimensional index of function, and is just one of a number of important functional properties of muscles (see Ch. 4, Fig. 4.1). Thus weakness and dysfunction are multi-dimensional, and can be primary (sub-normal performance) and functional (inadequate for the prevailing demands). The overriding question is whether the muscles' capability is 'fit for purpose', or whether it induces a functional limitation. The latter can be defined as the inability to undertake a task that would be considered normal. For example, the inability of a middle-aged woman to walk on level ground at 3.96 km·h^{-1} (1.10 m·s^{-1}) (Bohannon & Williams Andrews, 2011) without the need to stop and 'catch her breath' defines her as being functionally limited by dyspnoea. In Chapter 1, the underlying physiology of dyspnoea and breathing effort was described. Although dyspnoea is a complex phenomenon, a major contributor to its magnitude is the relative intensity of inspiratory

muscle work. This is determined by two factors: (1) the prevailing respiratory system mechanics, and (2) the function of the respiratory muscles; in other words, the resistances and elastances that must be overcome during breathing, as well as the capacity of the respiratory muscles to meet these mechanical demands. An exacerbating factor with respect to this relationship is the prevailing ventilatory demand, which is affected by a wide range of factors including aerobic fitness, ventilation/perfusion matching, diffusing capacity and breathing pattern. To add a further layer of complexity to the demand/capacity relationship of the respiratory muscles, many of these factors are interdependent; for example, altered lung mechanics can precipitate a rapid shallow breathing pattern, which in turn increases the demand for minute ventilation because of its effect on the dead space/tidal volume relationship.

This chapter will explore how disease, exercise and posture interact to influence the demand/capacity relationship of the respiratory muscles. In doing so, a theoretical rationale for specific training will be offered. Evidence relating to the influence of respiratory muscle training upon clinical outcomes is considered in Chapter 4.

CHANGES IN RESPIRATORY MUSCLE FUNCTION AND BREATHING MECHANICS

In the various conditions described below there is either: (1) an imbalance in the demand/capacity relationship of the respiratory muscles that contributes to dyspnoea, exercise limitation and even to respiratory failure, or (2) a contribution to symptoms or morbidity that arises from the respiratory system, including the upper airway. This section will therefore describe the abnormalities of respiratory mechanics, respiratory muscle function and ventilatory demand in a range of situations and, in so doing, establish the rationale for training the respiratory muscles. A comprehensive overview of respiratory muscle disorders can also be found in the excellent review of Laghi & Tobin (2003).

This section is subdivided by 'condition', with five major chronic conditions affecting a large number of people presented under separate headings: *Respiratory disease, Chronic heart failure and pulmonary hypertension, Neurological and neuromuscular disease, Obesity* and *Ageing*. Conditions with lower population prevalence are listed under *Miscellaneous conditions*.

Respiratory disease

The primary symptom and exercise-limiting factor in respiratory disease is dyspnoea. In this section the impact of respiratory disease upon respiratory mechanics, respiratory muscle function and ventilatory demand will be described. Readers wishing to know more about the physiological basis of respiratory disease are referred to Hamid and colleagues' comprehensive text on the subject (Hamid et al, 2005).

Chronic obstructive pulmonary disease

The hallmark of chronic obstructive pulmonary disease (COPD) is expiratory flow limitation, which results from both reduced lung recoil and airway tethering (see Ch. 1), in addition to intrinsic airway narrowing. Although the most obvious repercussion of airway narrowing for the respiratory muscles is an increased flow resistive work of breathing, this is only the tip of the iceberg. In recent years, the phase 'dynamic hyperinflation' has emerged to describe how the loss of lung recoil and airway narrowing disrupt normal breathing mechanics during exercise. Hyperinflation is a pathophysiological manifestation of airway obstruction, and the consequent expiratory flow limitation, which lead to incomplete lung emptying, i.e., expiration is curtailed before the lungs have reached their equilibrium volume (functional residual capacity: FRC). The lungs therefore become hyperinflated. In severe COPD, hyperinflation is present at rest (static hyperinflation), but during exercise even mild obstruction results in a state of dynamic hyperinflation, the severity of which is proportional to the severity of flow limitation and the magnitude of the ventilatory demand.

Figure 3.1 illustrates how, during exercise, expiratory flow limitation stimulates migration of the tidal flow loop towards total lung capacity (TLC), increasing end-expiratory lung volume (EELV) and reducing inspiratory capacity (IC). Although dynamic hyperinflation serves to maximize tidal expiratory flow under conditions of expiratory flow limitation (by moving the tidal flow loop away

from the maximum envelope), the requirement to breathe at higher ranges of the TLC increases the elastic load presented to the inspiratory muscles by the lungs and chest wall. This creates a 'restrictive' pulmonary defect. The most important mechanical and sensory repercussions of expiratory flow limitation are therefore borne by the inspiratory muscles. However, the repercussions of hyperinflation and/or expiratory flow limitation are not limited to an increase in the elastic work of breathing; inspiratory muscle loading is exacerbated in three further ways:

- By inducing functional weakening of the inspiratory muscles (see inset to Fig. 3.1). Foreshortening of expiration alters diaphragm geometry, making it flatter and moving the inspiratory muscles to a weaker portion of their pressure–volume relationship (Decramer, 1997).
- By generating intrinsic positive end-expiratory pressure (PEEP$_i$). Expiration ends before all of the forces acting on the lung are in equilibrium, so inspiration is initiated under a positive expiratory load.
- By forcing inspiratory time to shorten. This is another adaptive response, in this case to allow more time for expiration. The cost is to move the inspiratory muscles to a weaker portion of their force–velocity relationship (the faster a muscle contracts, the lower is its force-generating capacity).

Hyperinflation has also been shown to impair respiratory muscle blood flow in a dog model (Kawagoe et al, 1994); in this study, despite an almost two-fold increase in the work of breathing, diaphragm blood flow remained unchanged and accessory muscle blood flow fell during acute hyperinflation. It is not clear whether hyperinflation exerts the same effect in human beings with COPD, but impaired accessory muscle perfusion in the face of an increased demand for muscle work would predispose these muscles to fatigue and/or accumulation of metabolic by-products (see section 'Respiratory muscle involvement in exercise limitation').

Thus, COPD-induced changes in respiratory mechanics exert a very potent influence upon dyspnoea because they affect both the demand for inspiratory pressure generation and the capacity of the inspiratory muscles to generate sufficient pressure to meet that demand (see Fig. 3.1). Both phenomena increase the requirement for inspiratory motor drive and intensify dyspnoea (O'Donnell, 2001). However, the inspiratory muscle dysfunction of COPD is not confined to the functional (secondary) weakening precipitated by hyperinflation (Similowski et al, 1991; Polkey et al, 1996). There is also primary dysfunction due to abnormalities within the muscle tissue itself, which lead to declines in strength and endurance (Levine et al, 2003; Barreiro et al, 2005; Ottenheijm et al, 2005). This deterioration of muscle may be in part due to disuse (sedentary lifestyles), but is more likely to be the result of oxidative stress (Barreiro et al, 2005) resulting from the systemic manifestations of COPD, including the chronic inflammatory state.

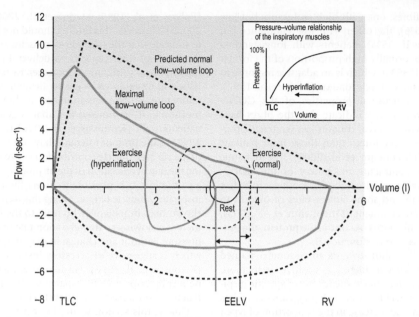

Figure 3.1 Comparison of the response of the exercise tidal flow volume in a person with expiratory flow limitation (EFL) (solid lines), compared with that predicted for someone with normal lungs (dashed lines). Note that in the presence of EFL there is encroachment upon the inspiratory capacity in order to increase minute ventilation (flow volume loop shifts to the left and end-expiratory lung volume (EELV) increases). The person with normal lungs (dashed lines) is able to increase minute ventilation by utilizing both their inspiratory and expiratory reserve volumes (EELV decreases). The inset illustrates the pressure–volume relationship of the inspiratory muscles showing that, as lung volume increases from residual volume (RV) towards total lung capacity (TLC) (as occurs in hyperinflation) the inspiratory muscles become weaker.

Furthermore, malnutrition causes generalized muscle weakness, which may exacerbate disease-specific respiratory muscle weakness (Decramer, 2001). Finally, the use of oral corticosteroids has been shown to have a myopathic influence upon the respiratory muscles of patients without respiratory disease, who show significant reductions in strength (∼30%) and endurance (∼50%) over the treatment period (Weiner et al, 1993; Weiner et al, 1995). Although these changes show some reversal following cessation of corticosteroid treatment, function may take as long as 6 months to normalize (Weiner et al, 1993). Since primary and secondary dysfunction coexist, there is a significant impairment in the capacity of the inspiratory muscles to deliver changes in intrathoracic pressure and tidal volume. Indeed, disease severity correlates negatively with respiratory muscle function (Terzano et al, 2008). Furthermore, hyperinflation leads to changes in chest wall geometry, inducing functional weakening of the accessory inspiratory muscles, which also contributes to a global reduction in the ability of the respiratory pump to generate inspiratory pressure (De Troyer & Wilson, 2009).

Much has been made in recent years of the adaptations that occur within the inspiratory muscles in response to the mechanical changes and increased physical demands described above. The chronically hyperinflated, flattened state of the diaphragm in COPD appears to lead to shortening of the total diaphragm length by around 15% to 25%, depending upon whether this is assessed at functional residual capacity FRC or residual volume (RV) respectively (McKenzie et al, 2009). This adaptation reduces the ability of the diaphragm to shorten during contraction, and thus limits its ability to generate inspiratory flow. However, the adaptations in diaphragm geometry and length appear to have some functional benefits in terms of maintaining its ability to deliver volume excursion, as well as its pressure-generating capacity (McKenzie et al, 2009). In respect of the latter, at equivalent absolute lung volumes the diaphragm pressure-generating capacity of patients with COPD is equal, or superior, to that of control participants (Similowski et al, 1991). However, despite this, the ability of the diaphragm to generate changes in volume at high lung volumes is diminished (McKenzie et al, 2009). It is important to keep in mind that diaphragm function at the same relative lung volumes is impaired in patients with COPD (see above), and that they have a reduced reserve capacity for volume and flow generation.

Change in diaphragm length is not the only chronic adaptation to hyperinflation and chronic inspiratory loading in patients with COPD. There are also changes in diaphragm biochemistry that appear to result from chronic loading (Levine et al, 1997; Ottenheijm et al, 2005). The healthy diaphragm is composed predominantly of two types of muscles fibres: one with high endurance but low power (type I, 45%), the other with low endurance but high power (type II, 55%). Patients with long-standing COPD have an abnormally high proportion of the former (type I 64%, type II 36%), which is an adaptive response to continuous inspiratory muscle loading (Levine et al, 1997).

Studies of the functional properties of the COPD-adapted diaphragm *in vitro* indicate that the fibres have a smaller cross-sectional area, contain less contractile protein and generate lower forces than those from patients without COPD (Ottenheijm et al, 2005). The dynamic properties of the contractile machinery of the COPD-adapted fibres are also impaired; the fibres appear to be less sensitive to calcium and show slower rates of myosin to actin attachment/detachment (Ottenheijm et al, 2005). Thus there is not only a loss of contractile protein; the protein that remains is also dysfunctional.

On the face of it, a shift towards an endurance-trained phenotype might be considered a positive adaptation; indeed it is cited as a reason for the futility of specific inspiratory muscle training (Polkey et al, 2011). However, it has been suggested that the increase in the proportion of type I fibres might, at least in part, explain the reduction in force-generating capacity (Clanton & Levine, 2009). Thus, depending upon the specific demands placed upon the inspiratory muscles, this adaptation can be either advantageous or disadvantageous. For example, it is advantageous for prolonged, low-intensity work, but disadvantageous for short, high-intensity work. The former is encountered at rest, whereas the latter is encountered during exercise. The diaphragm in patients with COPD therefore appears to be well adapted to generating low flow rates for long periods of time, but this adaptation robs them of the ability to generate the high pressures and flow rates required during exercise.

This suggestion is confirmed by studies of the *in vivo* strength and endurance of the inspiratory muscles of patients with COPD. For example, compared with control individuals, evoked diaphragm twitch pressure, maximal inspiratory pressure and a measure of endurance during inspiratory loading were all lower in patients with COPD (Barreiro et al, 2005). Furthermore, impairments were proportional to the severity of disease, despite the fact that a concomitant increase in type I fibres, and decrease in capillary to fibre ratio, were also proportional to disease severity. Thus, the shift towards a more endurance-trained phenotype reduced strength and did not appear to protect the inspiratory muscles from global fatigue under conditions of inspiratory loading (Barreiro et al, 2005). This is probably because weaker muscles must operate at a greater proportion of their maximum capacity, which predisposes them to fatigue.

Notwithstanding this apparent predisposition to fatigue, studies have so far failed to demonstrate evidence of exercise-induced contractile fatigue of the diaphragm in patients with COPD using low-frequency phrenic nerve stimulation (Polkey et al, 1995; Mador et al, 2000a; Mador et al, 2000b). However, this finding should not be misinterpreted to indicate that the inspiratory muscles are working within the limits of their capacity to deliver $\dot{V}_E$, or that they do not impose any limitation upon exercise tolerance. The latter issue will be explored in greater detail in the section 'Respiratory muscle involvement in exercise limitation', but in the meantime it is noteworthy that studies where COPD patients walk (Kyroussis et al, 1996) or cycle (Yan et al, 1997) to the limit of tolerance have found a predominance of the rib cage muscle contribution to breathing. By measuring the rate of relaxation of the inspiratory muscles following a sniff effort, it is possible to detect the presence of global inspiratory muscle fatigue. Using this technique, it has been shown that, in patients who walk to the limit of tolerance, there is a slowing of the relaxation rate of oesophageal sniff pressure without any change in diaphragm twitch pressure, which is suggestive of accessory inspiratory muscle fatigue (Kyroussis et al, 1996). Furthermore, there does appear to be a subgroup of COPD patients who display diaphragm fatigue post-exercise (see below) (Hopkinson et al, 2010).

Finally, this section would be incomplete without mentioning the expiratory muscles, as well as contextualizing the changes in muscle function induced by COPD. As has already been alluded to, there is generalized muscle weakness, which also affects the expiratory muscles (Gosselink et al, 2000). In COPD patients the voluntary force-generating capacity of the expiratory muscles (maximal expiratory pressure: MEP) is ~30% lower than in healthy elderly people (Gosselink et al, 2000). This compares with differences in maximal inspiratory pressure (MIP), handgrip and quadriceps strength of ~40%, ~20% and 25%, respectively (Gosselink et al, 2000). The slightly larger effect of COPD upon MIP than MEP is most likely a manifestation of the additional influence of secondary weakness, due to the effects of hyperinflation (Gosselink et al, 2000). A recent study examined the influence of symptom limited cycling upon non-voluntary measures of expiratory and inspiratory muscle strength in patients with COPD; a significant exercise-induced fatigue of the abdominal muscles (7.2% fall in twitch gastric pressure) was found, but no change in diaphragm function (Hopkinson et al, 2010). Interestingly, only around one-third of the group exhibited expiratory muscle fatigue (twitch gastric pressure, 21%), and this subgroup also exhibited a significant fall in twitch diaphragm pressure (7.9%). The non-fatiguers exhibited no change in twitch gastric pressure, but a 7.7% increase in twitch diaphragm pressure. Unfortunately, the group was not subdivided to examine the diaphragm fatiguers in more detail. These data suggest that: (1) there is both inspiratory and expiratory muscle overload in at least some patients with COPD, and (2) diaphragm fatigue may be masked by lack of reliability in baseline measurements of twitch diaphragm pressure.

Patients with COPD also experience an increase in the demand for inspiratory muscle work, which arises from an elevated demand for minute ventilation ($\dot{V}_E$), especially during exercise. Ventilation/perfusion mismatching and a higher than normal ratio of dead space to tidal volume (V_D/V_T) both necessitate an increase in $\dot{V}_E$ in order to minimize changes in blood gases, but hypoxaemia is nevertheless a common finding. Furthermore, patients with COPD also have poor aerobic fitness, which increases the ventilatory demand of exercise (Casaburi et al, 1991), and thus increases inspiratory muscle work still further. Needless to say, these increased ventilatory flow requirements also exacerbate hyperinflation (Somfay et al, 2002).

In summary, patients with COPD have a dramatically increased demand for inspiratory muscle work, but a reduced capacity to supply this demand due to muscle dysfunction. In other words, the demand/capacity relationship is stacked in completely the wrong direction. In the section 'Respiratory muscle involvement in exercise limitation', respiratory muscle-induced limitations to exercise tolerance will be considered, and Chapter 4 will review the evidence supporting specific respiratory muscle training for patients with COPD.

Asthma

The mechanical abnormalities in patients with asthma mimic closely those described in COPD; however, there are important differences. For example, there is less reduction in static lung recoil pressure and more widespread intrathoracic airway narrowing in asthma (Pride & Macklem, 1986). In addition, the increased airway collapsibility in patients with COPD is not seen in asthmatics. Furthermore, the reversible nature of airways obstruction in asthma results in relatively short-lived periods of stress upon the inspiratory muscles. The latter means that patients with asthma do not show the same changes in inspiratory muscle length or fibre composition that are expressed in patients with COPD (see above).

There is no clear consensus regarding the presence of primary weakness of the inspiratory muscles in patients with asthma compared with healthy people, as no biopsy data exists. However, the finding that steroid-dependent patients receiving oral corticosteroids show lower inspiratory muscle strength, but similar severity of hyperinflation, suggests that there may be myopathy in steroid-dependent patients with asthma (Akkoca et al, 1999). Generally, respiratory muscle strength and endurance are relatively normal in patients with stable asthma (Hill, 1991).

However, it is accepted universally that bronchoconstriction-induced hyperinflation is associated with secondary weakness of the inspiratory muscles (Fig. 3.1 inset) (Weiner et al, 1990; Perez et al, 1996; Akkoca et al, 1999; Stell et al, 2001; Weiner et al, 2002). As is the case in COPD, the major mechanical consequences of airway narrowing are increased flow resistive work, increased elastic work and $PEEP_i$ (resulting from dynamic lung hyperinflation), as well as reduced dynamic lung compliance (Martin et al, 1980; Lougheed et al, 1995). In a study

comparing inspiratory muscle function of patients with COPD and asthma, with equivalent severity of hyperinflation, endurance was impaired to a greater degree in patients with asthma (Perez et al, 1996). Interestingly, strength was lower in the COPD patients compared with those with asthma. These data suggest that some of the structural and biochemical adaptations that occur in response to chronic loading in COPD are absent in patients with asthma. Thus, where airway obstruction is present, patients with asthma experience the same acute functional defect in their pulmonary function as those with COPD. However, the reversible nature of the airway obstruction may place patients with asthma at a functional disadvantage, and thus greater vulnerability to functional overload.

In a study of histamine-induced bronchoconstriction (FEV_1 49% of baseline), the inspiratory work was found to increase 11-fold, 69% of the increase being due to the elastic component of the work of breathing (Martin et al, 1983). In addition, there also appears to be a prolonged activation of inspiratory muscles during exhalation in the presence of bronchoconstriction-induced hyperinflation (Muller et al, 1980; Muller et al, 1981), which suggests that the work of the total inspiratory muscles may be increased to an even greater extent than inspiratory work alone indicates.

The interrelationship between bronchoconstriction, hyperinflation and dyspnoea has also been studied. Multiple regression analysis indicates that, during methacholine-induced bronchoconstriction, change in inspiratory capacity (an index of dynamic hyperinflation) was the most powerful predictor of dyspnoea during bronchoconstriction – accounting for 74% of the variance in the perceptual rating (Lougheed et al, 1993). These observations are supported by more recent evidence confirming that hyperinflation is a major determinant of dyspnoea in patients with asthma (Martinez-Moragon et al, 2003).

As is the case in COPD, the mechanical changes associated with bronchoconstriction most likely increase the intensity of dyspnoea via their effect upon the magnitude of inspiratory neural drive (see Ch. 1). There is experimental support for this suggestion; Bellofiore et al (1996) found that the strongest determinant of dyspnoea during methacholine-induced bronchoconstriction was inspiratory neural drive ($P_{0.1}$, mouth occlusion pressure), which explained 82% of the total variance in dyspnoea. More recently, Binks et al (2002) reported that institution of mechanical ventilation during methacholine-induced bronchoconstriction and hyperinflation significantly reduced ratings of 'effort to breathe' in people with mild asthma. Furthermore, it has also been shown that gender differences in inspiratory muscle strength may underpin differences in dyspnoea perception, quality of life and consumption of β_2-agonist medication (Weiner et al, 2002). These data, along with data from inspiratory muscle training studies (see Ch. 4), support the notion that inspiratory muscle strength, and hence the relative intensity of inspiratory muscle work, makes a fundamental contribution to dyspnoea in people with asthma.

Because exercise is a trigger for asthma in around 90% of people with asthma (Wilkerson, 1998) there is an understandable anxiety regarding exercise that might translate into avoidance of physical activity, and poor aerobic fitness (Welsh et al, 2004). However, there remains no clear consensus regarding levels of physical activity and fitness, especially in children with asthma (Wilkerson, 1998), though there is some evidence to suggest that the aerobic fitness of adults with asthma is generally low (Satta, 2000). Thus, poor aerobic conditioning may exacerbate hyperinflation-related increases in the work of breathing during exercise by increasing the ventilatory requirement and exacerbating hyperinflation.

In summary, patients with asthma have an increased demand for inspiratory muscle work, which is proportional to the severity of their airway obstruction. It is not clear whether they have any primary weakness of their inspiratory muscles, but there is evidence of steroid-induced myopathy of the inspiratory muscles in steroid-dependent asthma. Furthermore, secondary weakness due to the influence of hyperinflation is well established, and linked strongly to dyspnoea. In the section 'Respiratory muscle involvement in exercise limitation', respiratory muscle-induced limitations to exercise tolerance will be considered, and Chapter 4 will review the evidence supporting specific respiratory muscle training for patients with asthma.

Bronchiectasis

Bronchiectasis is a chronic lung disease that is not normally included within the umbrella of COPD, but which overlaps with it (Neves et al, 2011); indeed one study found that 50% of patients with COPD also had bronchiectasis (Patel et al, 2004). It is characterized by irreversible widening of the medium-sized airways accompanied by inflammation, chronic infection and destruction of the bronchial walls (Neves et al, 2011). Both the pathology and the functional manifestations of bronchiectasis have similarities with those of COPD, including inflammatory cell profiles, protease release and consequent airway obstruction (Neves et al, 2011). In both conditions, these factors lead to detrimental changes in breathing mechanics, attendant exertional dyspnoea and exercise intolerance. Symptomology is also similar to COPD – including cough, sputum production and wheeze (Neves et al, 2011). Expiratory flow limitation (identified using the negative expiratory pressure technique) is present at rest in 39% of patients with bronchiectasis, which is a lower prevalence than in patients with COPD (Koulouris et al, 2003). The explanation for the latter finding may be that around half of patients had both obstructive and restrictive defects, i.e., restriction acted as a confounding influence; the presence of flow limitation was correlated with the MRC dyspnoea score, which in turn was correlated with exercise tolerance (Koulouris et al, 2003). Thus, the mechanical changes associated with bronchiectasis increase the demand for inspiratory muscle work, which is manifested symptomatically as exertional dyspnoea.

Compared with healthy people of a similar age, patients with moderate-to-severe bronchiectasis exhibit lower maximal inspiratory and expiratory muscle strength (around 20% and 40% lower, respectively) (Newall et al, 2005; Moran et al, 2010). The origin of this weakness is unclear, but is most likely due to a combination of primary weakness and functional weakness due to hyperinflation. Thus, in common with patients with COPD, patients with bronchiectasis have an imbalance in the demand/capacity relationship of the respiratory muscles. This imbalance will also be considered in the section 'Respiratory muscle involvement in exercise limitation', and Chapter 4 will review the evidence supporting specific respiratory muscle training for patients with bronchiectasis.

Cystic fibrosis

Respiratory failure is the most common cause of death in patients with cystic fibrosis (CF) (Taylor-Cousar, 2009), and dyspnoea is one of their main complaints (Leroy et al, 2011); it has also been suggested that the deterioration of lung function in patients with CF have is insufficient to explain their exertional dyspnoea. Patients with CF have an elevated work of breathing (Dunnink et al, 2009), and this has been identified as an important contributor to dyspnoea (Leroy et al, 2011). There appears to be no evidence of inspiratory muscle weakness in patients with CF; indeed, some authors have reported that patients with CF have superior strength (Dufresne et al, 2009; Dunnink et al, 2009) and diaphragm thickness (Dufresne et al, 2009). The elevated airway resistance of patients with CF appears to contribute to their diaphragm hypertrophy (Dufresne et al, 2009). However, patients with the lowest fat-free mass exhibit a loss of diaphragm thickness (Ionescu et al, 1998; Enright et al, 2007). Furthermore, although indices of inspiratory muscle strength have been found to be normal or superior in patients with CF, loss of maximal inspiratory muscle work capacity has been reported (Ionescu et al, 1998; Enright et al, 2007), suggesting that there is a deterioration in the metabolic properties of the inspiratory muscles. This finding is suggestive of an imbalance between demand and capacity since the preservation of inspiratory muscle strength is accompanied by an increased demand for inspiratory muscle work, and dyspnoea. The fact that respiratory failure is the primary cause of death highlights the important influence of the imbalance between demand and capacity. This will also be considered in the section 'Respiratory muscle involvement in exercise limitation', and Chapter 4 will review the evidence supporting specific respiratory muscle training for patients with CF.

Restrictive chest wall disorders

Conditions such as kyphoscoliosis, fibrothorax, thoracoplasty, flail chest and ankylosing spondylitis all induce chest wall restriction, creating a restrictive pulmonary defect in which total respiratory system elastance and resistance are elevated (Donath & Miller, 2009). In the case of severe kyphosis and/or scoliosis, thoracic volume may also be reduced by collapse of the vertebral column and the cranial displacement of the abdominal contents. As a consequence, breathing pattern tends to be rapid and shallow, creating a higher than normal ratio of dead space to tidal volume (V_D/V_T) ratio and necessitating an increase in $\dot{V}_E$. This exacerbates the already elevated work of inhalation (Donath & Miller, 2009), and attendant dyspnoea. Furthermore, inspiratory muscle function also tends to be impaired (Lisboa et al, 1985; Cejudo et al, 2009), owing to changes in chest wall and diaphragm configuration. In kyphoscoliosis, inspiratory muscle strength has been shown to correlate with forced vital capacity (FVC), as well as to arterial blood gases, such that weakest patients exhibited the worst FVC and blood gases (Lisboa et al, 1985). Ultimately, the outcome of these conditions can be respiratory failure and the requirement for mechanical ventilation. The imbalance in the demand/capacity relationship of the respiratory muscles will also be considered in the section 'Respiratory muscle involvement in exercise limitation'. See Chapter 4 for a description of the evidence supporting breathing exercises.

Interstitial lung disease (ILD) is an umbrella term for a group of lung disorders that share a number of pathophysiological characteristics and clinical features. The principal feature of ILD is exercise intolerance due to exertional dyspnoea and perceptions of fatigue. Exercise intolerance is correlated with quality of life (Holland, 2010), which makes it an important therapeutic target.

The reduced lung compliance in ILD leads to impairment of vital capacity, and a rapid and shallow breathing pattern that worsens during exercise (Javaheri & Sicilian, 1992). This pattern exacerbates the existing ventilation/perfusion ($\dot{V}/\dot{Q}$) mismatch, due to its effect upon the V_D/V_T ratio. There is also an impairment of diffusing capacity, and the combination with $\dot{V}/\dot{Q}$ mismatching can precipitate substantial arterial desaturation (Miki et al, 2003). These changes also increase the ventilatory demand of exercise and hence the work of breathing.

Sarcoidosis involves multiple organs, but pulmonary manifestations typically predominate (Lynch et al, 2007) in the form of an ILD. Dyspnoea is the most common presentation in patients with early to moderately advanced disease (Baydur et al, 2001). Sarcoidosis is associated with reduced inspiratory and expiratory muscle strength ($\sim 20\%$ reduction), as well as impaired endurance (Wirnsberger et al, 1997; Baydur et al, 2001; Spruit et al, 2005), and respiratory muscle function correlates more closely with dyspnoea during activities of daily living than pulmonary function (Baydur et al, 2001); indeed dyspnoea can be present in the absence of any lung function defects (Baydur et al, 2001). The underlying mechanisms for respiratory muscle dysfunction in sarcoidosis are unclear, but two case reports indicate that granulomatous involvement of respiratory muscles is present (Dewberry et al, 1993; Pringle & Dewar, 1997). At the time of writing there have been no studies of respiratory muscle training in patients with sarcoidosis or other ILD.

Chronic heart failure and pulmonary hypertension

Patients with chronic heart failure (CHF) present with dyspnoea, exercise intolerance and fatigue. Chronic heart failure is a complex condition that generates a number of interrelated pathophysiological changes that affect skeletal muscle, the vasculature, neurohormonal systems and the lungs (Brubaker, 1997).

Inspiratory muscle dysfunction has not been assessed as widely or with the same rigour in CHF as in COPD. For example, there are no biopsy studies of diaphragm composition, and only one study has examined diaphragm twitch pressure (Hughes et al, 1999). Notwithstanding this, the evidence of inspiratory muscle weakness is consistent and compelling (Ribeiro et al, 2009). It has been suggested that inspiratory muscle weakness may be part of the generalized atrophy that is common in CHF, but there is some evidence that there may be selective weakness of the inspiratory muscles (Ribeiro et al, 2009). Indeed, inspiratory muscle strength has been shown to have prognostic value (Frankenstein et al, 2008, 2009), which underscores its importance. Furthermore, inspiratory muscle weakness is correlated with a number of indices of haemodynamic dysfunction, including cardiac output and the severity of pulmonary hypertension (Filusch et al, 2011).

Patients with CHF tend to adopt a rapid, shallow and constrained breathing pattern during exercise (Johnson et al, 2000). This appears to be an adaptive response to changes in the demand/capacity relationship of the inspiratory muscles. Lung compliance is reduced by pulmonary oedema and pulmonary fibrosis (Wright et al, 1990), which increases the work of breathing (Cross et al, 2012). An interesting feature of the rapid, shallow breathing pattern is that it coexists with expiratory flow limitation and a reduction in end-expiratory lung volume. The result is an increase in both the elastic and resistive work of breathing, the latter being present during both phases of respiration, whilst the former is seen only during inspiration (Cross et al, 2012). Unlike patients with COPD and asthma, patients with CHF do not hyperinflate in order to decrease their expiratory flow limitation (Johnson et al, 2000). Instead, unpleasant breathing sensations are minimized by adopting a rapid, shallow breathing pattern. This strategy suggests that the sensations associated with hyperinflation are more unpleasant than those associated with expiratory flow limitation and rapid, shallow breathing. This is entirely reasonable, given that hyperinflation in the presence of pulmonary oedema and fibrosis would increase inspiratory elastic work considerably (Cross et al, 2012). The mechanisms underlying the greater resistive work of breathing in CHF are uncertain, but may be related to worsening of pulmonary congestions and/or bronchoconstriction during exercise (Cross et al, 2012).

There are also a number of abnormalities that increase the ventilatory requirement of exercise in CHF, and thus increase the demands imposed upon the respiratory muscles. For example, diffusion impairment is present in 67% of patients with severe CHF (Wright et al, 1990). This may be due to pulmonary fibrosis, but may also be due to the influence of an impaired cardiac output upon ventilation/perfusion mismatching (Lewis et al, 1996), which elevates the physiological dead space. Furthermore, rapid, shallow breathing increases dead space ventilation further, because it generates a higher than normal ratio of dead space to tidal volume (V_D/V_T). Higher dead space necessitates an increase in $\dot{V}_E$ in order to minimize changes in blood gases. A further corollary of rapid, shallow breathing is that the higher inspiratory flow rate increases the relative functional demands upon the inspiratory muscles, which must operate on a weaker part of their force–velocity relationship (see Ch. 4, Fig. 4.1).

Elevated peripheral chemoreflex sensitivity is found in as many as 40% of patients with CHF, and may contribute to the exaggerated exercise hyperpnoea, as well as sympatho-excitation (Chua et al, 1997). Recently, it was found that peripheral chemoreflex sensitivity to carbon dioxide is significantly higher in patients with CHF who have inspiratory muscle weakness than in those who do not (Callegaro et al, 2010). The study authors hypothesized that the elevated chemoreflex sensitivity was secondary to the sympathoexcitation resulting from metaboreflex activation in weakened/fatigued inspiratory muscles. This is consistent with the finding that ventilatory and cardiovascular responses to locomotor muscle metaboreflex activation are increased in patients with CHF (Piepoli et al, 1996). Thus, exaggerated responses to chemoreflex and metaboreflex stimulation during exercise most likely conspire to exacerbate an already elevated ventilatory demand.

For reasons that are not yet fully understood, MIP is an independent risk factor for myocardial infarction and cardiovascular disease death (van der Palen et al, 2004). One study has also shown that patient survival was lower in those patients with low MIP (Meyer et al, 2000).

Finally, pulmonary arterial hypertension (PAH) is worthy of mention at this point; the condition is associated with heart failure, but may also be idiopathic. The symptomatology and respiratory manifestations of PAH are similar to those of CHF, including respiratory muscle weakness (Meyer et al, 2005). Furthermore, there is evidence that inspiratory muscle strength may influence exercise tolerance in patients with PAH (Kabitz et al, 2008a).

Thus patients with CHF and/or PAH have an increased demand for inspiratory muscle work and a reduced capacity to supply this demand due to muscle dysfunction. In the section 'Respiratory muscle involvement in exercise limitation' the implications of this in the context of respiratory muscle-induced limitations to exercise tolerance will be considered, and Chapter 4 will review the evidence supporting specific respiratory muscle training for patients with CHF.

Neurological and neuromuscular disease

Neurological and neuromuscular diseases include conditions that affect the brain, spinal cord, nerves and muscles. Impairment can be the result of intrinsic muscle dysfunction, or arise indirectly via neurological/nerve dysfunction. The functional consequences are broadly divided into spasticity and paralysis. For simplicity, these conditions are considered collectively in this section under the terminology of neuromuscular disease (NMD), beginning with spinal cord injury.

Spinal cord injury

Respiratory complications remain a major cause of morbidity and mortality in people with spinal cord injury (SCI) (Schilero et al, 2009), the underlying cause for these complications is poor cough function, which leads to mucus retention, atelectasis and infections (Schilero et al, 2009). The extent and severity of respiratory system compromise following SCI depend upon a number of factors including the level of the lesion, the completeness of the lesion and the ensuing temporal adaptations to the lesion. Furthermore, there is an elevated prevalence of obstructive sleep apnoea (OSA) in people with high spinal cord lesions (see also the section on OSA below), which may precipitate an increase in cardiovascular disease risk (Schilero et al, 2009).

Figure 3.2 summarizes the spinal innervation levels of the respiratory muscles, as well as indicating the distinctions between paraplegia and tetraplegia. Lesions above the level of the phrenic motor neurons (C3–C5) induce paralysis of all respiratory muscles, whereas in lower cervical lesions (C5–C8) the functions of the diaphragm and sternocleidomastoid are preserved. However, in the latter there is still a loss of inspiratory accessory muscle function (external intercostals and scalenes), as well as the primary muscles of expiration (internal intercostals and abdominals). Lesions in the thoracic region result in progressively less extensive denervation of the intercostal muscles as the level becomes more caudal, but any lesion above T6 results in complete loss of anterior abdominal wall innervation. Lesions between T6 and L3 result in partial denervation of the anterior abdominal wall, becoming less extensive at more caudal levels. Innervation of the posterior abdominal wall originates between T12 and L4, but these muscles make only a minor contribution to breathing.

Muscles of breathing

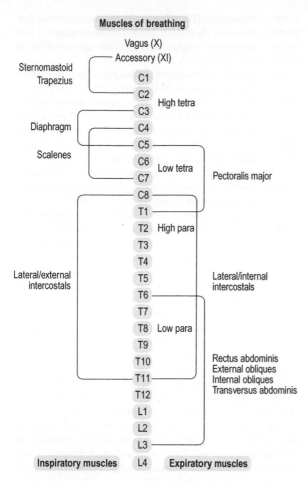

Figure 3.2 Levels of innervation of the respiratory muscles. Para = paraplegia; tetra = tetraplegia.

Maximal respiratory mouth pressures are correlated with the level of lesion for people with complete motor lesions, but not for those with incomplete lesions (Mateus et al, 2007). As one might expect, decrements in strength are greater for the expiratory muscles than for the inspiratory muscles, at equivalent lesion levels, the most severe compromise being for lesions at C4–C5 (maximal expiratory pressure 18% of predicted). In contrast, inspiratory muscle strength is least affected, and for lesions ranging from T1 to L6 is almost normal (85% predicted).

The loss of respiratory pressure-generating capacity has a predictable effect upon lung function, inducing a reduction in forced vital capacity (FVC) to between 49% (C4–C5) and 68% of predicted normal values (T7–L3) (Mateus et al, 2007). Forced expiratory volume in 1 second (FEV$_1$) is also reduced, but this is not an indication of obstruction but rather a reflection of a lower inspiratory capacity (initiating the expiratory effort from a lower lung volume). Indeed, the ratio of FVC to FEV$_1$ is supranormal (90–95%). Notwithstanding this, there is evidence of increased

bronchomotor tone, as well as airway hyperresponsiveness, which has been attributed to a loss of sympathetic innervation to the lungs (Schilero et al, 2005).

Respiratory mechanics are altered considerably, especially in tetraplegia. The systems that normally operate to optimize pressure and volume changes during breathing are disrupted, leading to mechanical inefficiency. For example, the normally efficient action of the diaphragm is impaired by paradoxical movement of the rib cage. This paradox may be reduced with time (Scanlon et al, 1989); the improvement has been attributed to ankylosis of the rib cage joints and intercostal spasticity (Estenne & De Troyer, 1985), but the penalty for this is an increased oxygen cost of breathing (Silver, 1963), increased breathing effort perception, a rapid shallow breathing pattern, and possibly increased diaphragm fatigability (Hopman et al, 1997). The increase in abdominal compliance also impairs the efficiency of the diaphragm by reducing the stability of the visceral fulcrum, and inducing a longer resting length. The former also reduces expansion of the lower ribs, generating inhomogeneity of changes in pleural pressure and gas distribution (Estenne & De Troyer, 1985), which is exacerbated by paradoxical movement of the rib cage (Hiraizumi et al, 1986). The resulting ventilation/perfusion mismatching may contribute to inefficient gas exchange.

As one might expect, decrements in pulmonary function are most severe during the acute phase, with some recovery of function over the 12 months following injury. However, recovery shows large inter-individual variation, and has been attributed to improvements in respiratory muscle function and changes in rib cage stability (Schilero et al, 2009).

Respiratory symptoms are common in patients with SCI, with dyspnoea being the most prevalent complaint. Dyspnoea is present in 73% of people with a lesion at C5, but only 29% in those with a lesion below T8 (Spungen et al, 1997). Other symptoms appear to be related to cough and phlegm, which are present in about a quarter of people with SCI, and with no correlation to level of injury. Increasing abdominal compliance, by means of a strapping, in people with lesions between C5 and T6 has been found to reduce breathing effort perception, most likely because of a concomitant increase in diaphragm length and function (Hart et al, 2005).

The prevalence of OSA in patients with SCI is at least twice that observed in the general population, is most prevalent in those with a cervical SCI, and also in the acute phase following injury (Schilero et al, 2009). A number of putative mechanisms have been suggested to explain the high prevalence of OSA in people with SCI, including disruption of the normal coordination between upper airway and respiratory pump muscles, thickening of the oropharyngeal wall and increased adiposity of the neck leading to reduced upper airway patency (Schilero et al, 2009).

The role of the respiratory muscle denervation in exercise tolerance will also be considered in the section 'Respiratory muscle involvement in exercise limitation', and Chapter 4 will review the evidence supporting specific respiratory muscle training for patients with SCI.

Other NMDs

The NMDs that affect breathing include amyotrophic lateral sclerosis (ALS), stroke, Parkinson's disease, multiple sclerosis, muscular dystrophy, myasthenia gravis, cerebral palsy, Guillain–Barré syndrome and post-polio syndrome. An understandable assumption is that the main deficit for patients with NMD is weakness of the respiratory muscles. However, there are a number of other detrimental changes to breathing that arise from respiratory muscle weakness, as well as from disease-specific factors, such as decreased chest wall mobility. Thus both sides of the demand/capacity relationship of the respiratory muscles are affected. Because of the diversity of conditions encompassed by NMD, this section focusses upon the principal deficits that affect breathing, citing a small number of examples of findings in specific conditions. A comprehensive description of the respiratory manifestations of NMDs is beyond the scope of this section; unfortunately, at the time of writing, such a review does not yet exist, so it is not possible to refer the reader elsewhere.

Weakness of both inspiratory and expiratory muscles is common in NMD, and leads to a restrictive pattern of pulmonary dysfunction, especially in advanced disease (Gibson et al, 1977). Because physical activity is limited by generalized deterioration of muscle function, dyspnoea is not always present. However, ventilatory limitation due to respiratory muscle weakness may be exacerbated by disease-specific factors that elevate the ventilatory demand, such as an early onset of the anaerobic threshold, particularly where mitochondrial myopathy is present (Flaherty et al, 2001). In addition, the adoption of a rapid, shallow breathing pattern generates a higher than normal ratio of dead space to tidal volume (V_D/V_T), increasing the demand for minute ventilation ($\dot{V}_E$), and the associated work of breathing. There may also be ventilation/perfusion mismatching and impaired gas exchange (Rochester, 1993). In advanced disease, respiratory muscle weakness, muscle fibrosis and microatelectasis may lead to chronic hypoventilation and hypercapnia. Under these conditions, there is a high risk of inspiratory muscle fatigue in response to small changes in the requirement for inspiratory muscle work, e.g., in the event of pulmonary complications (Kang, 2006). A recent study found that in patients with ALS, a supine Borg score ≥3 was associated with impaired inspiratory muscle strength and a lower vital capacity. The authors suggested that this simple assessment might provide a useful test of inspiratory muscle weakness in ALS (Just et al, 2010). Furthermore, respiratory muscle strength correlates with capability of daily living in the self-care and social function domains of a quality of life questionnaire (PEDI) in children with cerebral palsy (Wang et al, 2012), and with physical functioning domains of a quality of life questionnaire (SF-36) in patients with myotonic dystrophy (Araujo et al, 2010). These findings suggest a link between respiratory muscle strength and quality of life in children and adults with NMD.

Sleep-disordered breathing is also secondary to inspiratory muscle weakness via its influence upon vital capacity (Ragette et al, 2002). Furthermore, upper airway muscle involvement in NMD can result in obstructive respiratory events during sleep (Aboussouan, 2009). Aspiration and difficulties with swallowing are also related to the impairment of bulbar muscle function (Aboussouan, 2009). Poor cough function and respiratory muscle weakness conspire to make respiratory complications a leading cause of morbidity and mortality in NMD (Macklem, 1986).

Acute respiratory failure is a common complication of a number of acute onset neuromuscular conditions, such as Guillain–Barré syndrome, myasthenia gravis and polymyositis (Mehta, 2006), as well as in chronic conditions following development of respiratory complications. Multiple factors underlie the development of respiratory failure, but the principal contributors are weakness and fatigue of upper airway, inspiratory and expiratory muscles, as well as the influence that these impairments have upon cough efficacy and the development of infection (Mehta, 2006). See also the section 'Mechanical ventilation', below.

Thus, the picture in NMD is one of multifactorial defects in respiratory and upper airway function, and imbalance in the demand/capacity relationship of the respiratory muscles that can quickly result in respiratory failure (Macklem, 1986). In the section 'Respiratory muscle involvement in exercise limitation', the implications of these changes for exercise tolerance will be considered, and Chapter 4 will review the evidence supporting specific respiratory muscle training for patients with NMD.

Obesity

The influence of obesity upon respiratory muscle function stems primarily from the mechanical impedances imposed by fat deposition upon the movement of the chest wall and diaphragm (Salome et al, 2010). Fat deposited on the chest wall decreases respiratory system compliance, creating a restrictive pulmonary defect. Fat deposited within the abdominal cavity reduces its compliance and impedes diaphragm movement into the abdominal compartment. Respiratory system compliance of obese people is approximately half that of lean people, and reduces still further in obese people when supine (Naimark & Cherniack, 1960).

The effect of obesity upon lung volumes is primarily to reduce functional residual capacity (FRC) and end-expiratory lung volumes (EELV) (Babb et al, 2008b), owing to increased respiratory system recoil. This increases the likelihood of expiratory flow limitation (Ferretti et al, 2001). In addition, when breathing closer to residual volume, airway calibre is smaller and thus airway resistance is greater. For example, compared with overweight people (BMI 27 kg·m^{-2}), airway resistance was 56% greater in obese people (body mass index [BMI] 46 kg·m^{-2}); airway resistance was also correlated with the reduction in FRC (Zerah et al, 1993). Total lung capacity and residual volume tend to be preserved, but inspiratory reserve volume tends to increase and expiratory reserve volume to decrease (due to the reduction in EELV). However, in extreme obesity TLC may be impaired by the inability of the inspiratory muscles to overcome the increased compliance of the chest wall and abdominal compartment, or by a reduction in thoracic volume due to ingress of adipose tissue (Salome et al, 2010). Overall, the effects of obesity are to roughly double the work of breathing (Naimark & Cherniack, 1960; Pelosi et al, 1996; Kress et al, 1999), with most of the increase deriving from the increased elastic work (Pelosi et al, 1996).

The relative overloading of the respiratory pump in obesity is also reflected in a reduced maximum voluntary ventilation (MVV), the decline being greater with higher BMIs. However, this decline in MVV is greater than the declines in FEV$_1$ and FVC would predict (Weiner et al, 1998), which points strongly to a deficit in the function of the inspiratory muscles. Airway function is impaired slightly, with FEV$_1$ and FVC tending to decrease with increasing BMI (Salome et al, 2010). Since both indices decrease to the same extent, the impairment in FEV$_1$ is most likely secondary to the decrease in FVC, and not to a direct effect of obesity upon airway diameter (Salome et al, 2010). Changes in breathing mechanics mean that obesity leads to a reduction in EELV during exercise, with the consequence that some expiratory flow limitation may result (Rubinstein et al, 1990).

The effect of obesity upon the ventilatory requirement for exercise is self-evident, but the combination of an elevated oxygen and ventilatory cost of locomotion is exacerbated by poor aerobic fitness due to deconditioning. The latter leads to an early ventilatory compensation for metabolic acidosis. An important adaptive response during exercise is the adoption of a rapid and shallow breathing pattern, which increases the relative functional demands upon the inspiratory muscles, as well as the ventilatory requirement *per se* (by increasing the ratio of dead space ventilation to tidal volume). These factors conspire to create a huge increase in the requirement for respiratory muscle work to meet the elevated ventilatory requirement.

Respiratory muscle strength and endurance appear to be well preserved in some obese adults (Yap et al, 1995; Weiner et al, 1998; Collet et al, 2007), but studies have reported a small (~10%) impairment of respiratory muscle strength and endurance (Weiner et al, 1998; Chlif et al, 2005). Interestingly, even in those with relatively well-preserved respiratory muscle function, weight loss following bariatric surgery improves inspiratory and expiratory muscle strength by around 20% (Weiner et al, 1998). One thing is clear: inspiratory muscle function is inversely related to BMI. A significant negative correlation has been

observed by some investigators (Chlif et al, 2005), whilst others have noted that inspiratory muscle strength was slightly lower (~15%) in patients with a BMI >49 kg·m^{-2} than in those with a BMI <49 kg·m^{-2} (Collet et al, 2007).

Dyspnoea is a common complaint amongst obese individuals, both at rest and during exercise. This may be in part due to inspiratory muscle weakness (Chlif et al, 2007, 2009), but alterations in respiratory system mechanics also contribute. Breathing is associated with a rapid, shallow pattern, an increased ventilatory drive to the inspiratory muscles and an increased inspiratory muscle work (Chlif et al, 2007; Chlif et al, 2009). An increased oxygen cost of breathing has been implicated specifically in the dyspnoea associated with obesity (Babb et al, 2008a).

Another important factor to be borne in mind with regards to the influence of obesity upon breathing is the existence of co-morbidities. For example, it is increasingly common for obesity to be present with COPD (Franssen et al, 2008). There is also a well-established causal relationship between obesity and obstructive sleep apnoea (Schwartz et al, 2010), as well as hypoventilation syndrome (Anthony, 2008). Less well established, but an area of growing interest, is the apparent association between obesity and asthma, with some researchers suggesting that there may be a causal relationship between the two conditions (Sood, 2005), in which obesity is the antecedent (Ford, 2005). A putative underlying mechanism for the development of asthma, as well as the exacerbation of existing disease, is the production of pro-inflammatory cytokines by adipose tissue (Sood, 2010).

Thus, obese patients have an increased demand for inspiratory muscle work, which arises from complex changes in respiratory system mechanics. Furthermore, in those with inspiratory muscle weakness there is also a reduced capacity to supply this elevated demand. In the section 'Respiratory muscle involvement in exercise limitation', respiratory muscle-induced limitations to exercise tolerance will be considered, and Chapter 4 will review the evidence supporting specific respiratory muscle training for obese people.

Ageing

The process of normal ageing is associated with a number of changes that affect breathing (Janssens et al, 1999). Thus deterioration in pulmonary mechanics, lung function, locomotor efficiency and respiratory muscle function, as well as remodelling of pulmonary vasculature, all impact upon the demand/capacity relationship of the respiratory muscles.

The senescent changes to the pulmonary system have been dubbed 'senile emphysema' (Janssens et al, 1999) and are present from the age of 50 years, becoming most apparent at around 80 years (Britto et al, 2009). The most important of these changes are a decrease in the static recoil of the lung, a decrease in chest wall compliance and a reduction in the strength of the respiratory muscles (Janssens et al, 1999). Accordingly, many of the factors that increase the demand for inspiratory muscle pressure generation in COPD are also common to normal ageing. These include dynamic hyperinflation (Deruelle et al, 2008), and an increase in mechanical ventilatory constraints during exercise (DeLorey & Babb, 1999). Older people also adopt a rapid, shallow breathing pattern, and exhibit a greater dead space to tidal volume ratio (V_D/V_T), which necessitates an increase in $\dot{V}_E$ (DeLorey & Babb, 1999). There is also remodelling of the pulmonary vasculature, leading to increased vascular stiffness, resistance and pressure (Taylor & Johnson, 2010). These changes reduce pulmonary capillary blood volume and increase heterogeneity in the distribution of ventilation and perfusion. The resultant reduction in membrane diffusing capacity is consistent with a reduction in alveolar–capillary surface area (Taylor & Johnson, 2010). These changes make a small additional contribution to the ventilatory demand. In addition, the mechanical efficiency of exercise appears to be lower in older people (McConnell & Davies, 1992).

The term sarcopenia first appeared in the literature in the early 1990s to describe the age-related loss of muscle mass (Rogers & Evans, 1993). Respiratory muscles are also affected by this process, and their strength is correspondingly lower in older people (McConnell & Copestake, 1999); indeed, respiratory muscle strength is strongly and independently correlated with hand grip strength (Enright et al, 1994). Furthermore, respiratory muscle strength is also independently related to decline in mobility in older people (Buchman et al, 2008).

Finally, the influence of co-morbidities must also be borne in mind, since the majority of older people are not without disease. Accordingly, the age-related changes described above serve to exacerbate disease-related impairments. The picture in older people is therefore one of an emerging load/capacity imbalance within the respiratory muscles that worsens progressively with advancing age, and is exacerbated by chronic disease. In the section 'Respiratory muscle involvement in exercise limitation', the implications of these changes for exercise tolerance will be considered, and Chapter 4 will review the evidence supporting specific respiratory muscle training for older people.

Miscellaneous conditions

There are a number of other conditions that are associated with primary and functional respiratory muscle dysfunction, and/or imbalance of the demand/capacity relationship. These conditions have been less well studied from a respiratory perspective than those in the previous section, but are nevertheless worthy of consideration since specific training of the respiratory muscles could be considered as part of the management of these conditions. At best, functional weakness of the respiratory muscles impairs patients'

exercise tolerance; at worst, it can lead to life-threatening events or complications.

The underlying cause of respiratory muscle weakness in the conditions described below is diverse, ranging from the existence of a 'myopathic muscle milieu' (e.g., corticosteroid treatment), to profound disuse (mechanical ventilation). Where applicable, the evidence supporting the application of specific respiratory muscle training to these conditions will be described in Chapter 4.

Diabetes

Type 1 and 2 diabetes are associated with inspiratory and expiratory muscle weakness (~20% and ~10% impairment, respectively) (Heimer et al, 1990; Kaminski et al, 2011); in type 1, there is also impaired inspiratory muscle endurance (Heimer et al, 1990), vital capacity and FEV_1 (Innocenti et al, 1994). The reductions in lung volumes are at least partially explained by inspiratory muscle weakness (Wanke et al, 1991). However, loss of lung elasticity, and consequent airway collapse and obstruction, is also implicated (Goldman, 2003). The observation of a reduction in dynamic lung compliance is consistent with peripheral airway obstruction (Mancini et al, 1999). Biochemical changes in lung connective tissue have been suggested to underlie changes in elastic properties (Irfan et al, 2011). There is also a decrease in the pulmonary diffusing capacity, which may have its origins in pulmonary capillary damage induced by microvascular complications (Saler et al, 2009). Functionally, the structural changes to the lung parenchyma result in an elevated work of breathing (Wanke et al, 1992) and there is an increase in the magnitude of the ventilatory response to exercise, which is tachypnoeic in the presence of autonomic neuropathy (Tantucci et al, 1996). These factors most likely contribute to the greater intensity of dyspnoea during exercise (Wanke et al, 1992) and during hypoxia-induced hyperpnoea (Scano et al, 1999). Diabetic neuropathy has also been linked to inspiratory muscle weakness and autonomic dysfunction, as evidenced by a reduction in heart rate variability (Kaminski et al, 2011).

Putative underlying mechanisms for the inspiratory muscle weakness in patients with diabetes are divided broadly into two types: (1) biochemical and (2) neural. For example, inspiratory muscle strength is correlated with carnitine levels (Kilicli et al, 2010), which are lower in people with diabetes. In addition, there is evidence from rodent models of diabetes that the characteristics of resting membrane and action potentials are altered (van Lunteren & Moyer, 2003), and that responsiveness of the diaphragm to magnetic stimulation of the phrenic nerves is impaired in patients with diabetic polyneuropathy (Kabitz et al, 2008b). Impaired endurance of the inspiratory muscles may be explained by the many muscle metabolic abnormalities that arise because of insulin resistance and/or hyperglycaemia (Sun et al, 2008). In the section 'Respiratory muscle involvement in exercise limitation', the implications of these changes for exercise tolerance will be considered, and Chapter 4 will review the evidence supporting specific respiratory muscle training for patients with diabetes.

Renal failure

Respiratory system involvement in renal failure is extremely complex (Prezant, 1990), deriving from both the disease and its treatment. It has been known for many years that uraemic patients possess impaired inspiratory muscle strength and a restrictive pulmonary defect (Gomez-Fernandez et al, 1984). The latter is most likely due to the effects of hypervolaemia, which induces pulmonary hypertension and oedema. Impairment of vital capacity is reversible with dialysis, implicating hypervolaemia as a major contributory factor (Kovelis et al, 2008). Since respiratory muscle strength does not appear to improve post-dialysis, primary weakness is implicated. Furthermore, patients who have been receiving dialysis for the longest showed the most impaired inspiratory muscle function (Kovelis et al, 2008). This supports the notion of progressive development of primary weakness (Bark et al, 1988; Karacan et al, 2006; Kovelis et al, 2008). For this reason, estimates of the magnitude of impairment differ between studies, ranging from deficits of ~40% and 50% for inspiratory and expiratory muscle strength respectively (Bark et al, 1988), to ~10% (Kovelis et al, 2008). Interestingly, respiratory muscle dysfunction is partially reversible following renal transplantation (Guleria et al, 2005). Chapter 4 will review the evidence supporting specific respiratory muscle training for patients with renal failure.

Cancer

One of the most common chronic symptoms in patients with cancer is exertional dyspnoea, which is present in up to 10% of survivors of childhood cancers and up to 70% of patients with advanced cancer (Travers et al, 2008). Generally, pulmonary function is relatively normal in patients with cancer (Travers et al, 2008), and there are no major mechanical abnormalities. However, there are exceptions, and pulmonary function may be impaired in specific cancers affecting the thorax (e.g., lung and breast), especially following locoregional adjuvant radiotherapy (Spyropoulou et al, 2009). There are many ways in which cancer and/or its treatment might cause dyspnoea, but one unifying mechanism that has been suggested to underlie exertional dyspnoea in patients with cancer is respiratory muscle weakness (Feathers et al, 2003; Travers et al, 2008). Since pulmonary function does not correlate with dyspnoea, inspiratory muscle weakness is likely to be an important contributor to the symptom (Travers et al, 2008). In the section 'Respiratory muscle involvement in exercise limitation', the implications of these changes for exercise tolerance will be considered. At the time of writing

there have been no studies of respiratory muscle training in patients with cancer.

Anorexia nervosa

Anorexia nervosa is associated with generalized muscle wasting and specific weakness of the respiratory muscles (Birmingham & Tan, 2003; Gardini Gardenghi et al, 2009) including the diaphragm (Murciano et al, 1994). In addition, there is evidence of impaired spirometric function that is correlated with body mass (Ziora et al, 2008). Furthermore, malnourishment appears to induce changes to the lung parenchyma resulting in impaired diffusion capacity (Gardini Gardenghi et al, 2009) and/or emphysema-like changes to the lung structure (Coxson et al, 2004), as well as an increase in residual volume (Gonzalez-Moro et al, 2003). Functionally, there is impaired exercise tolerance (Biadi et al, 2001), perhaps due in part to dyspnoea (Birmingham & Tan, 2003). Case study evidence suggests that inspiratory muscle function may take longer to recover following refeeding than other muscles, leading to prolongation of dyspnoea symptoms and exercise intolerance (Birmingham & Tan, 2003).

The underlying causes for the spirometric changes are thought to be a combination of a restrictive defect caused by inspiratory muscle weakness (Ziora et al, 2008) and the effects of undernutrition on the lung parenchyma. Animal models of anorexia have demonstrated decreased production of lung surfactant (D'Amours et al, 1983), as well as the total protein, connective tissue and elastic content of the lungs of young animals (Sahebjami & MacGee, 1985), which is not completely reversible by refeeding (Sahebjami & Domino, 1992). In the section 'Respiratory muscle involvement in exercise limitation', the implications of these changes for exercise tolerance will be considered. At the time of writing there have been no studies of respiratory muscle training in patients with anorexia nervosa.

Myopathic pharmacological agents

The myopathic influence of orally administered corticosteroids was discussed briefly in relation to patients with COPD and asthma. Steroid-induced myopathy is a well-established phenomenon in patients receiving high doses of corticosteroids (Perkoff et al, 1959). The first study to examine the independent effects of costicosteroid treatment and disease progression demonstrated that, in non-respiratory patients, 1 to 1.5 mg·kg^{-1} per day of prednisolone induced significant reductions in the strength (~30%) and endurance (~50%) of the inspiratory muscles over an 8-week treatment period (Weiner et al, 1993; Weiner et al, 1995). Although these changes show some reversal following cessation of treatment, function may take as long as 6 months to normalize (Weiner et al, 1993).

There have also been a number of case reports of colchicine-induced myopathy following prolonged treatment (Wilbur & Makowsky, 2004) including one report in which the predominant clinical feature was respiratory muscle weakness, as indicated by severe dyspnoea, orthopnoea, tachypnoea and thoracoabdominal paradox (Tanios et al, 2004). Cessation of treatment resulted in an improvement in respiratory muscle function, which more than doubled from pre-cessation levels of ~25–$30 \, cmH_2O$ (Tanios et al, 2004).

Most recently, statin-induced myopathy has come under scrutiny, as it is estimated that 5–10% of patients receiving statins develop myopathy (Rallidis et al, 2011). At least one case study report has demonstrated an association between respiratory symptoms, inspiratory muscle dysfunction and statin administration (Chatham et al, 2009). See Chapter 4 for a description of the evidence supporting specific inspiratory muscle training.

Surgery

Post-operative pulmonary complications (PPC) are common in patients undergoing cardiothoracic, abdominal and other major surgeries. Because of variations in both the nature of surgeries and the definition of PPC, estimates of the incidence vary from 2% to 40% (Canet & Mazo, 2010). The substantial contribution made by PCC to the morbidity and mortality associated with surgery and anaesthesia has led to interest in predicting those patients at risk of developing a PPC. Three main factors contribute to risk, and their interaction appears to determine its level: (1) general health status, (2) effects of anaesthesia and (3) surgical trauma (Canet & Mazo, 2010).

General health status has a predictable influence upon risk, especially where patients have pre-existing respiratory and cardiovascular dysfunction (Canet & Mazo, 2010). Anaesthesia induces a range of pre- and post-operative changes that increase the risk of PCC (Canet & Mazo, 2010). For example, atelectasis is universal, arising from physical compression of the lungs, absorption of alveolar air and impairment of surfactant function. These changes induce ventilation/perfusion mismatching, which increases dead space and hypoxaemia (Canet & Mazo, 2010). Post-operative drugs such as anaesthetics and analgesics also affect upper airway and accessory muscle function, increasing the risk of PCC (Canet & Mazo, 2010). As one might expect, the site of surgery has a potent influence upon the development of PPC. Predictably, thoracic and abdominal surgeries are associated with the highest risk of PPC (10–40%; Duggan & Kavanagh, 2010), and give rise to post-operative respiratory muscle dysfunction. The origin of the resulting muscle dysfunction is complex, but includes factors such as changes in thoracoabdominal mechanics and loss of muscular integrity (Siafakas et al, 1999). In addition, post-operative pain can limit respiratory movements, which can also be impaired by reflex inhibition of respiratory

muscle activity, especially the diaphragm (Sharma et al, 1999). The latter arises because of feedback stimulated by mechanical disturbance of the viscera (Canet & Mazo, 2010). Finally, procedures lasting more than 3 hours have a higher risk of PCC (Duggan & Kavanagh, 2010), which may be partially due to the effects of inspiratory muscle inactivity during mechanical ventilation upon inspiratory muscle function (see the section 'Mechanical ventilation'). See Chapter 4 for a description of the evidence supporting specific inspiratory muscle training for the prevention of PPC.

Mechanical ventilation

The primary reason for admission to intensive care is the need for mechanical ventilation, which imposes a considerable burden upon both patients and healthcare systems (Bissett et al, 2012). Mechanical ventilation is a double-edged sword for the respiratory muscles. On the one hand it can provide much needed rest for overloaded muscles, but on the other the imposed rest can lead to rapid atrophy and loss of respiratory muscle function (Petrof et al, 2010). The latter can lead to prolongation of mechanical ventilation, and difficulty weaning patients from the ventilator (Callahan, 2009). Weaning typically accounts for 40–50% of the total duration of mechanical ventilation and 30% of patients fail to wean at the first attempt (Moodie et al, 2011). Indeed, patients who experience weaning failure are characterized by their rapid, shallow breathing pattern and a diaphragm tension–time index (TTI) that is close to the threshold for fatigue (Karakurt et al, 2011); multiple logistic regression analysis with the weaning outcome as the dependent variable has revealed TTI, and the ratio of breathing frequency to V_T, as significant predictors of weaning outcome (Vassilakopoulos et al, 1998). Patients who are weaned successfully from mechanical ventilation have been shown to possess higher MIP than those who do not (Epstein et al, 2002; Carlucci et al, 2009), and low MIP is an independent predictor of prolonged weaning (De Jonghe et al, 2007). However, a recent systematic review failed to find evidence that superior inspiratory muscle strength leads to a shorter duration of mechanical ventilation, improved weaning success or improved survival; the authors highlighted the need for further research (Moodie et al, 2011). It has been suggested that discrepancies relating to the influence of MIP upon these factors may reflect the inadequacy of MIP as a prognostic index of the respiratory muscle contribution to complex phenomena such as weaning (Bissett et al, 2012).

There is mounting evidence that mechanical ventilation leads to pathological changes to the respiratory system that may contribute to prolongation of ventilator dependence and difficulty in weaning (Bissett et al, 2012). The precise time course, as well as the prevalence and incidence of ventilator-acquired respiratory muscle dysfunction, remains unclear, but a primate model suggests a 46% loss of diaphragm strength and a 37% reduction in ventilator endurance after 11 days of mechanical ventilation (Anzueto et al, 1987). Human data are sparse, but one study has compared diaphragm fibre samples from mechanically ventilated brain-dead organ donors with those of control patients who were ventilated for less than 3 hours. Diaphragm fibre cross-sectional area (types I and II) was over 50% lower in the organ donor patients following just 18–69 hours of mechanical ventilation, compared with control (Levine et al, 2008). Interestingly, this atrophy was not present in control muscle biopsies (pectoralis major), suggesting that it was specific to diaphragm inactivity. In another study, twitch diaphragm pressure (TwP_{di}) was measured serially in mechanically ventilated patients to assess the time course of changes in diaphragm function (Hermans et al, 2010). Increasing duration of mechanical ventilation was associated with a logarithmic decline in TwP_{di}. This association was also found for cumulative dose of propofol and piritramide, suggesting a potential contribution from factors such as sedatives and analgesics (Hermans et al, 2010).

One of the reasons for the lack of information in this area is the difficulty of assessing respiratory muscle function in mechanically ventilated patients. Voluntary measures of strength such as MIP are considered too unreliable, although a technique in which the patient's tracheostomy tube is occluded using a one-way valve has been validated and found to be more reliable than conventional MIP (Caruso et al, 1999). Studies using non-volitional measures are difficult to obtain, and hence few and far between. Three such studies utilizing magnetic stimulation of the phrenic nerves found that TwP_{di} in mechanically ventilated patients was around 30% of that observed in normal people (Watson et al, 2001; Laghi et al, 2003; Hermans et al, 2010).

Underlying mechanisms for the development of ventilator-acquired inspiratory muscle weakness remain unclear. The picture is complex and, although it is one part of the polyneuropathy that has been described in critical illness (Latronico & Bolton, 2011), there appear to be factors that are specific to the respiratory muscles (Levine et al, 2008). These specific factors include the individual and combined effects of disuse atrophy/proteolysis, nutritional factors and pharmacological influences, as well as mechanical responses to positive end-expiratory pressure (PEEP) due to alterations in the length–tension relationship of the diaphragm (Bissett et al, 2012). See Chapter 4 for a description of the evidence supporting specific inspiratory muscle training.

Pregnancy

The increase in intra-abdominal mass during pregnancy impairs normal diaphragm movement, and the effect upon breathing is, to a limited extent, similar to that observed in obesity. The diaphragm is displaced cranially during the latter stages of pregnancy, but continues to move normally during tidal breathing (Laghi & Tobin, 2003). Similarly, respiratory muscle strength remains unchanged (Contreras et al, 1991). However, the hormonal milieu of pregnancy induces an increase in the drive to breathe, and in $\dot{V}_E$ (minute volume) (Jensen et al, 2007); the former is correlated with plasma progesterone levels (Contreras et al, 1991), whereas the latter is achieved exclusively via an increase in V_T (tidal volume) (Jensen et al, 2009b). These changes contribute to the increase in breathing effort and dyspnoea that are experienced by around three-quarters of pregnant women (Milne et al, 1978). Although several theories have been put forward to explain gestational dyspnoea, its aetiology remains poorly understood (see also the section 'Respiratory muscle involvement in exercise limitation', below), but recent evidence points to its being a 'normal awareness of increased ventilation' (Jensen et al, 2009b).

Another facet of pregnancy in which respiratory muscles play a key role is parturition, which has been shown to induce diaphragm fatigue (Nava et al, 1992). The action of the diaphragm during expulsive efforts plays a very important role in minimizing increases in intrathoracic pressure (which have detrimental haemodynamic effects) and maximizing increases in intra-abdominal pressure. The latter can exceed 150 cmH$_2$O, and is correlated with speed of delivery, i.e., the higher the intra-abdominal pressure that can be maintained the faster the delivery (Buhimschi et al, 2002). Since diaphragm fatigue occurs, it is reasonable to suggest that this may impair the effectiveness of expulsive efforts, which may prolong delivery.

In the section 'Respiratory muscle involvement in exercise limitation', the implications of these changes for exercise tolerance will be considered. At the time of writing there have been no studies of respiratory muscle training in pregnant women.

Obstructive sleep apnoea

The contraction of thoracic inspiratory muscles decreases intrapleural pressure, transmitting a sub-atmospheric pressure to the extrathoracic [upper] airways. This creates a transluminal pressure that tends to collapse the upper airways. The magnitude of the transluminal pressure gradient is determined by a number of factors including the airway wall elasticity, intrapleural pressure, as well as how resistance is distributed through the upper airway (Olson et al, 1988). In the absence of bony or cartilaginous structures to maintain upper patency at the pharyngeal level, upper airway patency is dependent entirely upon the activation of over 20 dilator muscles (see Ch. 1), which resist the collapsing effect of negative intraluminal pressure during inspiration (Series, 2002).

Dysfunctions in the coordinated activation of the upper airway and respiratory pump muscles, as well as of the neuromuscular tone of the upper airway muscles, have been identified as key factors in the pathogenesis of obstructive sleep apnoea (OSA) (Steier et al, 2010). Indeed, loss of neuromuscular tone in the upper airway dilator muscles initiates the cascade of events that culminate in airway occlusion (Hudgel & Harasick, 1990). According to the 'balance of pressures' concept, upper airway occlusion occurs when the positive dilating pressure from the upper airway musculature is unable to resist the negative intraluminal pressure caused by inspiratory effort (Brouillette & Thach, 1979). Whilst an index of airway dilator muscle function suggests patients with OSA have greater strength, this is accompanied by lower endurance (Eckert et al, 2011). Furthermore, the intrinsic, passive properties of the upper airway and pharynx also contribute to its propensity to collapse (Isono et al, 1997), i.e., the more compliant the walls of the airway, the smaller is the pressure gradient required to induce narrowing, and ultimately occlusion.

Thus, there are two mechanical mechanisms by which the collapsibility of the upper airway could be modified: firstly by improving active neuromuscular tone of the upper airway, and secondly by reducing the passive compliance of the upper airway. The former has two subcomponents, the first being reflex coordination of airway dilator muscles, and the second being the functional properties of these muscles (e.g., strength, fatigue resistance, rate of shortening). Both of these mechanical mechanisms can be influenced by specific training (Lindstedt et al, 2002; Demoule et al, 2008). See Chapter 4 for a description of the evidence supporting specific respiratory muscle training in OSA.

RESPIRATORY MUSCLE INVOLVEMENT IN EXERCISE LIMITATION

In the previous section, disease-related changes in the relationship between the demand for breathing and the capacity of the respiratory pump muscles to meet that demand were explored. A pragmatic method of defining 'weakness' was suggested, incorporating the context in which the respiratory pump operates. In this definition, if the demands that are placed upon a 'normal muscle' are excessive, then its capacity is inadequate, and it is rendered weak functionally. The following section will consider how the respiratory muscles contribute to exercise limitation in some of the conditions described in the previous section. However, it will begin by describing our current understanding of this limitation in healthy, athletic young people. The notion that the respiratory system limits exercise performance and tolerance in healthy people is relatively new, but it is nevertheless supported by a robust scientific evidence base.

Healthy people

In healthy young people, the physical work undertaken by the respiratory muscles during the task of pumping air in and out of the lungs can be immense (Harms & Dempsey, 1999), but even in non-athletes the work of breathing has been shown to influence exercise tolerance. Research suggests that this occurs via two mechanisms: (1) by contributing to perceived effort, and (2) by exacerbating the demands placed upon the circulatory system for blood flow. This section will consider how these factors contribute to exercise limitation, with an emphasis on the role and repercussions of respiratory muscle work.

An important premise in the argument that respiratory muscles limit exercise performance in healthy people is that the muscles operate at, or close to, the limits of their capacity. When muscles work in this way, they become fatigued (see Ch. 1, 'Mechanisms of fatigue'). Accordingly, without some evidence of exercise-induced respiratory muscle fatigue (RMF), the argument in favour of training these muscles is flimsy at best.

Respiratory muscles are separated functionally according to whether they have inspiratory or expiratory actions. Since breathing demands equal movement of inspiratory and expiratory air, one might predict that fatigue would be present in both groups of muscles under the same conditions. This is not the case. One reason for this is the fact that inspiratory muscle work is always greater than expiratory work (recall the party balloon analogy from Ch. 1 – the stretching of tissues on inhalation assists exhalation); a second reason is the differing training state of the muscles themselves (expiratory muscles are engaged in many postural activities that improve their training status); a third reason is that different exercise conditions overload the inspiratory and expiratory muscles to differing extents.

The earliest reports of inspiratory muscle fatigue (IMF) following competitive sports events appeared in the early 1980s. In this context fatigue was defined as a loss of voluntary force generating capacity post-exercise, and a significant decrease in inspiratory muscle strength (MIP) was measured following marathon running (Loke et al, 1982). Subsequent studies have confirmed this finding (Chevrolet et al, 1993; Ross et al, 2008), as well as showing IMF after ultramarathon (Ker & Schultz, 1996) and triathlon competitions (Hill et al, 1991).

Under laboratory and field-based research conditions, IMF has been demonstrated following rowing (Volianitis et al, 2001; Griffiths & McConnell, 2007), cycling (Romer et al, 2002b) and swimming (Lomax & McConnell, 2003), as well as a sprint triathlon (Sharpe et al, 1996) and treadmill marathon running (Ross et al, 2008). All of the studies cited above have evaluated IMF using maximal inspiratory pressure (MIP) measured at the mouth, which is a holistic, voluntary surrogate of inspiratory muscle force production (see Ch. 6 for a description of MIP assessment). Although MIP has its merits (being non-invasive, portable, quick and easy to administer, reliable and holistic), it can also be criticized for being susceptible to the influence of changes in effort. In other words, immediately after exercise a lower MIP might be the result of reduced effort, and not due to physiological factors. However, contractile fatigue of the diaphragm has also been confirmed in the laboratory following heavy exercise using electrical and magnetic stimulation of the phrenic nerves (Johnson et al, 1993; Mador et al, 1993; Babcock et al, 1997; Babcock et al, 1998). Thus, not only is there evidence of IMF following real world sports participation and laboratory simulations of competition, but rigorous laboratory trials also demonstrate specific contractile fatigue of the diaphragm after heavy exercise. The observation that the diaphragm was susceptible to exercise-induced fatigue initiated a process that has led to a complete rethink about the role of respiratory muscles in exercise limitation (Romer & Polkey, 2008).

But what of the expiratory muscles? The effect of real world sports activities upon expiratory muscle function has been studied much less extensively, and existing data are currently contradictory. Following marathon running that induced a fall in MIP, no change in maximal expiratory pressure (MEP) was observed post-exercise (Chevrolet et al, 1993; Ross et al, 2008). Similarly, following a triathlon that elicited a significant fall in MIP, there was no change in MEP (Hill et al, 1991). In contrast, following a rowing time trial that simulated a 2000-metre rowing race in the laboratory, a significant decline in MEP was observed (Griffiths & McConnell, 2007). Similarly, under laboratory conditions where cycling exercise was performed to the limit of tolerance (T_{lim}), MEP was shown to decline (Cordain et al, 1994). In contrast, some authors observed no change in MEP following maximal cycle ergometer exercise, but did observe a fall in MIP (Coast et al, 1999). Non-volitional assessment of expiratory muscle fatigue (EMF) using magnetic stimulation of abdominal muscles has recently demonstrated EMF occurring after high-intensity cycle ergometer exercise to T_{lim} (Taylor et al, 2006; Verges et al, 2006). Thus, it appears that EMF may be specific to certain exercise modalities and/or intensities of exercise. These conditions appear to be characterized by exercise at maximal intensity, and/or situations in which the expiratory muscles have a key role in propulsive force transmission, such as rowing.

Collectively, the literature points to IMF occurring in response to a wider range of activities than EMF, and possibly also at lower intensities and/or following shorter durations of activity.

The next question to consider is whether there are any functional repercussions of RMF. This has been studied using a variety of experimental designs, but principally by using two basic approaches: first by inducing RMF and studying its influence upon subsequent exercise, and second by manipulating the work of breathing during exercise to accelerate RMF (by adding a resistance to breathing) or to delay the time to RMF (by using a ventilator to undertake the work of breathing). The effects of prior IMF and EMF are to increase the intensity of breathing effort during subsequent whole-body exercise, and to lead to a shorter time to T_{lim} during constant power output exercise. For example, one of the first studies to examine the effect of prior IMF on exercise tolerance observed a 23% reduction in the ability to sustain cycling at 90% of maximal oxygen uptake (Mador & Acevedo, 1991). There was an increase in the sensation of effort during exercise, i.e., exercise after IMF felt harder. Using a slightly different experimental design, the effects of prior IMF on isolated plantar flexor exercise have been studied (McConnell & Lomax, 2006). In this case, a more rapid fatigue of the plantar flexor muscles was observed after IMF (the reasons for this are explained later).

More recently, the effects of prior EMF on cycling performance were assessed (Taylor & Romer, 2008). A decrease in T_{lim} (33%) was observed when exercise followed EMF, as well as an increase in the perceptions of both breathing and leg effort. Leg fatigue was also more severe after EMF. However, a note of caution is required in the interpretation of studies that have pre-fatigued the expiratory muscles. The same authors have also shown that expiratory loading induces simultaneous IMF and EMF (Taylor & Romer, 2009). In other words, the effect of EMF on subsequent exercise performance is 'contaminated' by accompanying IMF. This is because the inspiratory muscles are involved in the transmission of expiratory pressure. Thus, any effects of EMF on performance cannot be ascribed solely to the expiratory muscles.

On the face of it the observations that IMF, and possibly also EMF, exacerbates limb muscle fatigue defy logical explanation; after all, why should fatiguing the respiratory muscles exacerbate fatigue in the limb muscles? The answer lies in the findings of a series of studies that have examined the influence of manipulating the work of breathing during exercise. In theory, if respiratory muscle work limits exercise performance, then reducing the amount of work they undertake during exercise should improve performance. Similarly, increasing the work of breathing during exercise should impair performance. In a series of very elegant studies undertaken during the mid-1990s, a proportional assist ventilator was utilized to 'unload' the inspiratory muscles during exercise, whilst a flow resistor was used to increase inspiratory muscle work.

In the first study to explore the impact of the work of breathing on exercise tolerance, the influence of changes in the work of breathing upon leg blood flow during maximal cycle ergometer exercise was examined (Harms et al, 1997). A reciprocal relationship between leg blood flow and the work of breathing was observed, such that when the inspiratory work was undertaken by a ventilator there was a 4.3% increase in leg blood flow. In contrast, when inspiratory work was increased by a flow resistor the leg blood flow decreased by 7%. The changes in leg blood flow were mediated by changes in the neural input to the blood vessels in the limbs, resulting in vasoconstriction when inspiratory work was increased and dilatation when it was reduced. In a series of subsequent studies, it was shown that the stimulus for limb vasoconstriction was a cardiovascular reflex originating within the inspiratory muscles, which became known as the 'inspiratory muscle metaboreflex' (St Croix, 2000; Sheel et al, 2001; Sheel et al, 2002). The findings of these studies have been replicated and extended to provide compelling evidence that functional overload of the inspiratory muscles induces reflex cardiovascular adjustments that reduce exercising limb blood flow (McConnell & Lomax, 2006; Katayama et al, 2012). The exercise models employed by early studies suggested that only very-high-intensity exercise was associated with inspiratory muscle metaboreflex activation (Wetter et al, 1999). However, more recent studies have shown that moderate-intensity exercise combined with inspiratory muscle loading also leads to inspiratory metaboreflex activation (Katayama et al, 2012), suggesting that the critical factor is functional overload of the inspiratory muscles, not the whole body muscle intensity.

The 'inspiratory muscle metaboreflex' is activated when metabolite accumulation within the inspiratory muscles stimulates afferent nerve fibres (type III and IV) to increase their firing frequency. Stimulation of these fibres precipitates an increase in the strength of sympathetic efferent outflow, which induces a generalized vasoconstriction. Limiting blood flow restricts the supply of oxygen and impairs the removal of exercise metabolites from exercising muscles, with the result that muscles fatigue more quickly and exercise performance is impaired (McConnell & Lomax, 2006). Indeed, this is precisely what has been found; changes in leg blood flow elicited by increasing or reducing the work of inhalation are correlated with changes in the magnitude of exercise-induced leg fatigue (Romer et al, 2006). In other words, increasing the work of inspiration reduces leg blood flow, exacerbates leg fatigue and impairs exercise tolerance, whereas reducing the work of inhalation does the opposite. However, it is important to appreciate that contractile fatigue of the inspiratory muscles is not an essential prerequisite to metaboreflex activation; the prerequisite is metabolite accumulation, which may not necessarily induce contractile fatigue. Indeed, it has been argued that muscle feedback may provide an important protective mechanism that guards against fatigue (Gandevia, 2001). The findings summarized above complete the circle that links RMF with leg fatigue, i.e., metaboreflex activation precipitates limb vasoconstriction, reducing limb blood flow and accelerating limb fatigue. The evidence for an effect of IMT upon metaboreflex activation will be reviewed in Chapter 4.

Earlier, we touched briefly upon the effect of IMF and EMF on breathing and limb effort, i.e., RMF intensifies sense of effort during exercise (Mador & Acevedo, 1991; Taylor & Romer, 2008). The influence upon limb effort should now be clear: IMF reduces limb blood flow, thereby reducing oxygen delivery and accelerating limb fatigue. Although it

might seem self-evident that weak or fatigued muscles generate greater perception of effort than fresh or stronger muscles, the neurophysiological mechanism underpinning this reality merits a few words. The human brain is able to judge the size of the outgoing neural drive (McCloskey et al, 1983), and as muscles contract they return information to the brain about the amount of force that is being generated, as well as the speed and range of motion of the movement (Cafarelli, 1982). Heavy objects require high forces, they can be moved only slowly and may impose a limited range of motion; the opposite is true for light objects. The sensory area of the brain compares the size of the drive sent to the muscles with the sensory information coming from the muscles. In doing so, it formulates a perception of effort. The size of the neural drive required to generate a given external force is influenced by a number of factors, but principally by the strength of the muscle. A strong muscle requires a lower neural drive to generate a given force, which is why weights feel lighter after strength training. Similarly, a fatigued muscle requires a higher neural drive to generate a given force, which is why weights feel heavier when muscles are fatigued (Gandevia & McCloskey, 1978).

As was described in Chapter 1, the neurophysiological principles described above apply equally to the respiratory muscles (Campbell, 1966) as they do to other skeletal muscles. Thus, weakness, fatigue, or indeed strengthening, of the respiratory muscles modulates the perception of breathing effort and dyspnoea. Similarly, abnormalities of respiratory mechanics exacerbate perception of breathing effort (Scano et al, 2010). Recently, the term 'neuromechanical uncoupling' has been used to describe the imbalance between neural drive and the mechanical events that it produces (see Ch. 1).

Finally, it is worth mentioning some emerging evidence about the influence of group III and IV afferent feedback upon the central perception of effort and central fatigue. Group III and IV fibres project to a number of sites within the central nervous system. Most recently, Amann and colleagues employed a selective μ-opioid receptor agonist to demonstrate, for the first time, that afferent feedback from locomotor group III and IV fibres makes an 'essential contribution' to both cardiorespiratory control and perceptual responses in the exercising human being (Amann et al, 2010a). The latter finding is consistent with the observation that strengthening inspiratory muscles attenuates both respiratory and peripheral effort perception (Romer et al, 2002a), which may arise because of reduced feedback from group III and IV afferents in both respiratory and locomotor muscles.

Furthermore, feedback from group III and IV afferents is also implicated in central fatigue mechanisms, via inhibition of central motor output (Gandevia, 2001). It has been suggested that afferent feedback from exercising muscles protects locomotor and respiratory muscles from catastrophic fatigue (Gandevia, 2001). Indeed, Gandevia suggested, 'An extreme example [of central fatigue] occurs with exercise of the inspiratory muscles in which task failure can occur with minimal peripheral fatigue' (Gandevia, 2001). The importance of group III and IV afferent feedback in regulating integrated exercise responses was illustrated recently by a study in which a cycle time trial was undertaken with and without the selective μ-opioid receptor agonist fentanyl (Amann et al, 2009). During a self-paced 5 km time trial, intrathecal fentanyl was associated with greater quadriceps fatigue, a higher central motor output and greater perceived exertion compared with placebo. A higher power output in the first half of the fentanyl time trial was offset by a lower power output in the second, resulting in no change in performance time. However, compared with placebo, the decline in quadriceps twitch force was greater with fentanyl (45.6% vs 33.1%) and was associated with ambulatory problems post-exercise. The authors suggest their data 'emphasize the critical role of locomotor muscle afferents in determining the subject's choice of the "optimal" exercise intensity that will allow for maximal performance while preserving a certain level of locomotor muscle "functional reserve" at end-exercise' (Amann et al, 2009). The specific contribution of respiratory muscle group III and IV afferents to central fatigue during whole-body exercise awaits investigation. Given the importance of protecting diaphragm function, it is reasonable to speculate that the inhibitory feedback from diaphragm afferents during exercise influences both respiratory and locomotor central motor output.

Thus, the past decade has seen the emergence of evidence that respiratory muscle work has influences far beyond anything that was thought possible. The respiratory muscles can contribute to exercise limitation through their influence on cardiovascular reflex control, i.e., metaboreflex reduction of limb blood flow. In addition, the respiratory muscles make a potent contribution to the perception of effort during exercise, and may also play a role in central fatigue. The evidence that strengthening the respiratory muscles reduces effort perception and improves exercise tolerance is reviewed in Chapter 4.

In this section we have considered the limitation to exercise tolerance imposed by the respiratory muscles in healthy people. The following section will describe how disease-specific factors limit exercise by exacerbating the breathing-related limitations to exercise tolerance that exist in healthy people. In Chapter 4 we will consider the evidence that rebalancing the relationship between demand and capacity of the respiratory pump muscles using RMT induces beneficial adaptations to respiratory muscle structure and function, as well as clinical benefits.

Respiratory disease

Chronic obstructive pulmonary disease

Patients with chronic obstructive pulmonary disease (COPD) have a complex pattern of disease, and there is

an on-going debate regarding the precise exercise-limiting mechanisms(s) (Nici, 2008). However, what is not in doubt is that the primary symptom associated with exercise in patients with COPD is dyspnoea (O'Donnell & Webb, 2008a), the magnitude of which is influenced by both the pulmonary and systemic aspects of the disease (see 'Changes in breathing mechanics and respiratory muscle function', above). As O'Donnell & Webb so vividly put it, *'When you can't breathe nothing else matters!'* (O'Donnell & Webb, 2008a). Notwithstanding this, patients with COPD also exhibit significant exercise-induced locomotor muscle fatigue, to which they also appear to be more susceptible than healthy age-matched controls (Mador et al, 2003). Thus, peripheral factors also play an important role in exercise limitation, but, as will be discussed below, this influence is potentiated by the effect of elevated respiratory muscle work, which compromises limb oxygen delivery (Amann et al, 2010b).

In patients with COPD, the inspiratory muscle demand/capacity relationship is skewed such that the inspiratory muscles are severely overloaded (Moxham & Jolley, 2009). This imbalance not only affects limb blood flow during exercise (Vogiatzis et al, 2011), it is also a key contributor to dyspnoea via neuromechanical uncoupling (Moxham & Jolley, 2009). As was described in the previous section, COPD patients have primary inspiratory muscle weakness, which is exacerbated by the functional effects of hyperinflation. Hyperinflation increases the operating lung volume thereby raising the demand for inspiratory muscle work due to its influence upon the elastic work of breathing, as well as the inspiratory threshold load imposed by intrinsic positive end-expiratory pressure (PEEP$_i$). The overload of the inspiratory muscles is exacerbated still further during exercise by tachypnoea (rapid shallow breathing) due to tidal volume (V_T) restriction, caused by the mechanical consequences of hyperinflation (O'Donnell & Webb, 2008b; O'Donnell et al, 2012). The result of this rapid shallow breathing pattern is an increase in the ventilatory requirement ($\dot{V}_E$), and further functional weakening of the inspiratory muscles due to the increased velocity of inspiratory muscle shortening (O'Donnell & Webb, 2008b). In a retrospective analysis of data from two previous studies, O'Donnell and colleagues stratified patients into four levels of disease severity in order to examine the influence of hyperinflation upon ventilatory constraint and exertional dyspnoea. They observed a strong, negative influence of disease severity upon inspiratory capacity, V_T expansion, dyspnoea and exercise tolerance (O'Donnell et al, 2012). During incremental cycling, V_T expansion ceased at the same percentage of inspiratory capacity (73–77%), irrespective of disease severity, and dyspnoea escalated rapidly thereafter. The authors concluded that dyspnoea and exercise intolerance are associated with the attainment of 'critical constraints on V_T expansion and attendant increase in dyspnea at a progressively lower ventilation during exercise' (O'Donnell et al, 2012).

Hyperinflation induces extremely high levels of diaphragm activation during exercise in patients with COPD such that, at the end of an incremental exercise test to the limit of tolerance, diaphragm activation can reach 81% (Sinderby et al, 2001). This indicates that the diaphragm (and probably also accessory muscles), work at a very high relative intensity during exercise. Somewhat paradoxically, studies of diaphragm contractile fatigue using phrenic nerve stimulation have failed to demonstrate consistent evidence of diaphragm fatigue following symptom-limited exercise in patients with COPD (Mador et al, 2000a; Mador et al, 2000b), but have observed leg muscle fatigue (Mador et al, 2000a). This apparent paradox was mentioned in the previous section, and is explored further in the final paragraph of the present section.

Poor aerobic fitness and peripheral muscle myopathy also contribute to exercise limitation in COPD, as they lead to a rapid lactic acidosis and a greater ventilatory requirement for exercise. These factors also exacerbate hyperinflation, and its correlates such as inspiratory muscle work. It is therefore no surprise that dyspnoea intensity during exercise in COPD patients correlates significantly with the extent of hyperinflation (O'Donnell & Laveneziana, 2007). Several studies have noted significant decreases in dyspnoea following interventions that reduced the demand for inspiratory muscle work by reducing operational lung volumes, either pharmacologically, surgically or using non-invasive positive airway pressure ventilation (Ambrosino & Strambi, 2004). These studies suggest that modifying the demand side of the inspiratory muscles' demand/capacity relationship reduces dyspnoea (O'Donnell et al, 2007). It is therefore reasonable to suggest that modifying the capacity side of the relationship should evoke similar attenuation of dyspnoea, which is indeed the case, and the evidence for the latter will be reviewed in Chapter 4.

Reducing the demand for inspiratory muscle work also affects locomotor muscle performance in COPD patients. When the work of breathing is reduced by breathing heliox (a low-density gas), patients with COPD show an improvement in exercise tolerance and a reduction in the magnitude of exercise-induced leg fatigue (Butcher, 2008), which may be secondary to improved limb blood flow (Vogiatzis et al, 2011). Similarly, inspiratory muscle unloading using a proportional assist ventilator improves exercise tolerance, reduces leg effort and improves leg oxygenation in patients with COPD (Borghi-Silva et al, 2008b); the same group has made identical observations in patients with CHF. These data are entirely consistent with earlier observations in healthy young athletes during inspiratory muscle unloading (Harms et al, 1997). There is an emerging consensus that the inspiratory muscle metaboreflex described so extensively in healthy young athletes (Dempsey et al, 2006; see above) also operates to limit limb blood flow and exercise tolerance in patients with COPD (Dempsey et al, 2006; Scano et al, 2006).

These data may also explain the apparent paradox that contractile fatigue of the diaphragm has not been observed consistently in patients with COPD, yet limb fatigue has (Mador et al, 2000a). It is possible that high levels of inspiratory muscle work result in activation of the inspiratory muscle metaboreflex prior to any manifestations of overt diaphragm fatigue. This activation results in a generalized increase in sympathetic outflow that reduces limb blood flow, exacerbating limb fatigue (Romer et al, 2006), but preceding the development of diaphragm fatigue. Indeed, some researchers have suggested that the inspiratory muscle metaboreflex may be part of a protective reflex that preserves diaphragm oxygen delivery (Seals, 2001), sparing inspiratory muscles from fatigue. The emerging evidence that feedback from type III and IV afferents influences effort perception and central fatigue (see section 'Healthy people') provides a possible explanation for the absence of diaphragm contractile fatigue during exercise in some groups (Gandevia, 2001).

Another factor that may explain the apparent sparing of the diaphragm is that the work of the diaphragm is increasingly supported by the accessory muscles as exercise progresses, a strategy that is present in both healthy young athletes (Babcock et al, 1996) and patients with COPD (Yan et al, 1997). Unfortunately, there is only one study, in Polish, reporting post-exercise values for MIP, in COPD patients post-exercise; the abstract reports that both MIP and MEP were lower (11% and 10%, respectively) after an incremental treadmill exercise test (Maskey-Warzechowska et al, 2006). However, as mentioned previously, there is also evidence of global inspiratory muscle fatigue in COPD patients who walked to the limit of tolerance (slowing of the relaxation rate of oesophageal sniff pressure (Coirault et al, 1999), which is suggestive of accessory inspiratory muscle fatigue (Kyroussis et al, 1996). These data highlight the dangers of taking a reductionist approach to studying muscle fatigue specifically, and exercise tolerance generally. The inspiratory muscles cannot be discounted as a potential exercise-limiting factor because one, highly reductionist index of function, viz., diaphragm twitch pressure, does not appear to exhibit low-frequency fatigue post-exercise.

However, it is reasonable to ask why contractile fatigue of the diaphragm is present in healthy young adults, but not in patients with COPD. The relationship between diaphragm power output during exercise and subsequent fatigue suggests that the intensity of diaphragm work *per se* is only one of the factors that govern its propensity to fatigue (Babcock et al, 1995). It has been suggested that factors such as the competition for available blood flow, and the severity of the metabolic acidosis during exercise intensify the fatiguing stimulus of diaphragm work *per se* (Babcock et al, 1995). In other words, a given level of diaphragm work induces fatigue only in the presence of compromised blood flow and metabolic acidosis. In patients with COPD, dyspnoea limits exercise long before circulatory limitations and metabolic acidosis reach levels commensurate with those observed in healthy young people. Accordingly, although the relative intensity of diaphragm work is high during exercise in patients with COPD, diaphragm blood flow and the extracellular milieu of the muscle fibres may not be sufficiently compromised to induce diaphragm contractile fatigue.

Finally, it is worth considering that studies of exercise responses in patients with COPD have typically been undertaken using stationary cycling as the exercise modality. In a study comparing the ventilatory and metabolic responses of patients with COPD during incremental cycle ergometer exercise and incremental shuttle walking (Palange et al, 2000), the authors found that $\dot{V}_E$ was higher at all levels of $\dot{V}O_2$, and increased at a steeper rate during walking. There was also a lower V_T during walking. Given the role of the respiratory muscles in maintaining postural control and stability (see the section 'Non-respiratory functions of the respiratory muscles'), it is likely that the observed alterations in breathing pattern may have been secondary to a compromise to the respiratory function of the respiratory muscles, induced by the necessity for a contribution to postural control during walking. Inspiratory accessory muscles have been shown to contract out of synchrony with the diaphragm during walking in patients with COPD, and dyspnoea was the major symptom limiting exercise tolerance (Delgado et al, 1982). Gosselink and colleagues found that MIP was a significant contributor (along with quadriceps strength) to performance in a 6-minute walk test in patients with COPD (Gosselink et al, 1996), supporting the important contribution of inspiratory muscle function to walking tolerance. Thus, during activities of daily living, patients with COPD are likely to experience severe limitations to their mobility from respiratory muscle-related factors, including the exacerbating compromise to inspiratory muscle function that derives from their non-respiratory role as postural muscles. In Chapter 4 we will consider the evidence that rebalancing the relationship between demand and capacity of the respiratory pump muscles using RMT induces beneficial adaptations to respiratory muscle structure and function, as well as clinical benefits.

Asthma

Exercise limitation has been much less widely studied in patients with asthma than in those with COPD. However, where significant airway obstruction is present, and hyperinflation results, dyspnoea is a dominating symptom that curtails exercise. The underlying mechanisms have much in common with those present in patients with COPD, except perhaps that the imbalance within the demand/capacity relationship is not quite so severe, due to the relatively normal inspiratory muscle function that is present in asthma (Hill, 1991). Patients with asthma also tend to have better-preserved function of their locomotor muscles (de Bruin et al, 1997) than patients with COPD. Thus, in patients with stable asthma, and in the absence of any exercise-induced bronchoconstriction, the respiratory-related limitations to exercise are similar to those of healthy people. However, where the severity of the condition is less reversible, the respiratory-related limitations become similar to those of COPD. Chapter 4 will review the evidence that inspiratory muscle training improves exercise tolerance in these patients.

Bronchiectasis

The factors limiting exercise tolerance in patients with bronchiectasis are similar to those limiting patients with COPD. Symptomatically, the primary exercise-limiting factor is dyspnoea, which is secondary to expiratory flow limitation and attendant dynamic hyperinflation (Koulouris et al, 2003). As was described above for COPD, dynamic hyperinflation is accompanied by a number of mechanical changes that affect the inspiratory muscles, contributing to dyspnoea and exercise limitation. In addition to the overloading of the inspiratory muscles created by hyperinflation, there is also a contribution to inspiratory muscle work originating from the restrictive defect that is present.

Cystic fibrosis

Patients with cystic fibrosis (CF) have an elevated work of breathing (Dunnink et al, 2009), which is multifactorial in origin; increased dead space, air trapping and airway resistance, as well as decreased lung compliance, all contribute. Peripheral muscle deconditioning also reduces the lactate threshold, which elevates ventilatory demand during exercise. Not surprisingly, the work of breathing has been identified as an important contributor to exertional dyspnoea in patients with CF (Leroy et al, 2011). Whilst indices of inspiratory muscle strength can be normal, or even increased, in patients with CF, loss of maximal inspiratory muscle work capacity has been reported (Ionescu et al, 1998; Enright et al, 2007). In addition, impaired inspiratory muscle endurance has been linked to exertional dyspnoea and alveolar hypoventilation during exercise (Leroy et al, 2011). Thus, both sides of the demand/capacity relationship of the respiratory muscles may be affected during exercise, contributing to intolerance. In Chapter 4, the evidence that IMT improves exercise tolerance in patients with CF will be reviewed.

Restrictive chest wall disorders

Restrictive chest wall disorders influence both sides of the demand/capacity relationship of the respiratory muscles (see the section 'Changes in breathing mechanics and respiratory muscle function'). Furthermore, in conditions such as scoliosis there is a generalized muscle weakness that has been ascribed to the combined effects of deconditioning, nutritional factors and systemic inflammation (Martinez-Llorens et al, 2010). During the early stages of scoliosis, and in the presence of generalized muscle weakness, the principal exercise-limiting factor may be leg discomfort, particularly if cycle ergometry and incremental protocols are used (Martinez-Llorens et al, 2010). However, as has been mentioned previously, leg discomfort can also be a sign of inspiratory muscle overload due metaboreflex activation (see the section 'Lesson from the world of sport'). Interestingly, Martinez-Llorens et al (2010) found that maximal cycling performance was predicted most closely by an equation that incorporated both respiratory and peripheral muscle strength. This implies that, during the early stages of scoliosis, exercise limitation is multifactorial. However, as chest wall deformity increases, and the restrictive pulmonary manifestations of the disease(s) predominate, respiratory factors may become the primary exercise-limiting factors (Martinez-Llorens et al, 2010).

In patients with ankylosing spondylitis, exercise tolerance appears to be most closely linked to impairment of pulmonary function; specifically, multiple stepwise regression implicates vital capacity, which explains 55% of the variation in exercise tolerance (Ozdem Yr et al, 2011). It is unlikely that vital capacity *per se* has a bearing on exercise tolerance; rather, the interrelationship most likely exposes the association between the difficulty in expanding the chest and exercise intolerance. The former has a number of repercussions that can limit exercise tolerance, not least the sense of breathing effort and the repercussions of inspiratory muscle overload. Furthermore, inspiratory muscle strength and endurance have been shown to explain independently around 60% of the variance in peak cycle ergometer work rate and maximal oxygen uptake in patients with ankylosing spondylitis (van der Esch et al, 2004). This strongly suggests that the inspiratory muscles should be a therapeutic target. See Chapter 4 for a description of the evidence supporting breathing exercises for patients with restrictive chest wall disorders.

Sarcoidosis and interstitial lung disease

The pulmonary manifestations of sarcoidosis and interstitial lung disease (ILD) share many clinical features (see the section 'Changes in breathing mechanics and respiratory muscle function'), including exertional dyspnoea and exercise intolerance (Anderson & Bye, 1984). There are multiple factors underlying exercise intolerance (Markovitz & Cooper, 2010) and this complexity contributes to the poor relationship between resting pulmonary function and exercise intolerance (Cotes et al, 1988).

The exercise hyperpnoea of patients with ILD is tachypnoeic, which has been ascribed to reduced lung compliance (Agusti et al, 1991). Both features increase inspiratory muscle work and contribute to dyspnoea (see Ch. 1). Rapid shallow breathing is a behavioural adaptation to the discomfort associated with expansion of V_T during exercise, but the extent to which respiratory mechanics contribute to exercise limitation remains debatable, as not all studies have found

ventilatory limitation to be present (Markovitz & Cooper, 2010). However, the appearance of a 'breathing reserve' at end-exercise is misleading, and is not necessarily indicative that exercise is limited by non-respiratory factors (see the earlier section 'Healthy people').

Furthermore, the abnormally high ratio of dead space to tidal volume (V_D/V_T) resulting from rapid shallow breathing increases the ventilatory requirement of exercise, and contributes to other hallmarks of ILD, viz., exertional arterial oxygen desaturation and widening of the alveolar to arterial partial pressure gradient for oxygen. The principal underlying mechanism for these changes appears to be ventilation/perfusion ($\dot{V}/\dot{Q}$) mismatching, rather than diffusion limitation (Markovitz & Cooper, 2010). Furthermore, end-exercise V_D/V_T is highly correlated ($r = 0.909$) with arterial partial pressure of oxygen at end-exercise (Hansen & Wasserman, 1996), which highlights the complex interrelationships between potential exercise-limiting factors.

In the early stages of ILD, exercise is associated with pulmonary hypertension, which appears to be secondary to arterial hypoxaemia (Markovitz & Cooper, 2010). However, supplemental oxygen does not completely relieve the pulmonary vasoconstriction (Widimsky et al, 1977), which raises a question about whether factors such as muscle metaboreflex activation contribute to the increase in pulmonary arterial pressure (Lykidis et al, 2008). As was discussed in the earlier section 'Healthy people', high levels of inspiratory muscle work may be associated with activation of the inspiratory muscle metaboreflex, leading to premature locomotor muscle fatigue. This may be of particularly significance in patients with ILD, as peripheral muscle dysfunction has been demonstrated in patients with some ILDs, and quadriceps weakness is correlated with exercise limitation (Markovitz & Cooper, 2010). Similarly, in patients with sarcoidosis, granulomatous involvement of skeletal muscles contributes to both locomotor and respiratory muscle dysfunction, and quadriceps weakness is associated with exercise intolerance (Spruit et al, 2005). Thus, in patients with both ILD and sarcoidosis, inspiratory muscle weakness combined with high levels of inspiratory muscle work and activation of the inspiratory muscle metaboreflex may exacerbate peripheral muscle fatigue and exercise intolerance by inducing locomotor muscle vasoconstriction. At the time of writing there have been no studies of respiratory muscle training in patients with sarcoidosis or other ILD.

Chronic heart failure and pulmonary hypertension

Dyspnoea and exercise intolerance are hallmarks of chronic heart failure (CHF), with patients experiencing high levels of dyspnoea and limb discomfort at relatively low intensities of exercise (Wilson & Mancini, 1993). The complexity of the syndrome of CHF is such that the contribution of individual abnormalities to exercise intolerance is impossible to isolate. However, since dyspnoea is such a potent contributor to exercise intolerance in CHF, it is clear that the pulmonary contribution is extremely important. More specifically, evidence has emerged over the past decade implicating inspiratory muscle function and the demand/capacity relationship of the inspiratory muscles as important contributors to exercise intolerance in CHF (Ribeiro et al, 2012).

The causes of exertional dyspnoea in CHF and COPD have at least one common denominator: a high demand for inspiratory muscle work. As was described in the earlier section 'Changes in breathing mechanics and respiratory muscle function', this increased demand is multifactorial in CHF, being due to an exaggerated ventilatory response, tachypnoeic breathing pattern, increased lung compliance and expiratory flow limitation. Coupled to this increased demand is a reduced capacity for inspiratory muscle work, due to inspiratory muscle dysfunction (Ribeiro et al, 2012). In addition, patients with CHF also have to contend with a severely compromised cardiac output (Pina et al, 2003). The influence of CHF *per se* upon cardiac output and blood flow is not limited to the pulmonary circulation. During exercise, muscle blood flow is impaired leading to a reduction in oxygen delivery and metabolite removal, with the result that there is a greater reliance upon anaerobic metabolism. This has implications for the inspiratory muscles, as the resulting metabolic acidosis stimulates an increase in $\dot{V}_E$ (Franco, 2011). Patients with CHF also have greater chemoreflex sensitivity, causing an increase in the ventilatory response to chemoreflex activation as well as in muscle sympathetic nerve activity (Ribeiro et al, 2012). Furthermore, there is also evidence that competition for a share of the limited cardiac output results in underperfusion and deoxygenation within the inspiratory muscles during exercise (Mancini et al, 1991; Terakado et al, 1999).

In patients with CHF, the exercise hyperpnoea is associated with a high demand for inspiratory pressure relative to the capacity to generate pressure (MIP), as well as a high level of inspiratory neural drive (Vibarel et al, 1998). Given these conditions, and the evidence that accessory muscle perfusion is compromised (Mancini et al, 1991), one would predict a propensity for inspiratory muscle fatigue in patients with CHF. As is the case in COPD, exercise-related alterations in inspiratory muscle function have been studied relatively little in patients with CHF, and almost exclusively in terms of diaphragm contractile function. One study found no change in twitch diaphragm pressure (TwP$_{di}$) after a symptom-limited cycle ergometer test in patients with CHF (Kufel et al, 2002). In this study, four patients reported terminating exercise due to dyspnoea, whilst six stopped because of leg fatigue. The absence of post-exercise diaphragm fatigue was confirmed in a later study employing an incremental cycle test to the limit of tolerance (Dayer et al, 2006). However, these data need to be interpreted carefully as there is evidence that the work

of breathing most likely contributes to leg fatigue (Dempsey, 2010). Furthermore, the absence of diaphragm fatigue may also be explained by the support provided by inspiratory accessory muscles in delivering the required exercise hyperpnoea, thereby protecting the diaphragm from fatigue (see above section on COPD). As has been shown for patients with COPD, there is evidence to support the existence of accessory muscle fatigue following exercise in patients with CHF; furthermore, this fatigue appears to be related to their dyspnoea (Hughes et al, 2001). In a study of CHF patients who walked to the point of intolerable dyspnoea, inspiratory muscle relaxation rate was slowed, providing evidence for global inspiratory muscle fatigue (Hughes et al, 2001). These authors concluded that their observations were consistent with an imbalance between the demands placed on the inspiratory muscles and their capacity to meet this demand.

The limiting role of inspiratory muscles in patients with CHF is also supported by evidence that reducing the work of breathing during exercise improves exercise tolerance. When patients with CHF breathed heliox during an incremental exercise test, there was an increase in the time to the limit of tolerance (Mancini et al, 1997). Furthermore, when patients with CHF receive inspiratory assistance during exercise (partial inspiratory muscle unloading with pressure support), the time to the limit of tolerance during a constant load cycle test is increased (O'Donnell et al, 1999). The latter was also accompanied by a reduction in leg discomfort.

These data are similar to those in healthy athletes during assisted breathing, in whom improvements in exercise tolerance are ascribed to the absence of inspiratory muscle metaboreflex activation (Harms et al, 1997). Accordingly, a reduction in perception of leg effort during exercise with assisted breathing is due to improved leg blood flow. Indirect support for this comes from a study that confirmed the finding that inspiratory muscle unloading improves exercise tolerance and reduces leg effort in patients with CHF, but also found that these changes were associated with improved leg oxygenation (Borghi-Silva et al, 2008a). The same group has made identical observations in patients with COPD (Borghi-Silva et al, 2008b). Direct evidence comes from the improvement in limb blood flow observed when patients with CHF cycle (60% peak power) with inspiratory muscle unloading (Olson et al, 2010); however, unlike healthy people, when the inspiratory muscles of people with CHF were loaded, there was no reduction in limb blood flow above that observed during normal breathing. Thus, patients with CHF were unable to intensify the sympathetic output to limb vasculature when the work of breathing was increased, suggesting that this output is already maximal during normal breathing. These data provide support for the role of the inspiratory muscle metaboreflex in exercise limitation in patients with CHF. It is reasonable to suggest that, in patients with a compromised cardiac output, this reflex may play a particularly potent role in exercise limitation.

Resting indices of cardiac function have been shown to be poor predictors of exercise tolerance in patients with CHF; this is in contrast to the excellent predictive power of indices of respiratory function (Faggiano et al, 2001). The primary importance of inspiratory muscle function as a contributor to exercise intolerance in patients with CHF is supported by the observation that peak oxygen uptake is correlated with MIP (but not MEP) (Nishimura et al, 1994; Chua et al, 1995), as well as with inspiratory capacity (Nanas et al, 2003). Inspiratory capacity was also an independent predictor of exercise tolerance, and was correlated with pulmonary capillary wedge pressure (a determinant of lung compliance). The former study (Chua et al, 1995) illustrates the important role of inspiratory muscle capacity, and the latter (Nanas et al, 2003) of the demand for inspiratory muscle work in determining exercise tolerance in patients with CHF.

In Chapter 4, the evidence that inspiratory muscle training improves exercise tolerance in patients with CHF is reviewed.

Neurological and neuromuscular disease

Spinal cord injury

Respiratory symptoms are common in patients with SCI, and dyspnoea is present in 73% of people with a lesion at C5, but only 29% in those with a lesion below T8 (Spungen et al, 1997). However, the extent to which dyspnoea is an exercise-limiting factor is currently unclear.

As was described in the section 'Changes in breathing mechanics and respiratory muscle function', SCI induces profound changes to pulmonary and respiratory muscle function, as well as breathing mechanics. The extent of the impact upon breathing is influenced by the level and completeness of the lesion, and the time post-injury. People with high-level, acute lesions exhibit the greatest disruption to their breathing. The result of the changes in respiratory muscle function and breathing mechanics is the potential for an imbalance in the demand/capacity relationship of the inspiratory muscles, predisposing people to dyspnoea and exercise-induced inspiratory muscle fatigue (Taylor et al, 2010).

Peak exercise responses of cardiorespiratory variables are lower in absolute terms during upper body compared with whole-body exercise, owing to the smaller muscle mass involved. The crucial question in this regard is whether the smaller muscle mass involved in exercise imposes sufficient metabolic and ventilatory demands to overload the respiratory pump, rendering it a limiting factor during exercise.

Relatively few studies have compared directly the cardiorespiratory responses of SCI individuals with those of able-bodied people, but peak exercise values tend to be lower in untrained SCI injured people during arm-crank and wheelchair propulsion (Glaser et al, 1980; Keyser et al, 1999). This

may be indicative of the smaller amount of trunk muscle mass, and/or compromised respiratory mechanics. There is also an impairment in the ventilatory equivalent for oxygen, which is lower in people with SCI at equivalent oxygen uptakes, and is also proportional to the level of SCI (Lassau-Wray & Ward, 2000), indicating that the response of minute ventilation is compromised progressively as lesion level becomes more cranial. This impairment may influence the ability to make an effective respiratory compensation for a metabolic acidosis, thereby hastening fatigue (see Ch. 2).

The extent to which exercise is limited by ventilatory factors is unclear. In highly trained Paralympic athletes, cervical SCI did not induce any ventilatory constraint during constant power arm-crank exercise (90% peak power) to the limit of tolerance (Taylor et al, 2010). This was evidenced by a reserve capacity for delivery of volume and flow, as well as the absence of any evidence of inspiratory muscle fatigue. The lack of fatigue may stem from the absence of the normal competition for cardiac output during exercise. The smaller muscle mass involved in exercise in SCI most likely fails to compromise regional blood flow to the extent that oxygen delivery to respiratory muscles is impaired. The majority of the athletes (five of seven) rated arm discomfort greater than dyspnoea. Although none rated either sensation maximally at end-exercise, both ratings were similar in magnitude to those measured at the peak of incremental treadmill exercise in respiratory patients (Hamilton et al, 1996b). In addition, the ventilatory equivalent for oxygen was not reduced in the Paralympians, suggesting that their capacity to deliver minute ventilation was superior to that of non-athletes with cervical SCI (see above). Thus, the extent to which these Paralympic data are relevant to the general population of people with SCI is limited. See Chapter 4 for a description of the evidence supporting specific respiratory muscle training in SCI.

Other NMDs

Because physical activity is limited by generalized deterioration of muscle function in patients with neuromuscular diseases (NMD), dyspnoea is not always present, and may not therefore be the primary exercise-limiting factor (McCool & Tzelepis, 1995). However, this does not preclude respiratory-related limitation; as was discussed in the section 'Healthy people', high levels of inspiratory muscle work may be associated with activation of the inspiratory muscle metaboreflex, leading to swift fatigue of already compromised locomotor muscles.

The restrictive pattern of pulmonary dysfunction (Gibson et al, 1977) leads to a rapid, shallow breathing pattern and a higher than normal ratio of dead space to tidal volume (V_D/V_T). This increases the demand for minute ventilation ($\dot{V}_E$), and is exacerbated by an early metabolic acidosis, which increases the work of breathing during exercise. Although absolute $\dot{V}_E$ may not be high in patients with NMD, the relative work of breathing is elevated by respiratory muscle weakness, creating imbalance in the demand/capacity relationship. Thus, in patients with NMD, activation of the inspiratory muscle metaboreflex may contribute to peripheral muscle fatigue and exercise intolerance by inducing locomotor muscle vasoconstriction.

The inspiratory muscle metaboreflex may be a particularly important contributor to exercise limitation in NMD; impairment of the neuronal nitric oxide synthase system (nNOS), which opposes sympathetically mediated vasoconstriction, has been identified in a number of NMDs (Duchenne and Becker muscular dystrophies, as well as other muscle disorders involving limb-girdle muscular dystrophy, congenital muscular dystrophies, myositis and myopathy) (Kobayashi et al, 2008). Accordingly, dysfunction of the nNOS system has been suggested as a common mechanism of locomotor muscle fatigue in patients with NMD (Aboussouan, 2009). Thus, the inspiratory muscle metaboreflex may have a particularly potent effect in these patients, making these muscles an appealing therapeutic target.

In Chapter 4, the evidence that inspiratory muscle training improves exercise tolerance in patients with NMD is reviewed.

Obesity

Exertional dyspnoea is a common symptom in obese patients (Babb et al, 2008a), but it has been studied comparatively little from a mechanistic perspective. Extreme dyspnoea is not a limiting symptom in all obese patients, but a key underlying factor in determining the severity of dyspnoea appears to be the oxygen cost of breathing (Babb et al, 2008a). When the relationship between the oxygen cost of breathing and exertional dyspnoea was examined directly in obese women, the oxygen cost of breathing was found to be considerably and significantly higher (38–70%) in those who were breathless upon exertion (Babb et al, 2008a). Furthermore, around 65% of the variation in dyspnoea was explained by the variation in the oxygen cost of breathing. These findings are consistent with the notion that dyspnoea is directly related to the work of the respiratory muscles. Since work is elevated in the face of relatively normal inspiratory muscle strength, dyspnoea reflects an imbalance between the demand for inspiratory muscle work and the ability of the inspiratory muscles to meet that demand (Campbell, 1966).

An important factor that appears to influence the total oxygen cost of exercise in obese individuals is fat distribution. For example, obese women (mean BMI 40 $kg \cdot m^{-2}$) in whom fat was deposited in the upper body (UBD) had a greater oxygen cost of cycling, a higher $\dot{V}_E$, a more rapid and shallow breathing pattern and a lower anaerobic threshold than women whose fat was distributed in the lower body (Li et al, 2001). This suggests an underlying mechanism related to the higher work of breathing when fat is deposited in and around the trunk. Although dyspnoea was not assessed during this study (Li et al, 2001), it is reasonable to presume that it would have been higher in the UBD group.

The question then arises as to the extent of limitation imposed by dyspnoea and the relationship of this to the performance of the inspiratory muscles. In a study of obese men (mean BMI 42 $kg \cdot m^{-2}$), an index of the relative work of breathing has been created by referencing the work of breathing to the capacity of the inspiratory muscles to sustain work (Chlif et al, 2007). In addition, an index of the neural drive to the inspiratory muscles was assessed. The obese men had higher levels of inspiratory neural drive and dyspnoea at the same relative intensity of exercise compared with non-obese men. As is typical, the obese men also adopted a rapid shallow breathing pattern as part of their strategy to minimize respiratory discomfort. However, the strategy did not appear to normalize their dyspnoea, because the relative work of breathing remained too high for the inspiratory muscles, as evidenced by the inspiratory muscle fatigue that was present post-exercise. These data once again reinforce the fact that obese individuals have an imbalance between demand and capacity for inspiratory muscle work.

The inspiratory muscle fatigue observed in the study of Chlif et al (2007) and the high levels of inspiratory muscle work mean that the risk of inspiratory muscle metaboreflex activation is likely to be very high in obese individuals. The repercussions of this were described in the section 'Healthy people', and include a reduction in limb blood flow, leading to increased rate of development and magnitude of both limb discomfort and limb muscle fatigue.

To date, the interrelationships of dyspnoea, inspiratory muscle work and exercise tolerance in obesity have been studied only using cycle ergometer exercise. This modality is used because it minimizes the influence of the obese participants' body mass. However, in the real world, obese patients are required to walk, which not only requires them to cope with the increased metabolic and ventilatory demands imposed by their increased mass, but also increases the requirement to engage the postural role of the respiratory muscles. These factors are inescapable, exacerbating the demands placed upon these muscles, resulting in dyspnoea, inspiratory muscle overload and, perhaps, accelerated limb fatigue due to inspiratory muscle metaboreflex activation.

In Chapter 4, the evidence that respiratory muscle training improves exercise tolerance in patients with obesity is reviewed.

Ageing

The senescent changes to the pulmonary system have been dubbed 'senile emphysema' (Janssens et al, 1999). Accordingly, it is no surprise that exertional dyspnoea is a common complaint amongst the elderly, even in the absence of cardiopulmonary disease (Landahl et al, 1980). Furthermore, the intensity of dyspnoea is higher by 1 to 2 Borg units at a standardized submaximal oxygen uptake during incremental treadmill exercise in healthy elderly (60–80 years) adults compared with younger (40–59 years) adults (Ofir et al, 2008).

However, dyspnoea perception in healthy, active older people does not appear to be correlated with expiratory flow limitation or $\dot{V}_E$; instead it appears to be related to the relative load upon the inspiratory muscles, i.e., the inspiratory pressure requirement as a percentage of inspiratory pressure-generating capacity – in other words, the state of the demand/capacity relationship (Johnson et al, 1991). The requirement for inspiratory pressure generation during exercise is increased in healthy ageing by a number of factors, including a higher requirement for $\dot{V}_E$, dynamic lung hyperinflation and mechanical constraints on V_T expansion (Jensen et al, 2009a). Furthermore, inspiratory muscle strength declines with advancing age (McConnell & Copestake, 1999).

As was described in the earlier section 'Healthy people', inspiratory muscle overload can contribute to both respiratory and locomotor muscle fatigue. In healthy people, the symptoms leading to the cessation of exercise fall into two main categories: 'local' locomotor muscle fatigue and 'central' dyspnoea (Ekblom & Goldbarg, 1971). When the contributions of leg effort and dyspnoea to exercise limitation are assessed, over 60% of healthy people cease exercise because of the combined contribution of the two symptoms (Hamilton et al, 1996a). Interestingly, the Borg CR-10 rating of dyspnoea at exercise cessation in this healthy group was higher (6 units) than the rating in a similar group of patients with respiratory disease (5 units) (Hamilton et al, 1996a). These data indicate that, even in healthy people, dyspnoea is a troubling symptom that makes an important contribution to the decision to stop exercising.

In Chapter 4, the evidence that inspiratory muscle training improves exercise tolerance in healthy older people is reviewed.

Miscellaneous conditions

In the section 'Changes in breathing mechanics and respiratory muscle function' a wide range of disease conditions were considered, including some where respiratory limitation of exercise tolerance is irrelevant, e.g., mechanical ventilation. The following section is therefore limited to those conditions in which the demand/capacity relationship of the respiratory pump may limit exercise tolerance.

Diabetes

Patients with diabetes have inspiratory muscle weakness and an increased demand for inspiratory pressure generation during exercise (Wanke et al, 1992); accordingly, the demand/capacity relationship of the respiratory muscles is in a state of imbalance (see 'Changes in breathing mechanics and respiratory muscle function'). Exercise

tolerance is impaired during cycle ergometer exercise compared with healthy people, and the sense of respiratory effort is also elevated (Wanke et al, 1992). The ventilatory response to exercise in diabetes has been studied very little, so it is not clear whether dyspnoea is a primary exercise-limiting factor. However, evidence of neuromechanical uncoupling (see Ch. 1) during hypoxic ventilatory stimulation in diabetic patients (type 1) is indicative of an impairment of the mechanical response to inspiratory drive, and suggests that dyspnoea is a prominent feature of increased inspiratory muscle work (Scano et al, 1999). See Chapter 4 for a description of the evidence supporting specific inspiratory muscle training.

Cancer

One of the most common chronic symptoms in patients with cancer is exertional dyspnoea, which is present in up to 10% of survivors of childhood cancers and up to 70% of patients with advanced cancer (Travers et al, 2008). In general, cancer patients have been shown to have peripheral muscle weakness and a lower lactate threshold compared with healthy people (Travers et al, 2008). Cancer patients with chronic, unexplained exertional dyspnoea also have a lower symptom-limited peak oxygen uptake and minute ventilation compared with cancer patients without chronic dyspnoea, and controls; furthermore, dyspnoea is the primary exercise-limiting factor in ~70% of these dyspnoic patients (Travers et al, 2008). Dyspnoic cancer patients appear to be distinguishable by virtue of their rapid shallow breathing pattern during exercise, and their lower inspiratory capacity (Travers et al, 2008). The latter correlates with inspiratory muscle strength, suggesting a causal link (Travers et al, 2008).

The important contribution of inspiratory muscle strength to exercise intolerance was recently shown in patients with thoracic cancer (England et al, 2012). Of a range of physiological and psychological factors explored, only inspiratory muscle strength (MIP) and peripheral muscle power were found to be significant determinants of exercise tolerance (incremental shuttle walking). Dyspnoea made a contribution to exercise cessation in 92% of the patients, which perhaps explains why MIP was a stronger determinant of exercise tolerance than peripheral muscle power. The authors suggested that both factors should be considered as therapeutic targets. At the time of writing there have been no studies of respiratory muscle training in patients with cancer.

Anorexia nervosa

Unfortunately, much of the published literature relating to patients with anorexia nervosa is case study based. However, one study compared 19 young women with anorexia nervosa with matched 'thin' (BMI <19 $kg \cdot m^{-2}$) controls; it found that they had lower peak exercise values for all key cardiorespiratory parameters including maximal heart rate and oxygen uptake, lactate threshold, minute ventilation and oxygen pulse (Biadi et al, 2001). The extent to which dyspnoea contributes to exercise limitation is unclear, but case study evidence supports a link between inspiratory muscle weakness, dyspnoea and exercise intolerance (Birmingham & Tan, 2003).

The rationale for training the inspiratory muscles in patients with anorexia nervosa is to restore strength, thereby improving pulmonary function and reducing exertional dyspnoea. At the time of writing there have been no studies of respiratory muscle training in patients with anorexia nervosa.

Pregnancy

An increase in breathing effort and dyspnoea are experienced by around three-quarters of pregnant women (Milne et al, 1978). A recent study characterized the ventilatory, metabolic and perceptual response to cycle ergometer exercise in women in their third trimester, and compared these data to those collected 5 months postpartum. The participants were divided into two groups: those with 'clinically significant activity-related dyspnoea' (CSB), and those without. The work of breathing was, on average, 43% higher in the third trimester, yet dyspnoea was only higher (45%) in the group with CSB. The CSB group also had an exaggerated ventilatory response to cycle ergometer exercise, both in their third trimester and 5 months post-partum (Jensen et al, 2009b). As there were no differences in central ventilatory control or breathing mechanics, the increase in dyspnoea intensity in the CSB group was ascribed to a 'normal awareness of increased ventilation'. What is perhaps more intriguing is that a substantial increase in the work of breathing was not accompanied by an increased sense of breathing effort in the group without CSB. At the time of writing there have been no studies of respiratory muscle training in pregnant women.

Vocal cord dysfunction and inspiratory stridor

The upper airway muscles, including the larynx, are important accessory muscles of respiration. During normal resting breathing, the vocal cords abduct during inhalation in order to widen the laryngeal glottic opening, permitting unobstructed air flow through the larynx. This occurs via reflex activation of the posterior cricoarytenoid muscle, and without it the vocal cords would collapse across that laryngeal opening, causing an increase in upper airway flow resistance, increased breathing effort, dyspnoea and sudden exercise intolerance.

Inspiratory stridor is an external sign of vocal cord dysfunction (VCD) during exercise. The prevalence of the condition is between 5% and 15%, and it is frequently mistaken for exercise-induced asthma (Kenn & Hess, 2008). However, the fact that symptoms occur suddenly *during* exercise, and with a *loud, rasping, inspiratory* wheeze, are cardinal signs of VCD. Notwithstanding this, VCD and asthma can and do coexist (Kenn & Hess, 2008). The precise causes of inspiratory stridor remain unknown, and it probably has a multifactorial aetiology. However, one possible mechanism is fatigue of the muscles that abduct the vocal cords and maintain the upper airway opening.

Since the upper airway musculature is activated in proportion to the magnitude of inspiratory effort, the addition of an external inspiratory load induces increased metabolic activity, and thus a potential training stimulus to the upper airway muscles (How et al, 2007; Cheng et al, 2011). Accordingly, it is possible to train the upper-airway-stabilizing muscles using a resistive inspiratory muscle trainer. See Chapter 4 for a description of the evidence supporting specific respiratory muscle training in VCD.

NON-RESPIRATORY FUNCTIONS OF THE RESPIRATORY MUSCLES

How many patients find walking makes them more breathless than riding a stationary ergometer? The answer is most, if not all. The role of the respiratory muscles extends far beyond that of driving the respiratory pump. However, their contribution to postural control (balance) and core stabilization is almost completely overlooked in a rehabilitation context. This is surprising because these non-respiratory roles have profound implications for how we *should* train these muscles to optimize their function and minimize the unpleasant symptoms that they generate.

At this point, it is helpful to define the difference between the concepts of stability and control, as these are revisited many times:

*   *Core stability:* actions that maintain stability of the trunk and lumbopelvic region, protecting the spine from damage and creating a stable platform from which to generate limb movements.
*   *Postural control:* actions that maintain balance in response to destabilizing forces acting upon the body.

These non-respiratory roles of the trunk muscles are often brought into conflict with their role in breathing, with the result that none of these roles are undertaken optimally. When functional conflicts occur within the muscular system, the risk of system failure can be mitigated by providing the muscles in question with reserve capacity, and by establishing (as routine) specific neural activation patterns with training. In this section, the role of the respiratory muscles as postural controllers and core stabilizers is considered in order to develop the rationale for such functional respiratory muscle training.

Before beginning our discussion, it is helpful to develop our earlier definition of core stability slightly. In simple terms, core stability provides a stable platform from which the limbs can perform movements. Without the stable platform provided by the core muscles, we are just *'shooting a cannon from a canoe'* (Tsatsouline, 2000), with very similar results!

As mentioned above, the core acts anatomically as a stable base from which the limbs perform movements, and it comprises the spine, pelvis and a myriad of muscles that stabilize these bony structures. The majority of the prime movers and stabilizing muscles of the limbs attach to the pelvis and spine. It has been recognized for many years that breathing is linked functionally to trunk-loading tasks such as lifting, lowering and pushing/pulling. Human beings instinctively take a breath immediately before such movements, and use this to generate a pneumatic stabilizing pressure within the thorax, as well as increasing intra-abdominal pressure (see below). Typically, inspired volume prior to loading is proportional to the magnitude of the load (Hagins & Lamberg, 2006), and people with lower levels of physical fitness appear to require a higher preparatory inspired volume (Lamberg & Hagins, 2012). It is reasonable to suggest that in untrained people, with weaker trunk and abdominal muscles, there is a greater reliance upon intracompartmental pneumatic pressure for stabilization.

The abdominal muscles (transversus abdominis, internal/external obliques, rectus abdominis) are a group of large, relatively superficial muscles that act to stiffen the abdominal compartment and/or increase intra-abdominal pressure, thereby stiffening and stabilizing the spine and pelvis (Hodges et al, 2005). When contracted, these muscles form a rigid cylinder (or 'corset') and their ability to increase intra-abdominal pressure is influenced by the state of contraction of the pelvic floor and the diaphragm, which can be considered as the base and lid to the rigid cylinder formed by the abdominal muscles. The increase in intra-abdominal pressure resulting from contraction of the walls of the cylinder is dissipated if the lid (diaphragm) is not held in place. Conversely, if the lid moves downwards into the cylinder the increase in pressure can be magnified (Hodges & Gandevia, 2000). Hence the diaphragm makes a substantial and important contribution to the development of intra-abdominal pressure, and thus to core stability. This role is confirmed by the observations that a programme of weightlifting exercises induces an increase in diaphragm thickness and strength (DePalo et al, 2004) and that weightlifters have thicker, stronger diaphragms than non-weightlifters (McCool et al, 1997). Furthermore, diaphragm contribution to weightlifting tasks is proportional to the weight lifted, and greatest in tasks that induce spinal loading (Al-Bilbeisi & McCool, 2000). Imaging of the diaphragm using MRI (magnetic resonance imaging) during a variety of tasks suggests that human beings are able to voluntarily contract the diaphragm during breath holding, which contributes to stabilization (Kolar et al, 2009). However, this ability varies between individuals, and may explain why some develop low back pain (Kolar et al, 2009). A further interesting finding was that diaphragm contraction was heterogeneous, suggesting that different parts of the diaphragm were involved in stabilization under different conditions, possibly reflecting variations in the interplay between the diaphragm and abdominal musculature (Kolar et al, 2009).

Both the transversus abdominis and the diaphragm are involved in postural control, and contract automatically in anticipation of actions that destabilize and/or load the trunk (Hodges et al, 1997a; Hodges et al, 1997b). The contractions occur irrespective of the phase of breathing, and appear to be superimposed upon the respiratory state of the diaphragm. These feedforward contractions occur approximately 20 milliseconds before EMG (electromyogram) activity is detected in prime mover muscles (Hodges et al, 1997a; Hodges et al, 1997b), acting to stiffen the trunk as part of a strategy to protect the spine, and to exert postural control. The postural challenge employed by Hodges and colleagues was rapid flexion of the shoulder. It is well known that patients with COPD, for example, become breathless during activities of daily living that involve unsupported arm elevation (Breslin, 1992), especially if the movements are overhead, e.g., hair washing. It is not unreasonable to postulate that this may be related to the involvement of the respiratory muscles in stabilizing and balancing tasks. This being the case, it is not surprising that isolated arm resistance training has little effect upon dyspnoea in these patients (Janaudis-Ferreira et al, 2011).

Research has shown that, in situations of increased breathing demand, the diaphragm's role in breathing always takes precedence over its role in posture (Hodges et al, 2001). So in situations such as exercise the postural role of diaphragm may become compromised, which may lead to an increased risk of injury and/or an increased risk of falling or loss of balance. This has important implications for any activity where breathing demands are high. The conflicting demands of the respiratory and non-respiratory roles of the respiratory muscles are also evidenced by the fact that patients with COPD are able to generate higher respiratory mouth pressures and maximum voluntary ventilation, when the postural role of these muscles has been reduced by leaning forward and taking weight through the arms (Cavalheri et al, 2010). This latter observation also helps to explain why this posture relieves dyspnoea.

Many chronic diseases, including cardiovascular disease and COPD, are associated with an increased falling risk (Lawlor et al, 2003). Furthermore, a recent prospective study by Lawlor and colleagues (2003) found that around one-third of patients with COPD reported a fall during the 6-month trial. The authors concluded that patients with COPD have a high susceptibility to falls, which others have shown is also associated with a worsening of dyspnoea perception (Roig et al, 2011). Intrinsic risk factors for falling in patients with COPD include well-established contributors such as lower limb muscle weakness and deficits of gait and balance (Roig et al, 2009). With respect to the latter factor, specific balance deficits have been identified in patients with COPD, e.g., an increased body sway (Butcher et al, 2004; Chang et al, 2008; Smith et al, 2010), and an impaired ability to maintain balance whilst reaching with the arms (Butcher et al, 2004; Eisner et al, 2008). Hitherto the assumption has been that limb muscle weakness is the source of balance deficits in patients with COPD. However, a recent study suggests that patients with COPD also have an impaired postural control strategy, relying to a greater extent upon ankle proprioceptive feedback (Janssens et al, unpublished work). This strategy is also observed in people with low back pain (Brumagne et al, 2008b), but it is suboptimal and less efficient than the normal, multi-segmental strategy that includes knees, hips and spine (Butcher et al, 2004). Interestingly, when the inspiratory muscles are fatigued, healthy participants experienced larger postural sway when standing on an unstable surface, abandoning their normal multi-segmental strategy in favour of one that relied upon adjustments made around the ankle (Janssens et al, 2010). Thus, in the presence of inspiratory muscle fatigue (IMF), the postural control strategy of healthy people became the same as that of patients with chronic low back pain and COPD. Collectively, these data suggest that people revert to ankle-steered postural control strategy when the contribution of trunk muscles is impaired. In the case of patients with COPD, this may be due to an impaired postural contribution of the inspiratory muscles to balance. This may explain the greater falls risk in this population (Janssens et al, unpublished work).

The interrelationship of multiple factors related to the trunk muscle function was highlighted in a cross-sectional study of over 38 000 Australian women (Smith et al, 2006). Women with disorders of continence and respiration showed a higher prevalence of back pain than women who did not have these disorders. These findings are supported by earlier physiological data showing that the postural function of the diaphragm, abdominal and pelvic floor muscles is reduced by incontinence (Deindl et al, 1994) and respiratory disease (Hodges et al, 2000). Furthermore, people with chronic low back pain exhibit greater breathing-related postural sway than people without back pain (Hamaoui et al, 2002). In addition, when the inspiratory muscles are fatigued in healthy people prior to an isometric trunk extension test (a modified Biering-Sørensen test), fatigue of the back muscles occurs more quickly (Brumagne et al, 2008a). This suggests that inhibiting the contribution of the inspiratory muscles to trunk extension places greater demands upon the back musculature. Collectively, these data support the notion that the 'discrete' functions of the trunk muscles (breathing, continence, stabilization, balance) are in fact far from discrete, and are in fact interdependent.

Finally, it is also pertinent to remember that movements of the trunk, such as flexion and rotation, are brought about by muscles that also have respiratory functions. For example, trunk rotation involves not only the oblique muscles, but also the rib cage. Furthermore, movements of the upper limbs not only necessitate an increase in intra-abdominal pressure, they also require stabilizing contractions of the rib cage muscles. Stiffening and stabilizing the rib cage makes it harder to expand, necessitating more forceful contractions of the inspiratory muscles and greater inspiratory effort. This may be another reason that patients with COPD feel dyspnoeic during unsupported arm movements, or when carrying even light objects.

It will be clear by now that both inspiratory and expiratory muscles are fundamental to providing postural control and core stabilization. However, although the abdominal muscles are an integral part of most core stabilization training, the same is not true of the diaphragm or other inspiratory muscles. Perhaps more importantly for dyspnoeic patients, the non-respiratory roles of the respiratory muscles exacerbate the functional overload of these muscles, exacerbating symptoms and impairing effective postural control and stabilization.

Chapter 7 will consider how to implement functional respiratory muscle training that incorporates both respiratory and stabilizing/postural control challenges.

THE RATIONALE FOR RESPIRATORY MUSCLE TRAINING

The preceding sections have described a range of conditions in which there is an imbalance between the demand for respiratory muscle work, and the capacity of the respiratory muscles to meet that demand. This imbalance can be created by: (1) acute clinical and/or environmental changes, e.g., bronchoconstriction, exercise, a change of posture, (2) chronic disease-related changes to the condition of the respiratory muscles, the mechanics of breathing, the efficiency of gas exchange and (3) a combination of acute and chronic influences, e.g., an exacerbation of COPD.

The section 'Changes in breathing mechanics and respiratory muscle function' provided an overview of the pathophysiology of a range of conditions where demand/capacity imbalance exists. In each case, a theoretical rationale for respiratory muscle training (RMT) was offered. Similarly, in the section 'Respiratory muscle involvement in exercise limitation', the contribution of the respiratory muscles to exercise limitation was presented where appropriate, thereby establishing the theoretical rationale for RMT in improving exercise tolerance. Finally, the non-respiratory functions of the respiratory muscles were considered, as these increase the demand for respiratory muscle work, thereby exacerbating any demand/capacity imbalance. In all circumstances, the fundamental rationale of RMT is amelioration of the demand/capacity imbalance. The benefits of this to individual patients will depend upon the clinical manifestations of the imbalance – be they exercise intolerance or respiratory failure. In Chapter 4, the specific evidence for an influence of RMT upon the repercussions of the demand/capacity imbalance is presented. Indications for RMT are considered in Chapter 6 ('General principles of foundation IMT').

REFERENCES

Aboussouan, L.S., 2009. Mechanisms of exercise limitation and pulmonary rehabilitation for patients with neuromuscular disease. Chron. Respir. Dis. 6, 231–249.

Agusti, A.G., Roca, J., Gea, J., et al., 1991. Mechanisms of gas-exchange impairment in idiopathic pulmonary fibrosis. Am. Rev. Respir. Dis. 143, 219–225.

Akkoca, O., Mungan, D., Karabiyikoglu, G., et al., 1999. Inhaled and systemic corticosteroid therapies: Do they contribute to inspiratory muscle weakness in asthma? Respiration 66, 332–337.

Al-Bilbeisi, F., McCool, F.D., 2000. Diaphragm recruitment during nonrespiratory activities. Am. J. Respir. Crit. Care Med. 162, 456–459.

Amann, M., Proctor, L.T., Sebranek, J.J., et al., 2009. Opioid-mediated muscle afferents inhibit central motor drive and limit peripheral muscle fatigue development in humans. Am. J. Physiol. 587, 271–283.

Amann, M., Blain, G.M., Proctor, L.T., et al., 2010a. Group III and IV muscle afferents contribute to ventilatory and cardiovascular response to rhythmic exercise in humans. J. Appl. Physiol. 109, 966–976.

Amann, M., Regan, M.S., Kobitary, M., et al., 2010b. Impact of pulmonary system limitations on locomotor muscle fatigue in patients with COPD. Am. J. Physiol. Regul. Integr. Comp. Physiol. 299, R314–R324.

Ambrosino, N., Strambi, S., 2004. New strategies to improve exercise tolerance in chronic obstructive pulmonary disease. Eur. Respir. J. 24, 313–322.

Anderson, S.D., Bye, P.T., 1984. Exercise testing in the evaluation of diffuse interstitial lung disease. Aust. N. Z. J. Med. 14, 762–768.

Anthony, M., 2008. The obesity hypoventilation syndrome. Respir. Care 53, 1723–1730.

Anzueto, A., Tobin, M.J., Moore, G., et al., 1987. Effect of prolonged mechanical ventilation on diaphragmatic function, a preliminary study of a baboon model. Am. Rev. Respir. Dis. 135, A201.

Araujo, T.L., Resqueti, V.R., Bruno, S., et al., 2010. Respiratory muscle strength and quality of life in myotonic dystrophy patients. Rev. Port. Pneumol. 16, 892–898.

Babb, T.G., Ranasinghe, K.G., Comeau, L.A., et al., 2008a. Dyspnea on exertion in obese women: association with an increased oxygen cost of breathing. Am. J. Respir. Crit. Care Med. 178, 116–123.

Babb, T.G., Wyrick, B.L., DeLorey, D.S., et al., 2008b. Fat distribution and end-expiratory lung volume in lean and obese men and women. Chest 134, 704–711.

Babcock, M.A., Pegelow, D.F., McClaran, S.R., et al., 1995. Contribution of diaphragmatic power output to exercise-induced diaphragm fatigue. J. Appl. Physiol. 78, 1710–1719.

Babcock, M.A., Pegelow, D.F., Johnson, B.D., et al., 1996. Aerobic fitness effects on exercise-induced low-frequency diaphragm fatigue. J. Appl. Physiol. 81, 2156–2164.

Babcock, M.A., Harms, C.A., Pegelow, D.F., et al., 1997. Effects of mechanical unloading of inspiratory muscles on exercise-induced diaphragm fatigue. Am. Rev. Respir. Dis. 152, 178.

Babcock, M.A., Pegelow, D.F., Taha, B.H., et al., 1998. High frequency diaphragmatic fatigue detected with paired stimuli in humans. Med. Sci. Sports Exerc. 30, 506–511.

Bark, H., Heimer, D., Chaimovitz, C., et al., 1988. Effect of chronic renal failure on respiratory muscle strength. Respiration 54, 153–161.

Barreiro, E., de la Puente, B., Minguella, J., et al., 2005. Oxidative stress and respiratory muscle dysfunction in severe chronic obstructive pulmonary disease. Am. J. Respir. Crit. Care Med. 171, 1116–1124.

Baydur, A., Alsalek, M., Louie, S.G., et al., 2001. Respiratory muscle strength, lung function, and dyspnea in patients with sarcoidosis. Chest 120, 102–108.

Bellofiore, S., Ricciardolo, F.L., Ciancio, N., et al., 1996. Changes in respiratory drive account for the magnitude of dyspnoea during bronchoconstriction in asthmatics. Eur. Respir. J. 9, 1155–1159.

Biadi, O., Rossini, R., Musumeci, G., et al., 2001. Cardiopulmonary exercise test in young women affected by anorexia nervosa. Ital. Heart J. 2, 462–467.

Binks, A.P., Moosavi, S.H., Banzett, R.B., et al., 2002. 'Tightness' sensation of asthma does not arise from the work of breathing. Am. J. Respir. Crit. Care Med. 165, 78–82.

Birmingham, C.L., Tan, A.O., 2003. Respiratory muscle weakness and anorexia nervosa. Int. J. Eat. Disord. 33, 230–233.

Bissett, B., Leditschke, I.A., Paratz, J.D., et al., 2012. Respiratory dysfunction in ventilated patients, can inspiratory muscle training help? Anaesth Intensive Care 40, 236–246.

Bohannon, R.W., Williams Andrews, A., 2011. Normal walking speed: a descriptive meta-analysis. Physiotherapy 97, 182–189.

Borghi-Silva, A., Carrascosa, C., Oliveira, C.C., et al., 2008a. Effects of respiratory muscle unloading on leg muscle oxygenation and blood volume during high-intensity exercise in chronic heart failure. Am. J. Physiol. Heart Circ. Physiol. 294, H2465–H2472.

Borghi-Silva, A., Oliveira, C.C., Carrascosa, C., et al., 2008b. Respiratory muscle unloading improves leg muscle oxygenation during exercise in patients with COPD. Thorax 63, 910–915.

Breslin, E.H., 1992. Dyspnea-limited response in chronic obstructive pulmonary disease: reduced unsupported arm activities. Rehabil. Nurs. 17, 12–20.

Britto, R.R., Zampa, C.C., de Oliveira, T.A., et al., 2009. Effects of the aging process on respiratory function. Gerontology 55, 505–510.

Brouillette, R.T., Thach, B.T., 1979. A neuromuscular mechanism maintaining extrathoracic airway patency. J. Appl. Physiol. 46, 772–779.

Brubaker, P.H., 1997. Exercise intolerance in congestive heart failure: a lesson in exercise physiology. J. Cardiopulm. Rehabil. 17, 217–221.

Brumagne, S., Janssen, L., Polspoel, K., et al., 2008a. Inspiratory muscle fatigue and back muscle fatiguability in persons with and without low back pain. European Respiratory Society, Berlin, 2205. Eur. Respir. J. 32, 726S.

Brumagne, S., Janssens, L., Janssens, E., et al., 2008b. Altered postural control in anticipation of postural instability in persons with recurrent low back pain. Gait Posture 28, 657–662.

Buchman, A.S., Boyle, P.A., Wilson, R.S., et al., 2008. Respiratory muscle strength predicts decline in mobility in older persons. Neuroepidemiology 31, 174–180.

Buhimschi, C.S., Buhimschi, I.A., Malinow, A.M., et al., 2002. Pushing in labor: performance and not endurance. Am. J. Obstet. Gynecol. 186 (6), 1339–1344.

Butcher, S.J., 2008. Modulation of ventilatory mechanics during exercise in ventilation-limited populations. Appl. Physiol. Nutr. Metab. 33, 536–537.

Butcher, S.J., Meshke, J.M., Sheppard, M.S., 2004. Reductions in functional balance, coordination, and mobility measures among patients with stable chronic obstructive pulmonary disease. J. Cardiopulm. Rehabil. 24, 274–280.

Cafarelli, E., 1982. Peripheral contributions to the perception of effort. Med. Sci. Sports Exerc. 14, 382–389.

Callahan, L.A., 2009. Invited editorial on 'acquired respiratory muscle weakness in critically ill patients: what is the role of mechanical ventilation-induced diaphragm dysfunction?' J. Appl. Physiol. 106, 360–361.

Callegaro, C.C., Martinez, D., Ribeiro, P.A., et al., 2010. Augmented peripheral chemoreflex in patients with heart failure and inspiratory muscle weakness. Respir. Physiol. Neurobiol. 171, 31–35.

Campbell, E.J.M., 1966. The relationship of the sensation of breathlessness to the act of breathing. In: Howell, J.B.L. (Ed.), Breathlessness. Blackwell Scientific, London, pp. 55–64.

Canet, J., Mazo, V., 2010. Postoperative pulmonary complications. Minerva Anestesiol. 76, 138–143.

Carlucci, A., Ceriana, P., Prinianakis, G., et al., 2009. Determinants of weaning success in patients with prolonged mechanical ventilation. Crit. Care 13 (3), R97.

Caruso, P., Friedrich, C., Denari, S.D., et al., 1999. The unidirectional valve is the best method to determine maximal inspiratory pressure during weaning. Chest 115, 1096–1101.

Casaburi, R., Patessio, A., Ioli, F., et al., 1991. Reductions in exercise lactic acidosis and ventilation as a result of exercise training in patients with obstructive lung disease. Am. Rev. Respir. Dis. 143, 9–18.

Cavalheri, V., Camillo, C.A., Brunetto, A.F., et al., 2010. Effects of arm bracing posture on respiratory muscle strength and pulmonary function in patients with chronic obstructive pulmonary disease. Rev. Port. Pneumol. 16, 887–891.

Cejudo, P., Lopez-Marquez, I., Lopez-Campos, J.L., et al., 2009. Factors associated with quality of life in patients with chronic respiratory failure due to kyphoscoliosis. Disability Rehabilitation 31, 928–934.

Chang, A.T., Seale, H., Walsh, J., et al., 2008. Static balance is affected following an exercise task in chronic obstructive pulmonary disease. Journal of Cardiopulmonary Rehabilitation and Prevention 28, 142–145.

Chatham, K., Gelder, C.M., Lines, T.A., et al., 2009. Suspected statin-induced respiratory muscle myopathy during long-term inspiratory muscle training in a patient with diaphragmatic paralysis. Phys. Ther. 89 (3), 257–266.

Cheng, S., Butler, J.E., Gandevia, S.C., et al., 2011. Movement of the human upper airway during inspiration with and without inspiratory resistive loading. J. Appl. Physiol. 110, 69–75.

Chevrolet, J.C., Tschopp, J.M., Blanc, Y., et al., 1993. Alterations in inspiratory and leg muscle force and recovery pattern after a marathon. Med. Sci. Sports Exerc. 25, 501–507.

Chlif, M., Keochkerian, D., Mourlhon, C., et al., 2005. Noninvasive assessment of the tension-time index of inspiratory muscles at rest in obese male subjects. Int. J. Obes. (Lond.) 29, 1478–1483.

Chlif, M., Keochkerian, D., Feki, Y., et al., 2007. Inspiratory muscle activity during incremental exercise in obese men. Int. J. Obes. (Lond.) 31, 1456–1463.

Chlif, M., Keochkerian, D., Choquet, D., et al., 2009. Effects of obesity on breathing pattern, ventilatory neural drive and mechanics. Respir. Physiol. Neurobiol. 168, 198–202.

Chua, T.P., Anker, S.D., Harrington, D., et al., 1995. Inspiratory muscle strength is a determinant of maximum oxygen consumption in chronic heart failure. Br. Heart J. 74, 381–385.

Chua, T.P., Ponikowski, P., Webb-Peploe, K., et al., 1997. Clinical characteristics of chronic heart failure patients with an augmented peripheral chemoreflex. Eur. Heart J. 18, 480–486.

Clanton, T.L., Levine, S., 2009. Respiratory muscle fiber remodeling in chronic hyperinflation: dysfunction or adaptation? J. Appl. Physiol. 107, 324–335.

Coast, J.R., Haverkamp, H.C., Finkbone, C.M., et al., 1999. Alterations in pulmonary function following exercise are not caused by the work of breathing alone. Int. J. Sports Med. 20, 470–475.

Coirault, C., Chemla, D., Lecarpentier, Y., 1999. Relaxation of diaphragm muscle. J. Appl. Physiol. 87, 1243–1252.

Collet, F., Mallart, A., Bervar, J.F., et al., 2007. Physiologic correlates of dyspnea in patients with morbid obesity. Int. J. Obes. (Lond.) 31, 700–706.

Contreras, G., Gutierrez, M., Beroiza, T., et al., 1991. Ventilatory drive and respiratory muscle function in pregnancy. Am. Rev. Respir. Dis. 144, 837–841.

Cordain, L., Rode, E.J., Gotshall, R.W., et al., 1994. Residual lung volume and ventilatory muscle strength changes following maximal and submaximal exercise. Int. J. Sports Med. 15, 158–161.

Cotes, J.E., Zejda, J., King, B., 1988. Lung function impairment as a guide to exercise limitation in work-related lung disorders. Am. Rev. Respir. Dis. 137, 1089–1093.

Coxson, H.O., Chan, I.H., Mayo, J.R., et al., 2004. Early emphysema in patients with anorexia nervosa. Am. J. Respir. Crit. Care Med. 170, 748–752.

Cross, T.J., Sabapathy, S., Beck, K.C., et al., 2012. The resistive and elastic work of breathing during exercise in patients with chronic heart failure. Eur. Respir. J. 39, 1449–1457.

D'Amours, R., Clerch, L., Massaro, D., 1983. Food deprivation and surfactant in adult rats. J. Appl. Physiol. 55, 1413–1417.

Dayer, M.J., Hopkinson, N.S., Ross, E.T., et al., 2006. Does symptom-limited cycle exercise cause low frequency diaphragm fatigue in patients with heart failure? Eur. J. Heart Fail. 8, 68–73.

de Bruin, P.F., Ueki, J., Watson, A., et al., 1997. Size and strength of the respiratory and quadriceps muscles in patients with chronic asthma. Eur. Respir. J. 10, 59–64.

Decramer, M., 1997. Hyperinflation and respiratory muscle interaction. Eur. Respir. J. 10, 934–941.

Decramer, M., 2001. Respiratory muscles in COPD: regulation of trophical status. Verh. K. Acad. Geneeskd. Belg 63, 577–602; discussion 602–574.

Deindl, F.M., Vodusek, D.B., Hesse, U., et al., 1994. Pelvic floor activity patterns: comparison of nulliparous continent and parous urinary stress incontinent women: A kinesiological EMG study. Br. J. Urol. 73, 413–417.

De Jonghe, B., Bastuji-Garin, S., Durand, M.C., et al., 2007. Respiratory weakness is associated with limb weakness and delayed weaning in critical illness. Crit. Care Med. 35, 2007–2015.

Delgado, H.R., Braun, S.R., Skatrud, J.B., et al., 1982. Chest wall and abdominal motion during exercise in patients with chronic obstructive pulmonary disease. Am. Rev. Respir. Dis. 126, 200–205.

DeLorey, D.S., Babb, T.G., 1999. Progressive mechanical ventilatory constraints with aging. Am. J. Respir. Crit. Care Med. 160, 169–177.

Demoule, A., Verin, E., Montcel, S.T., et al., 2008. Short-term training-dependent plasticity of the corticospinal diaphragm control in normal humans. Respir. Physiol. Neurobiol. 160, 172–180.

Dempsey, J.A., 2010. Cardiorespiratory responses to exercise in CHF: a conspiracy of maladaptation. J. Physiol. 588, 2683.

Dempsey, J.A., Romer, L., Rodman, J., et al., 2006. Consequences of exercise-induced respiratory muscle work. Respir. Physiol. Neurobiol. 151, 242–250.

DePalo, V.A., Parker, A.L., Al-Bilbeisi, F., et al., 2004. Respiratory muscle strength training with nonrespiratory maneuvers. J. Appl. Physiol. 96, 731–734.

Deruelle, F., Nourry, C., Mucci, P., et al., 2008. Difference in breathing strategies during exercise between trained elderly men and women. Scand. J. Med. Sci. Sports 18, 213–220.

De Troyer, A., Wilson, T.A., 2009. Effect of acute inflation on the mechanics of the inspiratory muscles. J. Appl. Physiol. 107, 315–323.

Dewberry, R.G., Schneider, B.F., Cale, W.F., et al., 1993. Sarcoid myopathy presenting with diaphragm weakness. Muscle Nerve 16, 832–835.

Donath, J., Miller, A., 2009. Restrictive chest wall disorders. Semin. Respir. Crit. Care Med. 30, 275–292.

Dufresne, V., Knoop, C., Van Muylem, A., et al., 2009. Effect of systemic inflammation on inspiratory and limb muscle strength and bulk in cystic fibrosis. Am. J. Respir. Crit. Care Med. 180, 153–158.

Duggan, M., Kavanagh, B.P., 2010. Perioperative modifications of respiratory function. Best Pract. Res. Clin. Anaesthesiol. 24, 145–155.

Dunnink, M.A., Doeleman, W.R., Trappenburg, J.C., et al., 2009. Respiratory muscle strength in stable adolescent and adult patients with cystic fibrosis. J. Cyst. Fibros. 8, 31–36.

Eckert, D.J., Lo, Y.L., Saboisky, J.P., et al., 2011. Sensori-motor function of the upper airway muscles and respiratory sensory processing in untreated obstructive sleep apnea. J. Appl. Physiol. 111 (6), 1644–1653.

Eisner, M.D., Blanc, P.D., Yelin, E.H., et al., 2008. COPD as a systemic disease: impact on physical functional limitations. Am. J. Med. 121, 789–796.

Ekblom, B., Goldbarg, A.N., 1971. The influence of physical training and other factors on the subjective rating of perceived exertion. Acta Physiol. Scand. 83, 399–406.

England, R., Maddocks, M., Manderson, C., et al., 2012. Factors influencing exercise performance in thoracic cancer. Respir. Med. 106, 294–299.

Enright, P.L., Kronmal, R.A., Manolio, T.A., et al., 1994. Respiratory muscle strength in the elderly Correlates and reference values. Cardiovascular Health Study Research Group. Am. J. Respir. Crit. Care Med. 149, 430–438.

Enright, S., Chatham, K., Ionescu, A.A., et al., 2007. The influence of body composition on respiratory muscle, lung function and diaphragm thickness in adults with cystic fibrosis. J. Cyst. Fibros. 6, 384–390.

Epstein, C.D., El-Mokadem, N., Peerless, J.R., 2002. Weaning older patients from long-term mechanical ventilation: a pilot study. Am. J. Crit. Care 11, 369–377.

Estenne, M., De Troyer, A., 1985. Relationship between respiratory muscle electromyogram and rib cage motion in tetraplegia. Am. Rev. Respir. Dis. 132, 53–59.

Faggiano, P., D'Aloia, A., Gualeni, A., et al., 2001. Relative contribution of resting haemodynamic profile and lung function to exercise tolerance in male patients with chronic heart failure. Heart 85, 179–184.

Feathers, L.S., Wilcock, A., Manderson, C., et al., 2003. Measuring inspiratory muscle weakness in patients with cancer and breathlessness. J. Pain Symptom. Manage. 25, 305–306.

Ferretti, A., Giampiccolo, P., Cavalli, A., et al., 2001. Expiratory flow limitation and orthopnea in massively obese subjects. Chest 119, 1401–1408.

Filusch, A., Ewert, R., Altesellmeier, M., et al., 2011. Respiratory muscle dysfunction in congestive heart failure – the role of pulmonary hypertension. Int. J. Cardiol. 150, 182–185.

Flaherty, K.R., Wald, J., Weisman, I.M., et al., 2001. Unexplained exertional limitation: characterization of patients with a mitochondrial myopathy. Am. J. Respir. Crit. Care Med. 164, 425–432.

Ford, E.S., 2005. The epidemiology of obesity and asthma. J. Allergy Clin. Immunol 115, 897–909; quiz 910.

Franco, V., 2011. Cardiopulmonary exercise test in chronic heart failure: beyond peak oxygen consumption. Curr. Heart Fail. Rep. 8, 45–50.

Frankenstein, L., Meyer, F.J., Sigg, C., et al., 2008. Is serial determination of inspiratory muscle strength a useful prognostic marker in chronic heart failure? Eur. J. Cardiovasc. Prev. Rehabil. 15, 156–161.

Frankenstein, L., Nelles, M., Meyer, F.J., et al., 2009. Validity, prognostic value and optimal cutoff of respiratory muscle strength in patients with chronic heart failure changes with beta-blocker treatment. Eur. J. Cardiovasc. Prev. Rehabil. 16 (4), 424–429.

Franssen, F.M., O'Donnell, D.E., Goossens, G.H., et al., 2008. Obesity and the lung: 5. Obesity and COPD. Thorax 63, 1110–1117.

Gandevia, S.C., 2001. Spinal and supraspinal factors in human muscle fatigue. Physiol. Rev. 81, 1725–1789.

Gandevia, S.C., McCloskey, D.I., 1978. Interpretation of perceived motor commands by reference to afferent signals. J. Physiol. 283, 493–499.

Gardini Gardenghi, G., Boni, E., Todisco, P., et al., 2009. Respiratory function in patients with stable anorexia nervosa. Chest 136, 1356–1363.

Gibson, G.J., Pride, N.B., Davis, J.N., et al., 1977. Pulmonary mechanics in patients with respiratory muscle weakness. Am. Rev. Respir. Dis. 115, 389–395.

Glaser, R.M., Sawka, M.N., Brune, M.F., et al., 1980. Physiological responses to maximal effort wheelchair and arm crank ergometry. J. Appl. Physiol. 48, 1060–1064.

Goldman, M.D., 2003. Lung dysfunction in diabetes. Diabetes Care 26, 1915–1918.

Gomez-Fernandez, P., Sanchez Agudo, L., Calatrava, J.M., et al., 1984. Respiratory muscle weakness in uremic patients under continuous ambulatory peritoneal dialysis. Nephron 36, 219–223.

Gonzalez-Moro, J.M., De Miguel-Diez, J., Paz-Gonzalez, L., et al., 2003. Abnormalities of the respiratory function and control of ventilation in patients with anorexia nervosa. Respiration 70, 490–495.

Gosselink, R., Troosters, T., Decramer, M., 1996. Peripheral muscle weakness contributes to exercise limitation in COPD. Am. J. Respir. Crit. Care Med. 153, 976–980.

Gosselink, R., Troosters, T., Decramer, M., 2000. Distribution of muscle weakness in patients with stable chronic obstructive pulmonary disease. J. Cardiopulm. Rehabil. 20, 353–360.

Griffiths, L.A., McConnell, A.K., 2007. The influence of inspiratory and expiratory muscle training upon rowing performance. Eur. J. Appl. Physiol. 99, 457–466.

Guleria, S., Agarwal, R.K., Guleria, R., et al., 2005. The effect of renal transplantation on pulmonary function and respiratory muscle strength in patients with end-stage renal disease. Transplant. Proc. 37, 664–665.

Hagins, M., Lamberg, E.M., 2006. Natural breath control during lifting tasks: effect of load. Eur. J. Appl. Physiol. 96, 453–458.

Hamaoui, A., Do, M., Poupard, L., et al., 2002. Does respiration perturb body balance more in chronic low back pain subjects than in healthy subjects? Clin. Biomech. (Bristol, Avon) 17, 548–550.

Hamid, Q., Shannon, J., Martin, J. (Eds.), 2005. Physiologic basis of respiratory disease. BC Decker, Hamilton.

Hamilton, A.L., Killian, K.J., Summers, E., et al., 1996a. Quantification of intensity of sensations during muscular work by normal subjects. J. Appl. Physiol. 81, 1156–1161.

Hamilton, A.L., Killian, K.J., Summers, E., et al., 1996b. Symptom intensity and subjective limitation to exercise in patients with cardiorespiratory disorders. Chest 110, 1255–1263.

Hansen, J.E., Wasserman, K., 1996. Pathophysiology of activity limitation in patients with interstitial lung disease. Chest 109, 1566–1576.

Harms, C.A., Dempsey, J.A., 1999. Cardiovascular consequences of exercise hyperpnea. Exerc. Sport Sci. Rev. 27, 37–62.

Harms, C.A., Babcock, M.A., McClaran, S.R., et al., 1997. Respiratory muscle work compromises leg blood flow during maximal exercise. J. Appl. Physiol. 82, 1573–1583.

Hart, N., Hawkins, P., Hamnegard, C.H., et al., 2002. A novel clinical test of respiratory muscle endurance. Eur. Respir. J. 19, 232–239.

Hart, N., Laffont, I., de la Sota, A.P., et al., 2005. Respiratory effects of combined truncal and abdominal support in patients with spinal cord injury.

Arch. Phys. Med. Rehabil. 86, 1447–1451.

Heimer, D., Brami, J., Lieberman, D., et al., 1990. Respiratory muscle performance in patients with type 1 diabetes. Diabet. Med. 7, 434–437.

Hermans, G., Agten, A., Testelmans, D., et al., 2010. Increased duration of mechanical ventilation is associated with decreased diaphragmatic force: a prospective observational study. Crit. Care 14, R127.

Hill, A.R., 1991. Respiratory muscle function in asthma. J. Assoc. Acad. Minor. Phys. 2, 100–108.

Hill, N.S., Jacoby, C., Farber, H.W., 1991. Effect of an endurance triathlon on pulmonary function. Med. Sci. Sports Exerc. 23, 1260–1264.

Hiraizumi, Y., Fujimaki, E., Hishida, T., et al., 1986. Regional lung perfusion and ventilation with radioisotopes in cervical cord-injured patients. Clin. Nucl. Med. 11, 352–357.

Hodges, P.W., Gandevia, S.C., 2000. Changes in intra-abdominal pressure during postural and respiratory activation of the human diaphragm. J. Appl. Physiol. 89, 967–976.

Hodges, P.W., Butler, J.E., McKenzie, D.K., et al., 1997a. Contraction of the human diaphragm during rapid postural adjustments. J. Physiol. 505 (pt 2), 539–548.

Hodges, P.W., Gandevia, S.C., Richardson, C.A., 1997b. Contractions of specific abdominal muscles in postural tasks are affected by respiratory maneuvers. J. Appl. Physiol. 83, 753–760.

Hodges, P.W., McKenzie, D.K., Heijnen, I., et al., 2000. Reduced contribution of the diaphragm to postural control in patients with severe chronic airflow limitation. Respirology 5 (Suppl.), A8.

Hodges, P.W., Heijnen, I., Gandevia, S.C., 2001. Postural activity of the diaphragm is reduced in humans when respiratory demand increases. J. Physiol. 537, 999–1008.

Hodges, P.W., Eriksson, A.E., Shirley, D., et al., 2005. Intra-abdominal pressure increases stiffness of the lumbar spine. J. Biomech. 38, 1873–1880.

Holland, A.E., 2010. Exercise limitation in interstitial lung disease – mechanisms, significance and therapeutic options. Chron. Respir. Dis. 7, 101–111.

Hopkinson, N.S., Dayer, M.J., Moxham, J., et al., 2010. Abdominal muscle fatigue following exercise in chronic obstructive pulmonary disease. Respir. Res. 11, 15.

Hopman, M.T., van der Woude, L.H., Dallmeijer, A.J., et al., 1997. Respiratory muscle strength and endurance in individuals with tetraplegia. Spinal Cord 35, 104–108.

How, S.C., McConnell, A.K., Taylor, B.J., et al., 2007. Acute and chronic responses of the upper airway to inspiratory loading in healthy awake humans: an MRI study. Respir. Physiol. Neurobiol. 157, 270–280.

Hudgel, D.W., Harasick, T., 1990. Fluctuation in timing of upper airway and chest wall inspiratory muscle activity in obstructive sleep apnea. J. Appl. Physiol. 69, 443–450.

Hughes, P.D., Polkey, M.I., Harrus, M.L., et al., 1999. Diaphragm strength in chronic heart failure. Am. J. Respir. Crit. Care Med. 160, 529–534.

Hughes, P.D., Hart, N., Hamnegard, C.H., et al., 2001. Inspiratory muscle relaxation rate slows during exhaustive treadmill walking in patients with chronic heart failure. Am. J. Respir. Crit. Care Med. 163, 1400–1403.

Innocenti, F., Fabbri, A., Anichini, R., et al., 1994. Indications of reduced pulmonary function in type 1 (insulin-dependent) diabetes mellitus. Diabetes Res. Clin. Pract. 25, 161–168.

Ionescu, A.A., Chatham, K., Davies, C.A., et al., 1998. Inspiratory muscle function and body composition in cystic fibrosis. Am. J. Respir. Crit. Care Med. 158, 1271–1276.

Irfan, M., Jabbar, A., Haque, A.S., et al., 2011. Pulmonary functions in patients with diabetes mellitus. Lung India 28, 89–92.

Isono, S., Feroah, T.R., Hajduk, E.A., et al., 1997. Interaction of cross-sectional area, driving pressure, and airflow of passive velopharynx. J. Appl. Physiol. 83, 851–859.

Janaudis-Ferreira, T., Hill, K., Goldstein, R.S., et al., 2011. Resistance arm training in patients with COPD: a randomized controlled trial. Chest 139, 151–158.

Janssens, J.P., Pache, J.C., Nicod, L.P., 1999. Physiological changes in respiratory function associated with ageing. Eur. Respir. J. 13, 197–205.

Janssens, L., Brumagne, S., Polspoel, K., et al., 2010. The effect of inspiratory muscles fatigue on postural control in people with and without recurrent low back pain. Spine 35, 1088–1094.

Javaheri, S., Sicilian, L., 1992. Lung function, breathing pattern, and gas exchange in interstitial lung disease. Thorax 47, 93–97.

Jensen, D., Webb, K.A., O'Donnell, D.E., 2007. Chemical and mechanical adaptations of the respiratory system at rest and during exercise in human pregnancy. Appl. Physiol. Nutr. Metab. 32, 1239–1250.

Jensen, D., Ofir, D., O'Donnell, D.E., 2009a. Effects of pregnancy, obesity and aging on the intensity of perceived breathlessness during exercise in healthy humans. Respir. Physiol. Neurobiol. 167, 87–100.

Jensen, D., Webb, K.A., Davies, G.A., et al., 2009b. Mechanisms of activity-related breathlessness in healthy human pregnancy. Eur. J. Appl. Physiol. 106, 253–265.

Johnson, B.D., Reddan, W.G., Seow, K.C., et al., 1991. Mechanical constraints on exercise hyperpnea in a fit aging population. Am. Rev. Respir. Dis. 143, 968–977.

Johnson, B.D., Babcock, M.A., Suman, O.E., et al., 1993. Exercise-induced diaphragmatic fatigue in healthy humans. J. Physiol. 460, 385–405.

Johnson, B.D., Beck, K.C., Olson, L.J., et al., 2000. Ventilatory constraints during exercise in patients with chronic heart failure. Chest 117, 321–332.

Just, N., Bautin, N., Danel-Brunaud, V., et al., 2010. The Borg dyspnoea score: a relevant clinical marker of inspiratory muscle weakness in amyotrophic lateral sclerosis. Eur. Respir. J. 35, 353–360.

Kabitz, H.J., Schwoerer, A., Bremer, H.C., et al., 2008a. Impairment of respiratory muscle function in pulmonary hypertension. Clin. Sci. (Lond.) 114, 165–171.

Kabitz, H.J., Sonntag, F., Walker, D., et al., 2008b. Diabetic polyneuropathy is associated with respiratory muscle impairment in type 2 diabetes. Diabetologia 51, 191–197.

Kaminski, D.M., Schaan, B.D., da Silva, A.M., et al., 2011. Inspiratory muscle weakness is associated with

autonomic cardiovascular dysfunction in patients with type 2 diabetes mellitus. Clin. Auton. Res. 21, 29–35.

Kang, S.W., 2006. Pulmonary rehabilitation in patients with neuromuscular disease. Yonsei Med. J. 47, 307–314.

Karacan, O., Tutal, E., Colak, T., et al., 2006. Pulmonary function in renal transplant recipients and end-stage renal disease patients undergoing maintenance dialysis. Transplant. Proc. 38, 396–400.

Karakurt, Z., Fanfulla, F., Ceriana, P., et al., 2011. Physiologic determinants of prolonged mechanical ventilation in patients after major surgery. J. Crit. Care 27 (2), 221 e9–221.e16.

Katayama, K., Iwamoto, E., Ishida, K., et al., 2012. Inspiratory muscle fatigue increases sympathetic vasomotor outflow and blood pressure during submaximal exercise. Am. J. Physiol. Regul. Integr. Comp. Physiol. 302, R1167–R1175.

Kawagoe, Y., Permutt, S., Fessler, H.E., 1994. Hyperinflation with intrinsic PEEP and respiratory muscle blood flow. J. Appl. Physiol. 77, 2440–2448.

Kenn, K., Hess, M.M., 2008. Vocal cord dysfunction: an important differential diagnosis of bronchial asthma. Deutsches Arzteblatt International 105, 699–704.

Ker, J.A., Schultz, C.M., 1996. Respiratory muscle fatigue after an ultra-marathon measured as inspiratory task failure. Int. J. Sports Med. 17, 493–496.

Keyser, R.E., Rodgers, M.M., Gardner, E.R., et al., 1999. Oxygen uptake during peak graded exercise and single-stage fatigue tests of wheelchair propulsion in manual wheelchair users and the able-bodied. Arch. Phys. Med. Rehabil. 80, 1288–1292.

Kilicli, F., Dokmetas, S., Candan, F., et al., 2010. Inspiratory muscle strength is correlated with carnitine levels in type 2 diabetes. Endocr. Res. 35, 51–58.

Kobayashi, Y.M., Rader, E.P., Crawford, R.W., et al., 2008. Sarcolemma-localized nNOS is required to maintain activity after mild exercise. Nature 456, 511–515.

Kolar, P., Neuwirth, J., Sanda, J., et al., 2009. Analysis of diaphragm movement during tidal breathing and during its activation while breath holding using MRI synchronized with spirometry. Physiol. Res. 58, 383–392.

Koulouris, N.G., Retsou, S., Kosmas, E., et al., 2003. Tidal expiratory flow limitation, dyspnoea and exercise capacity in patients with bilateral bronchiectasis. Eur. Respir. J. 21, 743–748.

Kovelis, D., Pitta, F., Probst, V.S., et al., 2008. Pulmonary function and respiratory muscle strength in chronic renal failure patients on hemodialysis. J. Bras. Pneumol. 34, 907–912.

Kress, J.P., Pohlman, A.S., Alverdy, J., et al., 1999. The impact of morbid obesity on oxygen cost of breathing (VO(2RESP) at rest. Am. J. Respir. Crit. Care Med. 160, 883–886.

Kufel, T.J., Pineda, L.A., Junega, R.G., et al., 2002. Diaphragmatic function after intense exercise in congestive heart failure patients. Eur. Respir. J. 20, 1399–1405.

Kyroussis, D., Polkey, M.I., Keilty, S.E., et al., 1996. Exhaustive exercise slows inspiratory muscle relaxation rate in chronic obstructive pulmonary disease. Am. J. Respir. Crit. Care Med. 153, 787–793.

Laghi, F., Tobin, M.J., 2003. Disorders of the respiratory muscles. Am. J. Respir. Crit. Care Med. 168, 10–48.

Laghi, F., Cattapan, S.E., Jubran, A., et al., 2003. Is weaning failure caused by low-frequency fatigue of the diaphragm? Am. J. Respir. Crit. Care Med. 167, 120–127.

Lamberg, E.M., Hagins, M., 2012. The effects of low back pain on natural breath control during a lowering task. Eur. J. Appl. Physiol. 112 (10), 3519–3524.

Landahl, S., Steen, B., Svanborg, A., 1980. Dyspnea in 70-year-old people. Acta Med. Scand. 207, 225–230.

Lassau-Wray, E.R., Ward, G.R., 2000. Varying physiological response to arm-crank exercise in specific spinal injuries. J. Physiol. Anthropol. Appl. Human Sci. 19, 5–12.

Latronico, N., Bolton, C.F., 2011. Critical illness polyneuropathy and myopathy: a major cause of muscle weakness and paralysis. Lancet Neurol. 10, 931–941.

Lawlor, D.A., Patel, R., Ebrahim, S., 2003. Association between falls in elderly women and chronic diseases and drug use: cross sectional study. BMJ 327, 712–717.

Leroy, S., Perez, T., Neviere, R., et al., 2011. Determinants of dyspnea and alveolar hypoventilation during exercise in cystic fibrosis: impact of inspiratory muscle endurance. J. Cyst. Fibros. 10, 159–165.

Levine, S., Kaiser, L., Leferovich, J., et al., 1997. Cellular adaptations in the diaphragm in chronic obstructive pulmonary disease. N. Engl. J. Med. 337, 1799–1806.

Levine, S., Nguyen, T., Kaiser, L.R., et al., 2003. Human diaphragm remodeling associated with chronic obstructive pulmonary disease: clinical implications. Am. J. Respir. Crit. Care Med. 168, 706–713.

Levine, S., Nguyen, T., Taylor, N., et al., 2008. Rapid disuse atrophy of diaphragm fibers in mechanically ventilated humans. N. Engl. J. Med. 358, 1327–1335.

Lewis, N.P., Banning, A.P., Cooper, J.P., et al., 1996. Impaired matching of perfusion and ventilation in heart failure detected by ^{133}xenon. Basic Res. Cardiol. 91 (Suppl. 1), 45–49.

Li, J., Li, S., Feuers, R.J., et al., 2001. Influence of body fat distribution on oxygen uptake and pulmonary performance in morbidly obese females during exercise. Respirology 6, 9–13.

Lindstedt, S.L., Reich, T.E., Keim, P., et al., 2002. Do muscles function as adaptable locomotor springs? J. Exp. Biol. 205, 2211–2216.

Lisboa, C., Moreno, R., Fava, M., et al., 1985. Inspiratory muscle function in patients with severe kyphoscoliosis. Am. Rev. Respir. Dis. 132, 48–52.

Loke, J., Mahler, D.A., Virgulto, J.A., 1982. Respiratory muscle fatigue after marathon running. J. Appl. Physiol. 52, 821–824.

Lomax, M.E., McConnell, A.K., 2003. Inspiratory muscle fatigue in swimmers after a single 200 m swim. J. Sports Sci. 21, 659–664.

Lougheed, M.D., Lam, M., Forkert, L., et al., 1993. Breathlessness during acute bronchoconstriction in asthma. Pathophysiologic mechanisms. Am. Rev. Respir. Dis. 148, 1452–1459.

Lougheed, D.M., Webb, K.A., O'Donnell, D.E., 1995. Breathlessness during induced lung hyperinflation in asthma: the role of the inspiratory threshold load. Am. J. Respir. Crit. Care Med. 152, 911–920.

Lykidis, C.K., White, M.J., Balanos, G.M., 2008. The pulmonary vascular response to the sustained activation of the muscle metaboreflex in man. Exp. Physiol. 93, 247–253.

Lynch 3rd, J.P., Ma, Y.L., Koss, M.N., et al., 2007. Pulmonary sarcoidosis. Semin. Respir. Crit. Care Med. 28, 53–74.

Macklem, P.T., 1986. Muscular weakness and respiratory function. N. Engl. J. Med. 314, 775–776.

Mador, M.J., Acevedo, F.A., 1991. Effect of respiratory muscle fatigue on subsequent exercise performance. J. Appl. Physiol. 70, 2059–2065.

Mador, M.J., Magalang, U.J., Rodis, A., et al., 1993. Diaphragmatic fatigue after exercise in healthy human subjects. Am. Rev. Respir. Dis. 148, 1571–1575.

Mador, J.M., Kufel, T.J., Pineda, L.A., 2000a. Quadriceps and diaphragmatic function after exhaustive cycle exercise in the healthy elderly. Am. J. Respir. Crit. Care Med. 162, 1760–1766.

Mador, M.J., Kufel, T.J., Pineda, L.A., et al., 2000b. Diaphragmatic fatigue and high-intensity exercise in patients with chronic obstructive pulmonary disease. Am. J. Respir. Crit. Care Med. 161, 118–123.

Mador, M.J., Bozkanat, E., Kufel, T.J., 2003. Quadriceps fatigue after cycle exercise in patients with COPD compared with healthy control subjects. Chest 123, 1104–1111.

Mancini, D.M., Ferraro, N., Nazzaro, D., et al., 1991. Respiratory muscle deoxygenation during exercise in patients with heart failure demonstrated with near-infrared spectroscopy. J. Am. Coll. Cardiol. 18, 492–498.

Mancini, D., Donchez, L., Levine, S., 1997. Acute unloading of the work of breathing extends exercise duration in patients with heart failure. J. Am. Coll. Cardiol. 29, 590–596.

Mancini, M., Filippelli, M., Seghieri, G., et al., 1999. Respiratory muscle function and hypoxic ventilatory control in patients with type I diabetes. Chest 115, 1553–1562.

Markovitz, G.H., Cooper, C.B., 2010. Rehabilitation in non-COPD: mechanisms of exercise limitation and pulmonary rehabilitation for patients with pulmonary fibrosis/restrictive lung disease. Chron. Respir. Dis. 7, 47–60.

Martin, J., Powell, E., Shore, S., et al., 1980. The role of respiratory muscles in the hyperinflation of bronchial asthma. Am. Rev. Respir. Dis. 121, 441–447.

Martin, J.G., Shore, S.A., Engel, L.A., 1983. Mechanical load and inspiratory muscle action during induced asthma. Am. Rev. Respir. Dis. 128, 455–460.

Martinez-Llorens, J., Ramirez, M., Colomina, M.J., et al., 2010. Muscle dysfunction and exercise limitation in adolescent idiopathic scoliosis. Eur. Respir. J. 36, 393–400.

Martinez-Moragon, E., Perpina, M., Belloch, A., et al., 2003. Determinants of dyspnea in patients with different grades of stable asthma. J. Asthma 40, 375–382.

Maskey-Warzechowska, M., Przybylowski, T., Hildebrand, K., et al., 2006. Maximal respiratory pressures and exercise tolerance in patients with COPD. Pneumonol. Alergol. Pol. 74, 72–76.

Mateus, S.R., Beraldo, P.S., Horan, T.A., 2007. Maximal static mouth respiratory pressure in spinal cord injured patients: correlation with motor level. Spinal Cord 45, 569–575.

McCloskey, D.I., Gandevia, S., Potter, E.K., et al., 1983. Muscle sense and effort: motor commands and judgments about muscular contractions. Adv. Neurol. 39, 151–167.

McConnell, A.K., Copestake, A.J., 1999. Maximum static respiratory pressures in healthy elderly men and women: issues of reproducibility and interpretation. Respiration 66, 251–258.

McConnell, A.K., Davies, C.T., 1992. A comparison of the ventilatory responses to exercise of elderly and younger humans. J. Gerontol. 47, B137–B141.

McConnell, A.K., Lomax, M., 2006. The influence of inspiratory muscle work history and specific inspiratory muscle training upon human limb muscle fatigue. J. Physiol. 577, 445–457.

McCool, F.D., Tzelepis, G.E., 1995. Inspiratory muscle training in the patient with neuromuscular disease. Phys. Ther. 75, 1006–1014.

McCool, F.D., Conomos, P., Benditt, J.O., et al., 1997. Maximal inspiratory pressures and dimensions of the diaphragm. Am. J. Respir. Crit. Care Med. 155, 1329–1334.

McKenzie, D.K., Butler, J.E., Gandevia, S.C., 2009. Respiratory muscle function and activation in chronic obstructive pulmonary disease. J. Appl. Physiol. 107, 621–629.

Mehta, S., 2006. Neuromuscular disease causing acute respiratory failure. Respir. Care 51, 1016–1021; discussion 1021–1013.

Meyer, F.J., Zugck, C., Haass, M., et al., 2000. Inefficient ventilation and reduced respiratory muscle capacity in congestive heart failure. Basic Res. Cardiol. 95, 333–342.

Meyer, F.J., Lossnitzer, D., Kristen, A.V., et al., 2005. Respiratory muscle dysfunction in idiopathic pulmonary arterial hypertension. Eur. Respir. J. 25, 125–130.

Miki, K., Maekura, R., Hiraga, T., et al., 2003. Impairments and prognostic factors for survival in patients with idiopathic pulmonary fibrosis. Respir. Med. 97, 482–490.

Milne, J.A., Howie, A.D., Pack, A.I., 1978. Dyspnoea during normal pregnancy. Br. J. Obstet. Gynaecol. 85, 260–263.

Moodie, L., Reeve, J., Elkins, M., 2011. Inspiratory muscle training increases inspiratory muscle strength in patients weaning from mechanical ventilation: a systematic review. Journal of Physiotherapy 57, 213–221.

Moran, F., Piper, A., Elborn, J.S., et al., 2010. Respiratory muscle pressures in non-CF bronchiectasis: repeatability and reliability. Chron. Respir. Dis. 7, 165–171.

Moxham, J., Jolley, C., 2009. Breathlessness, fatigue and the respiratory muscles. Clin. Med. 9, 448–452.

Muller, N., Bryan, A.C., Zamel, N., 1980. Tonic inspiratory muscle activity as a cause of hyperinflation in histamine-induced asthma. J. Appl. Physiol. 49, 869–874.

Muller, N., Bryan, A.C., Zamel, N., 1981. Tonic inspiratory muscle activity as a cause of hyperinflation in asthma. J. Appl. Physiol. 50, 279–282.

Murciano, D., Rigaud, D., Pingleton, S., et al., 1994. Diaphragmatic function in severely malnourished patients with anorexia nervosa Effects of renutrition. Am. J. Respir. Crit. Care Med. 150, 1569–1574.

Naimark, A., Cherniack, R.M., 1960. Compliance of the respiratory system and its components in health and obesity. J. Appl. Physiol. 15, 377–382.

Nanas, S., Nanas, J., Papazachou, O., et al., 2003. Resting lung function and hemodynamic parameters as predictors of exercise capacity in patients with chronic heart failure. Chest 123, 1386–1393.

Nava, S., Zanotti, E., Ambrosino, N., et al., 1992. Evidence of acute diaphragmatic fatigue in a 'natural' condition. The diaphragm during labor. Am. Rev. Respir. Dis. 146 (5 pt 1), 1226–1230.

Neves, P.C., Guerra, M., Ponce, P., et al., 2011. Non-cystic fibrosis bronchiectasis. Interactive Cardiovascular and Thoracic Surgery 13 (6), 619–625.

Newall, C., Stockley, R.A., Hill, S.L., 2005. Exercise training and inspiratory muscle training in patients with bronchiectasis. Thorax 60, 943–948.

Nici, L., 2008. The major limitation to exercise performance in COPD is inadequate energy supply to the respiratory and locomotor muscles vs. lower limb muscle dysfunction vs. dynamic hyperinflation. Difficulties in determining the primary physiological abnormality that limits exercise performance in COPD. J. Appl. Physiol. 105, 760–761.

Nishimura, Y., Maeda, H., Tanaka, K., et al., 1994. Respiratory muscle strength and hemodynamics in chronic heart failure. Chest 105, 355–359.

O'Donnell, D.E., 2001. Ventilatory limitations in chronic obstructive pulmonary disease. Med. Sci. Sports Exerc. 33, S647–S655.

O'Donnell, D.E., Laveneziana, P., 2007. Dyspnea and activity limitation in COPD: mechanical factors. Chronic Obstructive Pulmonary Disease 4, 225–236.

O'Donnell, D., Webb, K., 2008a. Last word on Point:Counterpoint: The major limitation to exercise performance in COPD is 1) inadequate energy supply to the respiratory and locomotor muscles, 2) lower limb muscle dysfunction, 3) dynamic hyperinflation. J. Appl. Physiol. 105, 765.

O'Donnell, D.E., Webb, K.A., 2008b. The major limitation to exercise performance in COPD is dynamic hyperinflation. J. Appl. Physiol 105, 753–755; discussion 755–757.

O'Donnell, D.E., D'Arsigny, C., Raj, S., et al., 1999. Ventilatory assistance improves exercise endurance in stable congestive heart failure. Am. J. Respir. Crit. Care Med. 160, 1804–1811.

O'Donnell, D.E., Banzett, R.B., Carrieri-Kohlman, V., et al., 2007. Pathophysiology of dyspnea in chronic obstructive pulmonary disease: a roundtable. Proc. Am. Thorac. Soc. 4, 145–168.

O'Donnell, D.E., Guenette, J.A., Maltais, F., et al., 2012. Decline of resting inspiratory capacity in COPD: the impact on breathing pattern, dyspnea, and ventilatory capacity during exercise. Chest 141, 753–762.

Ofir, D., Laveneziana, P., Webb, K.A., et al., 2008. Sex differences in the perceived intensity of breathlessness during exercise with advancing age. J. Appl. Physiol. 104, 1583–1593.

Olson, L.G., Fouke, J.M., Hoekje, P.L., et al., 1988. A biomechanical view of upper airway function. In: Mathew, O.P., Sant'Ambrogio, G. (Eds.), Respiratory function of the upper airway. Marcel Dekker, New York, pp. 359–389.

Olson, T.P., Joyner, M.J., Dietz, N.M., et al., 2010. Effects of respiratory muscle work on blood flow distribution during exercise in heart failure. J. Physiol. 588, 2487–2501.

Ottenheijm, C.A., Heunks, L.M., Sieck, G.C., et al., 2005. Diaphragm dysfunction in chronic obstructive pulmonary disease. Am. J. Respir. Crit. Care Med. 172, 200–205.

Ozdem Yr, O., Inanici, F., Hascelik, Z., 2011. Reduced vital capacity leads to exercise intolerance in patients with ankylosing spondylitis. European Journal of Physical and Rehabilitation Medicine 47, 391–397.

Palange, P., Forte, S., Onorati, P., et al., 2000. Ventilatory and metabolic adaptations to walking and cycling in patients with COPD. J. Appl. Physiol. 88, 1715–1720.

Patel, I.S., Vlahos, I., Wilkinson, T.M., et al., 2004. Bronchiectasis, exacerbation indices, and inflammation in chronic obstructive pulmonary disease. Am. J. Respir. Crit. Care Med. 170, 400–407.

Pelosi, P., Croci, M., Ravagnan, I., et al., 1996. Total respiratory system, lung, and chest wall mechanics in sedated-paralyzed postoperative morbidly obese patients. Chest 109, 144–151.

Perez, T., Becquart, L.A., Stach, B., et al., 1996. Inspiratory muscle strength and endurance in steroid-dependent asthma. Am. J. Respir. Crit. Care Med. 153, 610–615.

Perkoff, G.T., Silber, R., Tyler, F.H., et al., 1959. Studies in disorders of muscle. XII. Myopathy due to the administration of therapeutic amounts of 17-hydroxycorticosteroids. Am. J. Med. 26, 891–898.

Petrof, B.J., Jaber, S., Matecki, S., 2010. Ventilator-induced diaphragmatic dysfunction. Curr. Opin. Crit. Care 16, 19–25.

Piepoli, M., Clark, A.L., Volterrani, M., et al., 1996. Contribution of muscle afferents to the hemodynamic, autonomic, and ventilatory responses to exercise in patients with chronic heart failure: effects of physical training. Circulation 93, 940–952.

Pina, I.L., Apstein, C.S., Balady, G.J., et al., 2003. Exercise and heart failure: A statement from the American Heart Association Committee on exercise, rehabilitation, and prevention. Circulation 107, 1210–1225.

Polkey, M.I., Kyroussis, D., Keilty, S.E., et al., 1995. Exhaustive treadmill exercise does not reduce twitch transdiaphragmatic pressure in patients with COPD. Am. J. Respir. Crit. Care Med. 152, 959–964.

Polkey, M.I., Kyroussis, D., Hamnegard, C.H., et al., 1996. Diaphragm strength in chronic obstructive pulmonary disease. Am. J. Respir. Crit. Care Med. 154, 1310–1317.

Polkey, M.I., Moxham, J., Green, M., 2011. The case against inspiratory muscle training in COPD. Eur. Respir. J. 37, 236–237.

Prezant, D.J., 1990. Effect of uremia and its treatment on pulmonary function. Lung 168, 1–14.

Pride, N.B., Macklem, P.T., 1986. Lung mechanics in disease. In: Fishman, A.P. (Ed.), Handbook of physiology. American Physiological Society, Bethesda, MD, pp. 659–692.

Pringle, C.E., Dewar, C.L., 1997. Respiratory muscle involvement in severe sarcoid myositis. Muscle Nerve 20, 379–381.

Ragette, R., Mellies, U., Schwake, C., et al., 2002. Patterns and predictors of sleep disordered breathing in primary myopathies. Thorax 57, 724–728.

Rallidis, L.S., Fountoulaki, K., Anastasiou-Nana, M., 2011. Managing the underestimated risk of statin-associated myopathy. Int. J. Cardiol. 159 (3), 169–176.

Ribeiro, J.P., Chiappa, G.R., Neder, J.A., et al., 2009. Respiratory muscle function and exercise intolerance in heart failure. Curr. Heart Fail. Rep. 6, 95–101.

Ribeiro, J.P., Chiappa, G.R., Callegaro, C.C., 2012. The contribution of inspiratory muscles function to exercise limitation in heart failure: pathophysiological mechanisms. Revista Brasileira de Fisioterapia 16 (4), 261–267.

Rochester, D.F., 1993. Respiratory muscles and ventilatory failure: 1993 perspective. Am. J. Med. Sci. 305, 394–402.

Rogers, M.A., Evans, W.J., 1993. Changes in skeletal muscle with aging: effects of exercise training. Exerc. Sport Sci. Rev. 21, 65–102.

Roig, M., Eng, J.J., Road, J.D., et al., 2009. Falls in patients with chronic obstructive pulmonary disease: a call for further research. Respir. Med. 103, 1257–1269.

Roig, M., Eng, J.J., MacIntyre, D.L., et al., 2011. Falls in people with chronic obstructive pulmonary disease: an observational cohort study. Respir. Med. 105, 461–469.

Romer, L.M., Polkey, M.I., 2008. Exercise-induced respiratory muscle fatigue: implications for performance. J. Appl. Physiol. 104, 879–888.

Romer, L.M., McConnell, A.K., Jones, D.A., 2002a. Effects of inspiratory muscle training on time-trial performance in trained cyclists. J. Sports Sci. 20, 547–562.

Romer, L.M., McConnell, A.K., Jones, D.A., 2002b. Inspiratory muscle fatigue in trained cyclists: effects of inspiratory muscle training. Med. Sci. Sports Exerc. 34, 785–792.

Romer, L.M., Lovering, A.T., Haverkamp, H.C., et al., 2006. Effect of inspiratory muscle work on peripheral fatigue of locomotor muscles in healthy humans. J. Physiol. 571, 425–439.

Ross, E., Middleton, N., Shave, R., et al., 2008. Changes in respiratory muscle and lung function following marathon running in man. J. Sports Sci. 26, 1295–1301.

Rubinstein, I., Zamel, N., DuBarry, L., et al., 1990. Airflow limitation in morbidly obese, nonsmoking men. Ann. Intern. Med. 112, 828–832.

Sahebjami, H., Domino, M., 1992. Effects of repeated cycles of starvation and refeeding on lungs of growing rats. J. Appl. Physiol. 73, 2349–2354.

Sahebjami, H., MacGee, J., 1985. Effects of starvation on lung mechanics and biochemistry in young and old rats. J. Appl. Physiol. 58, 778–784.

Saler, T., Cakmak, G., Saglam, Z.A., et al., 2009. The assessment of pulmonary diffusing capacity in diabetes mellitus with regard to microalbuminuria. Intern. Med. 48, 1939–1943.

Salome, C.M., King, G.G., Berend, N., 2010. Physiology of obesity and effects on lung function. J. Appl. Physiol. 108, 206–211.

Satta, A., 2000. Exercise training in asthma. J. Sports Med. Phys. Fitness 40, 277–283.

Scanlon, P.D., Loring, S.H., Pichurko, B.M., et al., 1989. Respiratory mechanics in acute quadriplegia. Lung and chest wall compliance and dimensional changes during respiratory maneuvers. Am. Rev. Respir. Dis. 139, 615–620.

Scano, G., Seghieri, G., Mancini, M., 1999. Dyspnoea, peripheral airway involvement and respiratory muscle effort in patients with type I diabetes mellitus under good metabolic control. Clin. Sci. (Lond.) 96, 499–506.

Scano, G., Grazzini, M., Stendardi, L., et al., 2006. Respiratory muscle energetics during exercise in healthy subjects and patients with COPD. Respir. Med. 100, 1896–1906.

Scano, G., Innocenti-Bruni, G., Stendardi, L., 2010. Do obstructive and restrictive lung diseases share common underlying mechanisms of breathlessness? Respir. Med. 104, 925–933.

Schilero, G.J., Grimm, D.R., Bauman, W.A., 2005. Assessment of airway caliber and bronchodilator responsiveness in subjects with spinal cord injury. Chest 127, 149–155.

Schilero, G.J., Spungen, A.M., Bauman, W.A., et al., 2009. Pulmonary function and spinal cord injury. Respir. Physiol. Neurobiol. 166, 129–141.

Schwartz, A.R., Patil, S.P., Squier, S., et al., 2010. Obesity and upper airway control during sleep. J. Appl. Physiol. 108, 430–435.

Seals, D.R., 2001. Robin Hood for the lungs? A respiratory metaboreflex that 'steals' blood flow from locomotor muscles. J. Physiol. 537, 2.

Series, F., 2002. Upper airway muscles awake and asleep. Sleep. Med. Rev. 6, 229–242.

Sharma, R.R., Axelsson, H., Oberg, A., et al., 1999. Diaphragmatic activity after laparoscopic cholecystectomy. Anesthesiology 91, 406–413.

Sharpe, G.R., Hamer, M., Caine, M.P., et al., 1996. Respiratory muscle fatigue during and following a sprint triathlon in humans. J. Physiol. 165P.

Sheel, A.W., Derchak, P.A., Morgan, B.J., et al., 2001. Fatiguing inspiratory muscle work causes reflex reduction in resting leg blood flow in humans. J. Physiol. 537, 277–289.

Sheel, A.W., Derchak, P.A., Pegelow, D.F., et al., 2002. Threshold effects of respiratory muscle work on limb vascular resistance. Am. J. Physiol. Heart Circ. Physiol. 282, H1732–H1738.

Siafakas, N.M., Mitrouska, I., Bouros, D., et al., 1999. Surgery and the respiratory muscles. Thorax 54, 458–465.

Silver, J.R., 1963. The oxygen cost of breathing in tetraplegic patients. Paraplegia 1, 204–214.

Similowski, T., Yan, S., Gauthier, A.P., et al., 1991. Contractile properties of the human diaphragm during chronic hyperinflation. N. Engl. J. Med. 325, 917–923.

Sinderby, C., Spahija, J., Beck, J., et al., 2001. Diaphragm activation during exercise in chronic obstructive pulmonary disease. Am. J. Respir. Crit. Care Med. 163, 1637–1641.

Smith, M.D., Russell, A., Hodges, P.W., 2006. Disorders of breathing and continence have a stronger association with back pain than obesity and physical activity. Aust. J. Physiother. 52, 11–16.

Smith, M.D., Chang, A.T., Seale, H.E., et al., 2010. Balance is impaired in people with chronic obstructive pulmonary disease. Gait Posture 31, 456–460.

Somfay, A., Porszasz, J., Lee, S.M., et al., 2002. Effect of hyperoxia on gas exchange and lactate kinetics following exercise onset in nonhypoxemic COPD patients. Chest 121, 393–400.

Sood, A., 2005. Does obesity weigh heavily on the health of the human airway? J. Allergy Clin. Immunol. 115, 921–924.

Sood, A., 2010. Obesity, adipokines, and lung disease. J. Appl. Physiol. 108, 744–753.

Spruit, M.A., Thomeer, M.J., Gosselink, R., et al., 2005. Skeletal muscle weakness in patients with sarcoidosis and its relationship with exercise intolerance and reduced health status. Thorax 60, 32–38.

Spungen, A.M., Grimm, D.R., Lesser, M., et al., 1997. Self-reported prevalence of pulmonary symptoms in subjects with spinal cord injury. Spinal Cord 35, 652–657.

Spyropoulou, D., Leotsinidis, M., Tsiamita, M., et al., 2009. Pulmonary function testing in women with breast cancer treated with radiotherapy and chemotherapy. In Vivo 23, 867–871.

St Croix, C.M., Morgan, B.J., Wetter, T.J., et al., 2000. Fatiguing inspiratory muscle work causes reflex sympathetic activation in humans. J. Physiol. 529 (pt 2), 493–504.

Steier, J., Jolley, C.J., Seymour, J., et al., 2010. Increased load on the respiratory muscles in obstructive sleep apnea. Respir. Physiol. Neurobiol. 171, 54–60.

Stell, I.M., Polkey, M.I., Rees, P.J., et al., 2001. Inspiratory muscle strength in acute asthma. Chest 120, 757–764.

Sun, Z., Liu, L., Liu, N., Liu, Y., 2008. Muscular response and adaptation to diabetes mellitus. Front. Biosci. 13, 4765–4794.

Tanios, M.A., El Gamal, H., Epstein, S.K., et al., 2004. Severe respiratory muscle weakness related to long-term colchicine therapy. Respir. Care 49, 189–191.

Tantucci, C., Bottini, P., Dottorini, M.L., et al., 1996. Ventilatory response to exercise in diabetic subjects with autonomic neuropathy. J. Appl. Physiol. 81, 1978–1986.

Taylor, B.J., Johnson, B.D., 2010. The pulmonary circulation and exercise responses in the elderly. Semin. Respir. Crit. Care Med. 31, 528–538.

Taylor, B.J., Romer, L.M., 2008. Effect of expiratory muscle fatigue on exercise tolerance and locomotor muscle fatigue in healthy humans. J. Appl. Physiol. 104, 1442–1451.

Taylor, B.J., Romer, L.M., 2009. Effect of expiratory resistive loading on inspiratory and expiratory muscle fatigue. Respir. Physiol. Neurobiol. 166, 164–174.

Taylor, B.J., How, S.C., Romer, L.M., 2006. Exercise-induced abdominal muscle fatigue in healthy humans. J. Appl. Physiol. 100 (5), 1554–1562.

Taylor, B.J., West, C.R., Romer, L.M., 2010. No effect of arm-crank exercise on diaphragmatic fatigue or ventilatory constraint in Paralympic athletes with cervical spinal cord injury. J. Appl. Physiol. 109, 358–366.

Taylor-Cousar, J.L., 2009. Hypoventilation in cystic fibrosis. Semin. Respir. Crit. Care Med. 30, 293–302.

Terakado, S., Takeuchi, T., Miura, T., et al., 1999. Early occurrence of respiratory muscle deoxygenation assessed by near-infrared spectroscopy during leg exercise in patients with chronic heart failure. Jpn. Circ. J. 63, 97–103.

Terzano, C., Ceccarelli, D., Conti, V., et al., 2008. Maximal respiratory static pressures in patients with different stages of COPD severity. Respir. Res. 9, 8.

Travers, J., Dudgeon, D.J., Amjadi, K., et al., 2008. Mechanisms of exertional dyspnea in patients with cancer. J. Appl. Physiol. 104, 57–66.

Tsatsouline, P., 2000. Power to the people!: Russian strength training secrets for every American. Dragon Door Publications, St Paul, MN.

van der Esch, M., van 't Hul,, A.J., Heijmans, M., et al., 2004. Respiratory muscle performance as a possible determinant of exercise capacity in patients with ankylosing spondylitis. Aust. J. Physiother 50, 41–45.

van der Palen, J., Rea, T.D., Manolio, T.A., et al., 2004. Respiratory muscle strength and the risk of incident cardiovascular events. Thorax 59, 1063–1067.

van Lunteren, E., Moyer, M., 2003. Streptozotocin-diabetes alters action potentials in rat diaphragm. Respir. Physiol. Neurobiol. 135, 9–16.

Vassilakopoulos, T., Zakynthinos, S., Roussos, C., 1998. The tension-time index and the frequency/tidal volume ratio are the major pathophysiologic determinants of weaning failure and success. Am. J. Respir. Crit. Care Med. 158, 378–385.

Verges, S., Schulz, C., Perret, C., Spengler, C.M., 2006. Impaired abdominal muscle contractility after high-intensity exhaustive exercise assessed by magnetic stimulation. Muscle Nerve 34, 423–430.

Vibarel, N., Hayot, M., Pellenc, P.M., et al., 1998. Non-invasive assessment of inspiratory muscle performance during exercise in patients with chronic heart failure. Eur. Heart J. 19, 766–773.

Vogiatzis, I., Habazettl, H., Aliverti, A., et al., 2011. Effect of helium breathing on intercostal and quadriceps muscle blood flow during exercise in COPD patients. Am. J. Physiol. Regul. Integr. Comp. Physiol. 300, R1549–R1559.

Volianitis, S., McConnell, A.K., Koutedakis, Y., et al., 2001. Inspiratory muscle training improves rowing performance. Med. Sci. Sports Exerc. 33, 803–809.

Wang, H.Y., Chen, C.C., Hsiao, S.F., 2012. Relationships between respiratory muscle strength and daily living function in children with cerebral palsy. Res. Dev. Disabil. 33, 1176–1182.

Wanke, T., Formanek, D., Auinger, M., et al., 1991. Inspiratory muscle performance and pulmonary function changes in insulin-dependent diabetes mellitus. Am. Rev. Respir. Dis. 143, 97–100.

Wanke, T., Formanek, D., Auinger, M., et al., 1992. Mechanical load on the inspiratory muscles during exercise hyperpnea in patients with type 1 (insulin-dependent) diabetes mellitus. Diabetologia 35, 425–428.

Watson, A.C., Hughes, P.D., Louise Harris, M., et al., 2001. Measurement of twitch transdiaphragmatic, esophageal, and endotracheal tube pressure with bilateral anterolateral magnetic phrenic nerve stimulation in patients in the intensive care unit. Crit. Care Med. 29, 1325–1331.

Weiner, P., Suo, J., Fernandez, E., et al., 1990. The effect of hyperinflation on respiratory muscle strength and efficiency in healthy subjects and patients with asthma. Am. Rev. Respir. Dis. 141, 1501–1505.

Weiner, P., Azgad, Y., Weiner, M., 1993. The effect of corticosteroids on inspiratory muscle performance in humans. Chest 104, 1788–1791.

Weiner, P., Azgad, Y., Weiner, M., 1995. Inspiratory muscle training during treatment with corticosteroids in humans. Chest 107, 1041–1044.

Weiner, P., Waizman, J., Weiner, M., et al., 1998. Influence of excessive weight loss after gastroplasty for morbid obesity on respiratory muscle performance. Thorax 53, 39–42.

Weiner, P., Magadle, R., Beckerman, M., et al., 2002. The relationship among inspiratory muscle strength, the perception of dyspnea and inhaled beta$_2$-agonist use in patients with asthma. Can. Respir. J. 9, 307–312.

Welsh, L., Roberts, R.G., Kemp, J.G., 2004. Fitness and physical activity in children with asthma. Sports Med. 34, 861–870.

Wetter, T.J., Harms, C.A., Nelson, W.B., et al., 1999. Influence of respiratory muscle work on VO(2) and leg blood flow during submaximal exercise. J. Appl. Physiol. 87, 643–651.

Widimsky, J., Riedel, M., Stanek, V., 1977. Central haemodynamics during exercise in patients with restrictive pulmonary disease. Bull. Eur. Physiopathol. Respir. 13, 369–379.

Wilbur, K., Makowsky, M., 2004. Colchicine myotoxicity: case reports and literature review. Pharmacotherapy 24, 1784–1792.

Wilkerson, L.A., 1998. Exercise-induced asthma. J. Am. Osteopath. Assoc. 98, 211–215.

Wilson, J.R., Mancini, D.M., 1993. Factors contributing to the exercise limitation of heart failure. J. Am. Coll. Cardiol. 22, 93A–98A.

Wirnsberger, R.M., Drent, M., Hekelaar, N., et al., 1997. Relationship between respiratory muscle function and quality of life in sarcoidosis. Eur. Respir. J. 10, 1450–1455.

Wright, R.S., Levine, M.S., Bellamy, P.E., et al., 1990. Ventilatory and diffusion abnormalities in potential heart transplant recipients. Chest 98, 816–820.

Yan, S., Kaminski, D., Sliwinski, P., 1997. Inspiratory muscle mechanics of patients with chronic obstructive pulmonary disease during incremental exercise. Am. J. Respir. Crit. Care Med. 156, 807–813.

Yap, J.C., Watson, R.A., Gilbey, S., et al., 1995. Effects of posture on respiratory mechanics in obesity. J. Appl. Physiol. 79, 1199–1205.

Zerah, F., Harf, A., Perlemuter, L., et al., 1993. Effects of obesity on respiratory resistance. Chest 103, 1470–1476.

Ziora, K., Ziora, D., Oswiecimska, J., et al., 2008. Spirometric parameters in malnourished girls with anorexia nervosa. J. Physiol. Pharmacol. 59 (Suppl. 6), 801–807.

Chapter 4

Functional benefits of respiratory muscle training

The rationale for training any muscle is the presence of a functional overload. In Chapter 3 we explored the concept that particular disease conditions are associated with imbalance in the demand/capacity relationship of the respiratory pump muscles, i.e., a functional overload. Disease creates imbalance by altering the resistances and elastances that must be overcome during breathing, and the capacity of the respiratory muscles to meet these mechanical demands. For example, patients with chronic obstructive pulmonary disease (COPD) experience a 'double whammy' because their inspiratory muscles are weakened, and the demand for inspiratory work of breathing is increased. However, in other situations inspiratory muscle function may be normal, but the respiratory pump may be operating in the context of a transient increased demand, e.g., mild asthma. Thus, a muscle might be considered 'normal' in absolute terms, but if the demands that are placed upon a 'normal muscle' are supranormal then it is weak functionally. For example, a morbidly obese person with normal quadriceps muscle strength is functionally weak. Chapter 3 thus explored the rationale for specific training of the respiratory pump muscles in a range of conditions, as well as considering how the work of breathing contributes to exercise limitation in health and disease.

The purpose of the current chapter is to explore how respiratory muscles respond to specific training. It will begin by considering these responses at the structural and functional level of the muscle. A brief review of whole-body responses to respiratory muscle training (RMT) in healthy young athletes will follow, thereby helping to set the scene for responses to RMT in specific disease conditions. Detailed analysis of the different methods of RMT, and the specific adaptations that they elicit, can be found in Chapter 5.

RESPIRATORY MUSCLE RESPONSES TO RMT

Essentially, muscles adapt to training by changing their structure, the result of which is to induce changes in muscle function. For example, when weights are lifted the muscle fibres hypertrophy and the strength of the muscle increases. In contrast, if a muscle is subjected to prolonged, continuous bouts of low-intensity muscle loading, e.g., running, muscle fibres undergo structural and biochemical changes that increase their endurance (see Ch. 2). Broadly speaking, therefore, training can be subdivided into two main types: one that increases strength, and the other that increases endurance. However, there is a great deal of potential for hybridization of training responses in the middle ground between these extremes. In Chapter 5, the training principles of 'overload', 'specificity' and 'reversibility' will be considered in detail, as well as the methods and equipment used to implement respiratory muscle training (RMT). For the purposes of the current chapter, a very brief explanation of training methods follows.

As one might expect, the equipment and methods required to implement strength and endurance training of the respiratory muscles differ considerably. It is akin to comparing a leg press machine with a treadmill: both machines train the leg muscles, but the training and functional outcomes are very different. In the case of specific inspiratory and expiratory muscle strength training, devices are used to impose a resistance to the respiratory muscles at the mouth (like lifting a dumbbell). In contrast, respiratory muscle endurance training consists of hyperventilating for prolonged periods of time (like running on a treadmill). In the case of respiratory muscle endurance training, it is not possible to separate inspiratory and expiratory muscle contributions, so this method trains both sets of muscles simultaneously. Training principles, methods and equipment will be explored in greater detail in Chapter 5. However, in the mean time, the preceding explanation provides a working knowledge of specific RMT.

The following section explores the adaptations that have been measured in respiratory muscles. The evidence is derived from studies of human beings only, and includes evidence from both patients and healthy young adults. The differentiation of RMT as either inspiratory, expiratory or both is made very deliberately by referring to IMT, EMT or RMT, respectively. Thus, where the discussion relates to specifically to IMT or EMT, these terms are used; where the discussion is more generic, the term RMT is used.

Structural adaptations to RMT

The data pertaining to structural adaptations following RMT are derived from studies employing two forms of measurement: firstly, analysis of muscle biopsy samples taken from patients and secondly ultrasound measurements of muscle thickness derived from both patients and healthy people. This evidence is currently confined to inspiratory muscles following resistance training.

Patients

At the time of writing, the only study to have obtained inspiratory muscle biopsy samples pre- and post-RMT is that of Ramirez-Sarmiento and colleagues from patients with COPD (Ramirez-Sarmiento et al, 2002). Their randomized controlled trial sampled muscle fibres from the external (inspiratory) intercostal muscles before and after 5 weeks of pressure threshold IMT (see Ch. 5). The training regimen had an endurance training bias (30 minutes training, 5 days per week at a load of 40–50% of maximal inspiratory pressure [MIP]), and patients showed a corresponding increase in the proportion of type I muscle fibres (fatigue-resistant fibres), and a decrease in the proportion of type II fibres. Both fibre types showed an increase in fibre cross-sectional area (hypertrophy), especially the type II fibres. Patients' inspiratory muscle strength increased, as assessed by MIP (see Ch. 6, 'Assessment of respiratory muscle function'), as did the ability to breathe continuously against an external load (endurance).

The response of the diaphragm to IMT has also been studied using ultrasound imaging and measurement of diaphragm thickness in patients with chronic heart failure (CHF) and in those with cystic fibrosis (CF). In patients with CHF and inspiratory muscle weakness ($MIP \leq 60\%$

predicted), 4 weeks of pressure threshold IMT (30 minutes daily at 30% of MIP) elicited a 55% increase in diaphragm thickness and a 72% increase in MIP (Chiappa et al, 2008b). The fact that the patients had pre-existing weakness may explain the particularly large improvements observed following IMT in this group. Diaphragm thickness has also been shown to increase after IMT in patients with CF. After 8 weeks of high-intensity incremental flow-resistive loading (80% of MIP), diaphragm thickness increased by 19%, whilst MIP increased by 18% (Enright et al, 2004).

Healthy people

In healthy young people, the only data available on structural adaptations are derived from measuring diaphragm thickness using ultrasound. Contracted diaphragm thickness increases $\sim 12\%$ following 4 to 8 weeks of inspiratory muscle resistance training (Enright et al, 2006; Downey et al, 2007). As would be expected, the increase in thickness was accompanied by improvements in MIP (24% and 41% after 4 and 8 weeks of training, respectively). Interestingly, the same magnitude of change in diaphragm thickness was observed after 4 and 8 weeks of training, yet changes in MIP differed. This clearly indicates that diaphragm hypertrophy is not the only source of improvement in MIP, which can also improve through improvements in accessory muscle function as well as neural adaptations. These neural adaptations include an enhanced ability to coordinate the contraction of synergistic muscles, as well as an enhanced ability to maximize the activation of individual muscles. It should also be noted that the 4- and 8-week studies employed different training techniques, i.e., pressure threshold (Downey et al, 2007) and incremental flow-resistive loading (Enright et al, 2006), respectively. See Chapter 5 for details of each training method.

In keeping with its key role as a postural control and core-stabilizing muscle, diaphragm thickness and inspiratory muscle strength have also been shown to increase following 16 weeks of sit-up and bicep curl training (DePalo et al, 2004). The training stimulus to the diaphragm in this study derived from the increases in transdiaphragmatic pressure that resulted from its role as a postural and core-stabilizing muscle. Participants undertook sit-up and bicep curl training 3–4 times per week, for 16 weeks. Expiratory muscle strength increased 37%, which is to be expected as rectus abdominis is an important expiratory muscle. These data highlight the close interrelationship of the breathing and postural stabilizing functions of the trunk muscles, thereby reinforcing the potential benefits of applying functional training techniques to the respiratory muscles (see Ch. 3, 'Non-respiratory functions of the respiratory muscles'). Diaphragm thickness and respiratory muscle strength have also been shown to be greater in healthy active elderly people than in their more sedentary counterparts

(Summerhill et al, 2007). As expected, MIP correlated with diaphragm thickness. These data add further support to the notion that non-respiratory activities generate a training stimulus to the respiratory muscles.

Collectively, these data from patients and healthy people present a picture of the inspiratory muscles as a highly adaptable tissue showing hypertrophy and fibre-type shifts that are consistent with the well-established evidence relating to limb-muscle training. These changes appear to occur similarly in both healthy people and in patients. The data also indicate that respiratory muscles are trained by a variety of overloading stimuli (see also Ch. 5, 'Methods of respiratory muscle training'). In the following section the functional adaptations to RMT will be considered. The section is divided into subsections addressing different training types (resistance or endurance) and muscle groups (inspiratory, expiratory, or both).

Functional adaptations to RMT

Principally, muscles respond to training by improving their strength, speed of contraction, power output and/or endurance. Because muscles respond to training stimuli in highly specific ways (see Ch. 5, 'Methods of respiratory muscle training'), different training regimens tend to elicit slightly different changes in each property. For example, training that consists of maximal, static efforts with high force improves strength, but not contraction speed (Romer & McConnell, 2003). However, there is also a good

deal of cross-over, such that training regimens that are ostensibly strength orientated can also give rise to improvements in endurance, but generally not vice versa (see Ch. 5, 'Specificity'). The following section describes what is known about improvements in each functional property following resistance training.

A helpful method of characterizing the functional properties of muscles is to plot a graph of the relationship between strength and contraction speed; the so-called force–velocity relationship (see also Ch. 5, 'Specificity'). It is also possible to add a third dimension to this in the form of muscle power output, which is the product of force and velocity. Figure 4.1 illustrates these interrelationships for the inspiratory muscles, and encapsulates the three key and interrelated functional properties of muscles (strength, speed and power), all of which can be modified by appropriate training.

Inspiratory muscle adaptations to resistance training

The most widely studied muscles are those of inspiration, the functional properties of which have been characterized extensively. As was described above, inspiratory muscle training (IMT) elicits hypertrophy and improvements in strength, and the reader is referred elsewhere for systematic review of the extensive evidence base drawn from both patients and healthy people (Geddes et al, 2008; Gosselink et al, 2011; Hajghanbari et al, 2012; Illi et al,

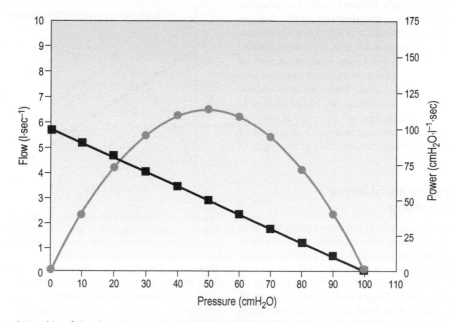

Figure 4.1 Interrelationship of the three key properties of inspiratory muscles: pressure (strength), flow (velocity) and power (strength × velocity). Squares = pressure/flow; circles = pressure/power.
(Adapted from McConnell AK, 2011. Breathe strong, perform better. Human Kinetics, Champaign, IL, with permission.)

2012; Plentz et al, 2012; Smart et al, 2012). When IMT is undertaken using moderate loads (~60% of MIP) that allow rapid muscle shortening, improvements in strength are accompanied in healthy people by increases in maximal shortening velocity (peak inspiratory flow rate) and maximal power (Tzelepis et al, 1994; Tzelepis et al, 1999; Romer & McConnell, 2003). Moderate loads can typically be sustained for ~30 breaths, and have also been shown to improve endurance significantly in healthy people (Caine & McConnell, 1998a). In most studies of resistance IMT a placebo has been used, which typically consists of 30 to 60 breaths at a load of 15% of MIP. The latter has been used repeatedly as an IMT placebo in healthy people as it creates a perceptible resistance, but does not elicit any significant changes in inspiratory muscle function (Volianitis et al, 2001; Romer et al, 2002a; Romer et al, 2002b; Bailey et al, 2010; Brown et al, 2011; Turner et al, 2011; Turner et al, 2012).

Figure 4.2 illustrates the significant changes in strength, peak inspiratory flow and power induced by different IMT regimens in healthy people. It is clear that different types of training induce changes in different functional properties, and this is explored in more detail in Chapter 5 (section on 'Specificity'), which describes the specificity principle of training, i.e., muscles adapt according to the nature of the training stimulus. For example, it is clear from Figure 4.2 that high-pressure training (maximum static muscle contractions) improves strength, but not velocity of shortening. The opposite was true for high-flow training (unloaded maximal inhalations). No such changes are observed after placebo IMT.

As mentioned earlier, strength training can also improve endurance. There is no single accepted method of assessing endurance, but, borrowing the methods used to assess whole-body exercise tolerance, IMT improves inspiratory muscle endurance measured using tests employing continuous incremental and fixed-intensity loading, as well as tests requiring the maintenance of maximal hyperventilation (see below and Ch. 6, section 'Assessment of respiratory muscle function'). In addition, an improvement in endurance after IMT can be implied from the absence or attenuation of fatigue following a task that had previously induced fatigue, which also occurs after IMT in healthy people (Romer et al, 2002d).

Expiratory muscle adaptations to resistance training

Expiratory muscle training (EMT) has been much less widely studied, but there is good-quality evidence, primarily from patients, that maximal expiratory pressure (MEP) improves significantly in response to specific EMT (19–56%) (Smeltzer et al, 1996; Sapienza et al, 2002; Weiner et al, 2003b; Baker et al, 2005; Chiara et al, 2007; Mota et al, 2007; Kim et al, 2008; Roth et al, 2010). In a particularly comprehensive study on patients with COPD, IMT, EMT

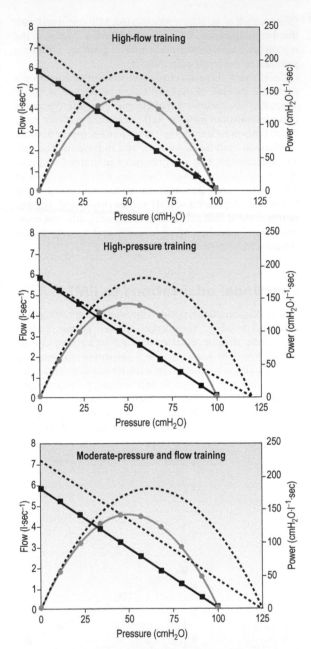

Figure 4.2 Changes in pressure (strength), flow (velocity) and power (strength × velocity) in response to different training stimuli. Dotted lines = post-training; straight lines = pressure/velocity; curved lines = pressure/power.
(Data derived from Romer LM, McConnell AK, 2003. Med. Sci. Sports Exerc. 35, 237–244. Adapted from McConnell AK, 2011. Breathe strong, perform better. Human Kinetics, Champaign, IL, with permission.)

and EMT + IMT were studied in three separate, matched groups of patients as well as a fourth placebo control group (Weiner et al, 2003a); this study is unique in that an identical training device and training regimen was used for all of the training. In addition, the IMT and EMT groups received placebo training immediately after their real training session in order to mimic the experience of the EMT + IMT group, who undertook EMT followed immediately by IMT. Following 3 months of IMT the MIP improved significantly by 25%, whereas following EMT the MEP improved significantly by 20%. In the group that undertook EMT + IMT, both MIP and MEP improved significantly by 33%, suggesting that there may be a small potentiation of the training effect when EMT is followed by IMT. Indeed, the IMT and EMT groups both showed small, non-significant increases in maximal pressures for the placebo phase of their training ($\sim$5%), suggesting a small training effect. In addition, expiratory endurance performance (breathing against an incremental pressure load) improved significantly by 31% following EMT, and significantly by 25% following EMT + IMT, whereas inspiratory endurance improved significantly by 25% following IMT, and significantly by 33% following EMT + IMT. Collectively, these data suggest that, in patients with COPD, expiratory muscles respond in an identical manner to inspiratory muscles when the same training stimulus is applied.

A caveat that is worthy of mention is the 'purity', or otherwise, of EMT. A number of studies on patients purporting to undertake EMT have documented improvements in MIP as well as MEP (Roth et al, 2010). On the face of it, this might imply a placebo effect in both groups; however, the effect has been demonstrated in placebo-controlled trials in which there were no significant changes in the placebo groups (Roth et al, 2010). Furthermore, a study that examined the acute responses of inspiratory and expiratory muscles to expiratory loading in healthy people found that it induced a significant decrease in both MIP and MEP, i.e., fatigue (Taylor & Romer, 2009). In other words, expiratory loading also loads the inspiratory muscles. This presumably occurs because of the requirement for inspiratory muscle activation during forceful expiratory efforts. In healthy people, this 'contamination' of the training stimulus does not appear to be present during inspiratory loading and IMT, where there is no change in MEP (Romer et al, 2002b; Griffiths & McConnell, 2007), but responses are more variable in patients. For example, patients with spinal cord injury and renal failure show no change in MEP after IMT (Rutchik et al, 1998; Silva et al, 2011), but patients with CHF and multiple sclerosis show a significant increase (Cahalin et al, 1997; Klefbeck & Hamrah Nedjad, 2003). It is possible that these discrepancies are explained by variations in the baseline strength of expiratory muscles and the extent to which they are recruited to lower end-expiratory lung volume during IMT.

Adaptations to simultaneous inspiratory and expiratory muscle resistance training

One might predict that combining IMT and EMT within the same breath cycle (concurrent IMT and EMT) would result in improvements in function in both muscle groups. However, the results of two studies in healthy people that have implemented concurrent training suggest that this approach impairs training responses. For example, a study in young swimmers found no significant change in MIP or MEP despite a strenuous, progressive training regimen (Wells et al, 2005). Similarly, a study on rowers found only modest changes at best in MIP and MEP (Griffiths & McConnell, 2007). Participants generally reported that they found the simultaneous loading of both breath cycles uncomfortable, and that it was impossible to train with maximal effort when both breathing phases are loaded. This may be because of the training stimulus 'contamination' effect described in the previous paragraph. However, one study of healthy elderly people has demonstrated significant increases of 22% and 30% in MIP and MEP, respectively, following 8 weeks of concurrent IMT and EMT (Watsford & Murphy, 2008).

Functional adaptations to respiratory endurance training

Pure endurance training of the respiratory muscles is undertaken using a sustained, high-intensity hyperpnoea task (see Ch. 5, 'Methods of respiratory muscle training'), and has been used much less widely than resistance training, especially in patients. Hyperpnoea training recruits both inspiratory and expiratory muscles simultaneously and, unlike IMT, its nature makes a true placebo difficult to implement. Accordingly, trials have typically included a 'no training' control group rather than a placebo group. In healthy people and patients, the training significantly improves the ability to sustain high levels of hyperventilation (an index of endurance) (Scherer et al, 2000; Illi et al, 2012). In healthy people, the training also improves the volume of air that can be respired during a brief maximal burst of hyperventilation, typically 15 seconds (an index of power output) (Verges et al, 2008; Illi et al, 2012). The latter finding is also consistent with improvements in peak velocity of muscle contraction, although there is no direct evidence of this to date. This type of training does not improve the strength of the respiratory muscles in healthy people (Verges et al, 2008; Illi et al, 2012), which is not surprising since the training stimulus required to improve strength must include an increase in the force of muscle contraction (see Ch. 5, section 'Specificity'). However, in patients with COPD, a small but significant increase in MEP has been shown in one study (Scherer et al, 2000). This may be explained by the presence of expiratory flow limitation in patients with COPD, which creates an expiratory flow resistive load during hyperpnoea. Thus, in the absence of expiratory flow limitation, functional adaptations are typically confined to flow, power and endurance.

Summary

Respiratory muscles respond to training stimuli in the same manner as other skeletal muscles, i.e., by undergoing adaptations to their structure and function that are specific to the training stimulus (see Ch. 5, section 'Specificity'). Depending upon the training protocol implemented, functional adaptations to respiratory muscle resistance training can include improvement in all four muscle properties, viz., strength, speed of shortening, power output and endurance. Training regimens employing moderate loads (50–60%) sustained to the limit of tolerance (typically 30 breaths) have been shown to generate the widest range of functional benefits (Romer & McConnell, 2003). Expiratory muscle adaptations have been less comprehensively studied, but it is likely that the expiratory muscles respond to training in a similar manner to the inspiratory muscles. Attempts to resistance train both inspiratory and expiratory muscles simultaneously have so far proved impractical, and appear to yield inferior results to loading inhalation and exhalation separately. Specific respiratory muscle endurance training improves speed, power and endurance, but not strength, unless expiratory flow limitation is present thereby creating an expiratory resistive load.

Improving the function of the respiratory muscles is only the first step on the road to a useful clinical intervention. The most important steps on this journey are the changes in functional and clinical outcomes that follow this first step. In the next section, the physiological changes that are stimulated by RMT in healthy young people will be considered. This will be followed by consideration of the disease-specific responses to RMT in a range of clinical conditions.

RESPONSES TO RMT IN HEALTHY PEOPLE

In the first section of this chapter, we considered the structural and functional adaptations elicited by specific training of the respiratory muscles. In Chapter 3 we discovered how breathing limits exercise performance in a range of disease conditions, including performance in sports people. In this section we will see how the muscle adaptations described above overcome the limitations to sports performance described in Chapter 3. This will set the scene for a review of the evidence relating to the clinical benefits of RMT for patients in the final section of this chapter.

To get the most from this chapter, it is desirable (but not essential) to have an understanding of breathing-related limitations to exercise performance in healthy people (as described in Ch. 3). In short, there appear to be two major influences arising from the respiratory pump muscles that can cause athletes to slow down or stop exercise: (1) the perception of breathing effort and (2) the consequences of activation of the group III and IV afferents within the inspiratory muscles. The former makes exercise feel more difficult, and it intensifies as the inspiratory muscles become fatigued; the latter reduces limb blood flow, hastens limb fatigue and exacerbates the perception of limb and whole-body effort.

Logically, making the respiratory muscles stronger and more fatigue resistant should delay or abolish the negative influences of breathing upon exercise tolerance. But what is the scientific evidence supporting this, how big are any improvements and what types of activities are improved? The following description of the published literature is subdivided into two subsections, depending upon the type of performance outcome measure tested: (1) time trials and test of endurance, and (2) tests of anaerobic endurance and sprinting. In addition, this section will consider a study of healthy young people in which the physiological responses to hypoxic conditions were examined before and after RMT. The latter has some bearing on patients with hypoxaemia such as those with COPD. For an overview of the entire evidence base relating to RMT in healthy people, readers are referred to Illi et al's (2012) systematic review of RMT. This detailed analysis of some 46 original studies of RMT included both strength and endurance RMT, revealing 'significant improvement in performance after RMT, which was detected by constant load tests, time trials, and intermittent incremental tests, but not by [continuous] incremental tests'. Below is a description of the types of performance tests employed in athletes, as well as a summary of the key papers that have evaluated RMT in athletes.

Influence of RMT upon time trials and tests of endurance

Most of the studies of respiratory muscle training (RMT) in healthy people have examined endurance sports, and two types of exercise tests have been used: fixed-intensity exercise undertaken to the limit of tolerance (T_{lim}) and time trials. The majority have been randomized placebo-controlled trials; unfortunately, some weaker studies with either a simple no-training control or no control at all have found their way into the literature (Illi et al, 2012). However, only placebo-controlled and controlled trials are considered within this section.

There are no competitive events that require athletes to keep going at the same intensity for as long as they can (a T_{lim} test), but this type of test does provide an excellent laboratory model for studying the effects of 'ergogenic aids' such as RMT (i.e., interventions that purport to improve performance). This is because T_{lim} tests are extremely sensitive to small physiological improvements, they yield large changes (typically greater than 30%) and they allow physiological and perceptual responses to be studied under identical conditions before and after the intervention. In contrast, the obvious advantage of using a time trial to assess performance is that it simulates a race. However, for this very reason the magnitude of the changes that are typically observed after ergogenic interventions is extremely small, typically less than 5% (Currell & Jeukendrup, 2008). In addition, it is impossible to compare physiological responses in a meaningful way before and after the intervention using a time trial because the exercise conditions are not identical. For example, if performance is enhanced post-RMT, athletes will be working at a greater intensity, which cannot then be compared with the pre-intervention test. Both types of tests have provided useful insights into the effects of RMT.

Typically T_{lim} tests are conducted at intensities that are just above the lactate threshold. The ability to sustain exercise above the lactate threshold is limited, and the more the intensity of exercise exceeds the lactate threshold the sooner is the onset of exercise intolerance. Studies on RMT have used exercise intensities that can be tolerated for 20 to 40 minutes. In contrast, time trials have varied considerably depending on the sport being studied; for example, studies have used as little as 1 minute for swimming, and as much as 1 hour for cycling.

Studies that have used resistance training of the respiratory muscles (see Ch. 5) have done so using cycling, rowing, swimming and running modalities. In the case of cycling and running, this has been undertaken using both T_{lim} tests and time trials. For rowing and swimming, only time trials have been used. Table 4.1 summarizes the findings of placebo-controlled studies. Many more studies than those presented have been conducted, but their quality is variable (Illi et al, 2012) so the table is limited to those with robust designs.

Table 4.1 indicates clearly that inspiratory muscle training (IMT) produces statistically significant improvements in performance, but that expiratory muscle training (EMT) does not. As demonstrated statistically by Illi et al (2012), performance improvements occur whether tested using time trials (1.7% to 4.6% improvement for tests lasting 1 to 60 minutes), or T_{lim} tests (greater than 30% improvement for a 30-minute test). For higher-intensity, shorter-duration T_{lim} tests, the improvements are smaller (~4% for a test lasting less than 4 minutes). This difference in the size of the improvements occurs because of differences in the factors that lead to people stopping exercise and the rate at which these factors accumulate and lead to intolerance (Currell & Jeukendrup, 2008).

Endurance training of the respiratory muscles involves hyperventilation at high levels for prolonged periods

(see Ch. 5). Table 4.2 summarizes the controlled and placebo-controlled trials using endurance RMT. Despite the profound difference in the training method, the results are strikingly similar to those for resistance IMT, a finding confirmed statistically by Illi and colleagues (Illi et al, 2012). Typically, T_{lim} increases by 20% to 50%, whereas a time trial shows ~4% improvement. This similarity is quite unlike the response to whole-body endurance and resistance training, which suggests that breathing muscle training taps into a unique and profoundly important mechanism. As was described in the Chapter 3, the most likely candidate mechanism for this effect is an increase in the threshold for activation of the inspiratory muscle metaboreflex.

It is impossible to separate the inspiratory and expiratory effects of hyperventilation training, but when this has been done for resistance training the independent roles of the two groups of muscles in performance changes become clear (Griffiths & McConnell, 2007): only IMT improves performance. Indeed, adding EMT to IMT during the same breath cycle seems to impair inspiratory muscle responses to IMT (Griffiths & McConnell, 2007) and to negate any performance benefits (Wells et al, 2005), which provides a strong argument against using this approach or, perhaps, undertaking EMT in healthy young people at all.

Tables 4.1 and 4.2 also summarize some of the physiological changes that accompany RMT, and these help to shed some light on the potential mechanisms that do, and do not, lead to the improvement in performance. Specifically, after IMT there are no changes in the 'usual suspects' underpinning improved exercise performance after training, viz., maximal oxygen uptake ($\dot{V}O_{2max}$) and lactate threshold (see Ch. 2). Since breathing does not limit oxygen diffusion (see Ch. 1), we would not expect $\dot{V}O_{2max}$ to improve. However, the absence of a change in lactate threshold is slightly puzzling given that IMT reduces blood lactate concentrations $[La]_b$ during exercise at equivalent intensities (see Tables 4.1 and 4.2). It seems that IMT reduces $[La]_b$, but not the intensity of exercise at which accumulation commences, or indeed the critical power, which is a functional correlate of the lactate threshold (Johnson et al, 2007). The mechanism by which steady state $[La]_b$ is reduced without an accompanying change in the lactate threshold is an intriguing one. It is common for different people to have different steady-state lactate concentrations but very similar lactate thresholds, so it is clear that the $[La]_b$ per se is not a determinant of the lactate threshold. There is good evidence that IMT increases the metabolic potential of the inspiratory muscles, and thus their ability to consume lactate during submaximal exercise (Brown et al, 2011). One might also hypothesize a lower production of lactate by locomotor muscles due to enhanced oxygen delivery, which could arise because of a reduction in sympathetic vasoconstriction. However, improving oxygen delivery in sub-elite athletes by inhaling an oxygen-rich inspirate does not enhance their lactate

Table 4.1 Placebo-controlled studies of the influence of resistance breathing muscle training upon endurance performance

Type of training	Exercise modality	Type of exercise test	Duration/intensity of test	Training duration (weeks)	Performance change (%)	Physiological changes in training group	Comments	Authors
Resistance IMT	Cycling	T_{lim}	21 min	4	33*	Attenuation of $[La]_b$* and RPE*		Caine & McConnell, 1998b
Resistance IMT	Cycling	TT	20 km and 40 km (~30 and ~60 min)	6	20 km = 3.8* 40 km = 4.6*	Attenuation of breathing* and leg effort*	Inspiratory muscle fatigue also attenuated*	Romer et al, 2002c
Resistance IMT	Cycling	T_{lim}	75% $\dot{V}O_{2max}$	10	36*	Attenuated f_c*, $\dot{V}_E$* and perception of effort*		Gething et al, 2004
Resistance IMT	Cycling	TT	25 km (36 min)	6	2.6*		Inspiratory muscle fatigue also attenuated*	Johnson et al, 2007
Resistance IMT	Cycling	T_{lim}	Severe Maximal	4	Severe = 39* Maximal = 18*	$\dot{V}O_2$ kinetics accelerated* and $[La]_b$* lower during severe exercise	Inspiratory muscle fatigue also attenuated*	Bailey et al, 2010
Resistance IMT	Running	T_{lim}	3.8 min	4	4*			Edwards & Cooke, 2004
Resistance IMT	Running	TT	5000 m (~20 min)	4	2*	Attenuation of RPE*		Edwards et al, 2008
Resistance IMT	Rowing	TT	6 min and ~20 min (~2 km and 5 km)	4 and 11	2 km = 1.9* 5 km = 2.2*	Attenuation of $[La]_b$* and breathing effort* and increased V_T*	Performance improved at 4 and ~1 weeks. Inspiratory muscle fatigue also attenuated	Volianitis et al, 2001
Resistance IMT + EMT	Rowing	TT	6 min (~2 km)	4 and 10	2.7*	Attenuated f_c*, $[La]_b$* and perception of breathing effort*	Performance and other outcomes only improved in response to IMT. Inspiratory muscle fatigue also attenuated*	Griffiths & McConnell, 2007
Resistance IMT	Swimming	TT	100 m (~1 min) 200 m (~2 min) 400 m (~4.4 min)	6	1.7* 1.5* No change	Attenuation of RPE*	No change in performance over 400 m	Kilding et al, 2010

IMT = inspiratory muscle training; EMT = expiratory muscle training; RMT = respiratory muscle training; T_{lim} = fixed intensity to the limit of tolerance; TT = time trial; $\dot{V}O_2$ = oxygen uptake; $\dot{V}O_{2max}$ = maximal oxygen uptake; f_c = heart rate; $\dot{V}_E$ = minute ventilation; V_T = tidal volume; $[La]_b$ = blood lactate concentration; RPE = rating of perceived exertion.

* $p < 0.05$.

Table 4.2 Controlled studies of the influence of endurance breathing muscle training upon endurance performance

Type of training	Exercise modality	Type of exercise test	Duration/ intensity of test	Training duration (weeks)	Performance change (%)	Physiological changes in training group	Comments	Author
Endurance RMT	Cycling	T_{lim}	70% peak power	15	24*		No placebo group, just non-RMT control group	Markov et al, 2001
Endurance RMT	Cycling	T_{lim}	70% peak power	15	24*		No placebo group, just non-RMT control group	Stuessi et al, 2001
Endurance RMT	Cycling	T_{lim}	85% peak power	4–6	~20*		No placebo group, just non-RMT control group	McMahon et al, 2002
Endurance RMT	Cycling	TT	40 min	6	4.70*			Holm et al, 2004
Endurance RMT	Running	TT and T_{lim}	TT = 4 miles T_{lim} = 80% $\dot{V}_{2max}$	4	TT = 4* T_{lim} = 50*	Attenuated $\dot{V}_E$*, $\dot{V}_{O_2}$*, $[La]_b$*		Leddy et al, 2007

RMT = respiratory muscle training; T_{lim} = fixed intensity to the limit of tolerance; TT = time trial; $\dot{V}_{O_2}$ = oxygen uptake; $\dot{V}_{O_2max}$ = maximal oxygen uptake; $\dot{V}_E$ = minute ventilation; $[La]_b$ = blood lactate concentration.

* $p < 0.05$.

threshold (Sadowsky et al, 1995). Thus the most likely explanation for the lower steady state $[La]_b$ without a change in the lactate threshold is enhanced consumption of lactate by the inspiratory muscles (Peter Brown & Graham Sharpe, personal communication). However, this does not imply that an improved muscle blood flow is redundant. Enhancing muscle blood flow by manipulating the work of breathing reduces exercise-induced locomotor muscle contractile fatigue (Romer et al, 2006). Furthermore, the removal of muscle metabolites may also influence the central contribution to fatigue (see Ch. 1, 'Mechanisms of fatigue').

So far as the factors that *do* change after IMT are concerned, these include reductions in $[La]_b$, heart rate, and perception of breathing and limb effort, as well as a speeding of oxygen uptake kinetics during heavy exercise. In addition, breathing becomes deeper and slower, as well as more metabolically efficient (Turner et al, 2012). Perhaps most importantly, IMT delays or abolishes the exercise-induced decrease in MIP observed post-exercise, i.e., IMT attenuates inspiratory muscle fatigue (Romer et al, 2002d). These changes are all consistent with the respiratory-related exercise-limiting factors described in Chapter 3. The attenuation of inspiratory muscle fatigue is indicative of an improvement in the functional capacity of the respiratory pump muscles. Since metabolite accumulation contributes to deficits in the ability to produce muscular force at both a peripheral and a central level (see Ch. 2, 'Mechanisms of fatigue'), the attenuation of inspiratory muscle fatigue is consistent with a reduction and/or delay in both metabolite accumulation and activation of the inspiratory muscle metaboreflex. Activation of this reflex induces vasoconstriction in the locomotor muscles, but IMT has been shown to increase the intensity of inspiratory muscle work required to activate this reflex (McConnell & Lomax, 2006; Witt et al, 2007; Bailey et al, 2010), and to reduce La production by the inspiratory muscles (Brown et al, 2011). As a result, muscle blood flow may be preserved, and limb fatigue attenuated or delayed (McConnell & Lomax, 2006). This mechanism may also explain the reduction in $[La]_b$, and leg effort, as better-perfused locomotor muscles generate less lactate and have lower levels of metabolites to stimulate the group III and IV afferents that contribute to effort perception (Amann et al, 2010) and fatigue (Gandevia, 2001; Amann et al, 2009) (see Ch. 3). In addition, if inspiratory muscle fatigue is attenuated the perception of breathing effort will be reduced, making it possible to maintain a more efficient deep, slow breathing pattern (Turner et al, 2012). In short, the physiological changes point strongly to the ergogenic effect of IMT being underpinned by preservation of limb blood flow and reduction in breathing effort. These effects are arguably even more important in patients, since exercise tolerance is frequently limited by dyspnoea and/or muscle dysfunctions that are exacerbated by impaired blood flow.

In respect of the inspiratory muscle metaboreflex, there is one particular study of IMT that is worthy of detailed scrutiny because it has particular relevance to patients. The study in question not only demonstrated that IMT extends T_{lim}, but it also demonstrated that oxygen uptake kinetics were hastened during 'severe'- and 'maximal'-intensity cycling (Bailey et al, 2010), a finding that has since been confirmed (Brown et al, 2011). The authors' interpretation was that their observations were due to 'increased blood flow to the exercising limbs', and that this arose because of the absence of inspiratory muscle metaboreflex activation post-IMT (Bailey et al, 2010). These findings are especially relevant to patients since the oxygen uptake kinetics of patients are slowed by disease and inactivity (Chiappa et al, 2008a). The speed of this 'on transient' of the oxygen uptake kinetics determines the size of the oxygen deficit during exercise, and thus the size of the anaerobic contribution at the onset of exercise (see Ch. 1). Enhancing the amount of energy liberated from aerobic sources minimizes the production of fatiguing metabolic by-products, and reduces the ventilatory requirement for exercise. In patients for whom walking constitutes 'severe'-intensity exercise, and who are consequently teetering on the edge of the 'anaerobic abyss', this effect on oxygen uptake kinetics may be particularly important and make a disproportionate contribution to improving exercise tolerance. Interestingly, reducing the work of breathing using a low-density inspirate (heliox) speeds oxygen uptake kinetics and improves exercise tolerance in patients with COPD (Chiappa et al, 2009); this response is strikingly similar to that observed in healthy people following IMT (Bailey et al, 2010; Brown et al, 2011).

Finally, there has long been speculation that IMT may enhance the mechanical efficiency of breathing, as some studies have shown small (often non-significant) decreases in the oxygen cost of exercise (Romer et al, 2002a; Griffiths & McConnell, 2007; Turner et al, 2011). A recent study found that 6 weeks of IMT (30 repetitions against a load equivalent to 50% of MIP) reduced the oxygen cost of hyperpnoea by 5–12% (Turner et al, 2012). The greatest decrement in oxygen cost was seen at the highest intensity of respiratory muscle work. This finding has important implications for patients in whom disease-related impairments of breathing mechanics increase the oxygen cost of breathing. Since the latter may account for a considerable proportion of available oxygen uptake, reducing this burden may release oxygen for use by other muscle groups, thereby enhancing exercise tolerance.

In summary, the research using time trials and tests of endurance indicates that, for bouts of exercise involving a sustained effort against the clock of 1 to 60 minutes duration, IMT improves performance significantly by 1.7% to 4.6%. Although there is no direct research evidence that similar improvements will be seen during longer events (e.g., marathons or triathlons), the fact that a decline in MIP has been demonstrated after such events means that performance in these events may be limited by breathing-related factors. Accordingly, there is every reason to believe that IMT will improve performance in events lasting more than 1 hour. The mechanisms that underlie the changes in performance described above are applicable universally and have equal, if not greater, relevance to exercise-limited patients. Indeed, Illi and colleagues' systematic review revealed that the ergogenic effect of RMT was greatest in the least fit participants (Illi et al, 2012).

Influence of RMT upon tests of anaerobic endurance and sprinting

Sprinting is such a brief activity that the benefits of IMT are not immediately obvious. However, the changes that IMT induces in underlying physiology appear to be so fundamental that it is now clear that performance in sprint tasks can also benefit from IMT. This is relevant to patients because the metabolic demands of activities of daily living can be akin to those of a sprint in a young healthy individual. In the previous section we have already discussed the fact that maximal cycling to the limit of tolerance is extended significantly following IMT, and that this was accompanied by a significant speeding up of oxygen uptake kinetics (Bailey et al, 2010; Brown et al, 2011). Repeated sprinting may not be something that many patients engage in during their everyday lives, but it is encountered in interval training, which is finding increasing favour within rehabilitation programmes (Mador et al, 2009). Thus, the results of studies on repeated sprinting suggest potential benefits of IMT for tolerance to repeated bouts of anaerobic exercise, such as interval training. Improving the tolerability of training interventions has the benefit of enhancing the potency of the training stimulus, and the resulting performance benefits. Indeed, it has been shown that athletes undertaking a period of IMT prior to a programme of interval training were able to train significantly harder, and showed significantly greater improvements in repeated sprint performance, compared with a group that did not receive prior IMT (Tong et al, 2010). Unfortunately, there was no placebo control within this trial.

In the context of team sports, a sense of increased breathing effort between sprints has a profound influence on a player's ability to sprint again, and in competition this has implications for the quality of the athlete's contribution to the match or game. For this reason, the first study to examine the effect of IMT on sprinting used perceived rate of recovery during continuous bouts of repeated sprinting (Romer et al, 2002b). The expectation was that IMT would reduce breathing effort between sprints and delay the onset of inspiratory muscle fatigue, thereby making the participants feel as if they had recovered more quickly. However, because the sprint was very brief (3.2 seconds) and punctuated with periods of recovery, there was no expectation that actual sprint performance would improve. These expectations were confirmed; after 6 weeks of IMT (30 repetitions against a load equivalent to 50% of MIP)

the athletes showed a significantly faster rate of recovery compared with baseline and placebo, but no change in sprint performance. The potential relevance of these findings for a patient who is limited acutely by dyspnoea is that IMT may reduce the duration that they must spend 'catching their breath'; this hypothesis awaits evaluation.

Using a slightly different approach, two controlled studies (one of which was placebo controlled) have explored the benefits of IMT to the ability to sustain repeated sprinting, with gradually escalating sprint speed, and short active recovery breaks between sprints (Yo-Yo test) (Bangsbo et al, 2008). Performance in a test of this kind is influenced by both effort perception and factors related to limb blood flow, such as oxygen delivery and metabolite removal. As has been explained previously, both of these factors are potentially influenced by IMT, via its hypothesized effects upon breathing effort and activation of the inspiratory muscle metaboreflex. After 5–6 weeks of IMT (30 repetitions against a load equivalent to 50% of MIP), both studies found that performance in the Yo-Yo test improved significantly by ~17% (Tong et al, 2008; Nicks et al, 2009). Accompanying the improvement in performance were significant reductions in perception of breathing and whole-body effort, as well as markers of metabolic stress. In a more recent study, the distribution of blood flow to the legs and respiratory muscles during repeated sprinting has been studied (Tong et al, 2012). As the sprint test progressed, minute ventilation showed a progressive increase and, at the point where respiratory compensation for the developing metabolic acidosis commenced, there was a clear reduction in the oxygenation of both the respiratory and leg muscles. The timing of the two events was correlated significantly. These data are consistent with activation of the inspiratory muscle metaboreflex by the escalating ventilatory demand, followed by vasoconstriction of both the respiratory and leg muscle vasculature. Thus, as suggested for endurance exercise, IMT may improve performance during repeated sprinting by increasing the intensity of respiratory muscle work required to activate the metaboreflex, thereby preserving limb blood flow (McConnell & Lomax, 2006; Witt et al, 2007; Bailey et al, 2010).

Most recently, the effects of combining IMT with a specific inspiratory muscle warm-up (see Ch. 6) have been tested in a placebo-controlled trial on semi-professional football players (Lomax et al, 2011). The same IMT protocol and repeated sprint test were used as in previous studies; after 4 weeks of IMT, sprint performance increased significantly by 12%. At baseline, the warm-up increased sprint performance significantly by 5–7% in both groups, which is consistent with previous findings (Tong & Fu, 2006). When an inspiratory muscle warm-up was added after IMT, performance increased significantly by a further 2.9%. Thus, the benefit of the inspiratory muscle warm-up and IMT were additive (14.9%).

In summary, IMT was once thought to be of benefit only for performance in activities dominated by aerobic metabolism. However, studies now suggest that IMT is more versatile, and that the fundamental nature of the underlying mechanisms makes it an effective tool for enhancing tolerance to both prolonged moderate-intensity exercise and brief intense exercise. The similarity between the physiological changes observed following IMT during sprint and endurance exercise in healthy people is to be expected, given that IMT is probably operating via the same underlying mechanisms in both situations, i.e., attenuation of breathing effort and enhancement of limb blood flow.

Influence of RMT under hypoxic conditions

The addition of an hypoxic drive to breathe during exercise places a large additional demand upon the respiratory muscles. Therefore, the potential benefits of RMT are arguably even greater to people exercising in an hypoxic environment, or those who have hypoxaemia due to the effects of disease. To date, only one placebo-controlled study has assessed the influence of IMT on exercise tolerance and physiological responses to exercise in hypoxia (Downey et al, 2007). The results of the randomized controlled study were both impressive and surprising. The IMT group trained for 40 breaths, 5 days per week at a load of $\sim$50% of MIP, whilst the placebo group used the same regimen at a load of 15% of MIP. The hypoxic environment simulated an altitude of $\sim$3500 metres ($\sim$12000 feet), which was sufficient to reduce arterial saturation to $\sim$93% at rest and $\sim$77% at end of exercise. Following 4 weeks of IMT, minute ventilation, cardiac output and oxygen uptake of hypoxic treadmill exercise were reduced significantly in the IMT group by 25%, 14% and 8–12% respectively. Despite the lower minute ventilation, arterial oxygen saturation (S_aO_2) and lung-diffusing capacity were increased by 4% and 22%, respectively. Perceived exertion and dyspnoea were also reduced significantly. No such changes were observed in the placebo group. The changes in minute ventilation and S_aO_2 appear to be completely at odds with one another, as an increase in S_aO_2 normally requires an increase in minute ventilation. The clue to resolving this paradox resides in the improvement in the diffusing capacity of the lungs, which can increase only if the lung diffusion surface area increases. The pulmonary vasculature is responsive to muscle metaboreflex activation (Lykidis et al, 2008). Thus, if IMT were to delay or abolish activation of the inspiratory muscle metaboreflex, it is conceivable that blood flow would be preserved in the pulmonary circulation. Should this occur, an increase in diffusion surface area would result, thereby increasing S_aO_2. The effect of IMT upon S_aO_2 in hypoxic conditions has been confirmed under resting conditions in a randomized controlled study of military personnel during an expedition to the Nepali Himalayas (Lomax, 2010). At altitudes of 4880–5550 metres, the resting S_aO_2 was 6% higher in the IMT group compared with the control

group. This protective effect upon S_aO_2 was not observed at 1400 metres.

High altitude is the only environment where the lungs limit oxygen transport in healthy people. However, there are many disease states that result in hypoxaemia and pulmonary vasoconstriction, both at rest and during exercise. Under these conditions, patients may be particularly sensitive to an additional vasoconstrictor input to the pulmonary vasculature from the inspiratory muscle metaboreflex. Accordingly, IMT may provide even greater benefits to these patients than those observed in normoxic, healthy people. In the following section, the evidence relating to the influence of RMT upon patients with a range of conditions will be reviewed.

DISEASE-SPECIFIC FUNCTIONAL RESPONSES TO RMT

In most of the literature that is reviewed below, the mode of RMT has been inspiratory resistance training. However, there have been a handful of studies using EMT, or endurance RMT, and these are identified accordingly.

Respiratory disease

Chronic obstructive pulmonary disease

Respiratory muscle training has been studied most extensively in patients with COPD, and the type of intervention implemented has overwhelmingly been inspiratory muscle resistance training (IMT). The first published studies appeared in the late 1970s and the number of studies appearing each year has grown steadily, such that the most recent meta-analysis of this literature included a total of 32 studies (Gosselink et al, 2011); however, these studies represent only the [high-quality] tip of an IMT research iceberg. As was explained in Chapter 3, the rationale for IMT in patients with COPD is the restoration of balance in the demand/capacity relationship of the respiratory pump muscles. Patients with COPD have primary weakness of inspiratory muscles, which is exacerbated by functional weakness. In addition, there is an increased demand for inspiratory muscle work, owing to changes in breathing mechanics and the elevated ventilatory requirement for exercise. The primary exercise-limiting symptom under these conditions is dyspnoea.

The extensive nature of the literature addressing IMT means that there has been a systematic review (Shoemaker et al, 2009) and two meta-analyses (Geddes et al, 2008; Gosselink et al, 2011) published since 2008. Accordingly, it is possible to draw conclusions about the usefulness of IMT in patients with COPD based upon statistical evidence. The three reviews are in agreement, indicating that IMT improves: inspiratory muscle strength (MIP) and endurance, exercise capacity (6-minute walk distance), dyspnoea, and quality of life. Gosselink et al (2011) found the effect sizes of these responses to be 'medium to large'. In sub-analyses, inspiratory muscle strength training was found to be superior to endurance training for improving exercise capacity and dyspnoea. In addition, patients with the lowest MIP at baseline showed the greatest improvements in MIP and exercise capacity.

An area that has so far received very little attention is the impact of IMT upon the use of healthcare resources. As part of a 12-month placebo-controlled trail of IMT, Beckerman et al (2005) not only noted improvements in MIP, exercise capacity, dyspnoea and quality of life, but also observed significant differences between the IMT group and the placebo group in the number of primary care consultations and days spent in hospital across the intervention. There was also a difference in the number of patients admitted and the total number of admissions, but these failed to reach significance. These data suggest that IMT may reduce the number of exacerbations and hasten recovery from exacerbations. However, further research is needed in order to clarify these potential benefits.

A question that remains unclear at present is the best way to incorporate IMT into a rehabilitation programme. As was described above, there is robust evidence that IMT can be used as a stand-alone intervention to improve inspiratory muscle strength and endurance, exercise capacity, dyspnoea and quality of life. However, it remains unclear whether IMT provides additional improvements when added to a rehabilitation programme that includes whole-body exercise. Nevertheless, based upon the evidence of Lotters et al (2002) and O'Brien et al (2008), addition of IMT to a general exercise programme for patients with inspiratory muscle weakness is recommended by the joint BTS/ACPRC Guidelines (Bott et al, 2009).

A recent systematic review comparing IMT and rehabilitation revealed that, compared with exercise alone, improvement in MIP and one index of exercise tolerance were superior if IMT was added to exercise (O'Brien et al, 2008). Interestingly, when comparing IMT with exercise training, the study also found 'no significant difference in effect for outcomes of MIP and exercise tolerance among patients with COPD who engage in IMT compared with exercise' (O'Brien et al, 2008). In other words, IMT appears to improve exercise tolerance as much as exercise. Furthermore, a systematic review of home-based physiotherapy interventions for patients with COPD found that home-based IMT significantly improved dyspnoea (on the Transitional Dyspnoea Index) by 2.36 units compared with the control (Thomas et al, 2010). These findings suggest that IMT is almost certainly a more cost-effective intervention than exercise for improving dyspnoea, as it can be implemented in a domiciliary setting with minimal supervision. It is also pertinent to recall that, in healthy people, implementing IMT prior to whole-body training improved the outcome of the whole-body training (Tong et al, 2010); thus IMT might be considered as 'pre-habilitation' for patients awaiting commencement of exercise training.

Expiratory muscle training has received very little attention. To date, there have been only two placebo-controlled studies examining the effect of EMT in patients with COPD: one using specific EMT (Weiner et al, 2003b), and the other comparing responses with EMT, IMT and combined IMT and EMT (Weiner et al, 2003a). In the EMT study, expiratory muscle strength (MEP) and endurance increased significantly, as did exercise capacity. There was no significant change in the sensation of dyspnoea during daily activities. In the second of the two studies (Weiner et al, 2003a), eight patients were assigned to receive EMT, eight received IMT, eight received EMT + IMT and a group of eight was assigned to be a placebo group. There were no changes in the placebo group, but training induced statistically significant, specific increases in MEP and endurance (in the EMT and in the EMT + IMT groups) and in MIP and endurance (in the IMT and EMT + IMT groups). Exercise capacity increased in all three training groups. However, the increase in the IMT and the EMT + IMT groups was significantly greater than that in the EMT group. There was also a decrease in dyspnoea in the IMT and in the EMT + IMT groups, but not in the EMT or placebo groups. It was concluded that the inspiratory and expiratory muscles can be trained specifically to improve both strength and endurance. However, there appears to be no additional benefit gained by combining IMT + EMT, compared with IMT alone.

Finally, there are two specific, less obvious applications of IMT that are worthwhile mentioning. The first relates to the observation that repeated, deep inhalations against an inspiratory load have been found to be twice as effective (as measured by sputum weight) as standardized physiotherapy consisting of postural drainage and the active cycle of breathing technique (Chatham et al, 2004). Thus IMT may also facilitate airway clearance. The second application is in promoting the ability of patients to use inhalers. Dry-powder inhalers (DPI) have been suggested to be more appropriate for patients with coordination difficulties. However, these often have a much higher inherent flow resistance, thus rendering them unusable by very weak patients; one study found that 20% of patients with COPD were unable to generate the required inspiratory flow rate to generate the required flow rate via the Turbohaler® DPI (Weiner & Weiner, 2006). Furthermore, the flow rates achieved through the DPI were correlated with MIP. After the patients had received an 8-week period of IMT, all were able to generate the required flow rate via the Turbohaler®. Thus IMT may be a useful to tool enable and improve DPI use by very weak patients.

In summary, the strength of evidence supporting the efficacy of RMT, and in particular IMT, in patients with COPD has achieved a level where it is possible to recommend IMT as a stand-alone treatment. Improvements in inspiratory muscle strength and endurance, exercise capacity, dyspnoea and quality of life can be expected. Questions remain regarding whether the addition of IMT to exercise training provides any supplemental benefits, but the preliminary indications are that outcomes such as dyspnoea are improved to a greater extent by implementing the two interventions in parallel. The role of EMT is much less clear, owing to a lack of studies. Patients with the weakest inspiratory muscles appear to show the greatest improvements following IMT, but there is no minimum threshold above or below which benefits can, or cannot, be anticipated. Furthermore, acute bouts of loaded breathing may also facilitate airway clearance. For specific recommendations regarding implementation of IMT see Chapters 5 and 6.

Asthma

Inspiratory muscle training has been studied less extensively in patients with asthma than in those who have COPD. As was presented in Chapter 3, the rationale for IMT in patients with asthma is the restoration of balance in the demand/capacity relationship of the respiratory pump muscles, which are overloaded when airway obstruction is present. The primary symptom under these conditions is dyspnoea. To date, there has been one attempt at a Cochrane systematic review (Ram et al, 2003), which included just five studies. The review concluded that there were insufficient data, and further research was required. However, the analysis was able to confirm that IMT yielded significant improvements in MIP. Unfortunately, since 2003 there has been only one further study of IMT in people with asthma. The findings of the available literature are summarized below, and are also placed in a mechanistic context.

A notable feature of airway obstruction in asthma is the large inter-subject variation in the intensity of dyspnoea for a given fall in FEV_1 (Lougheed et al, 1993). Furthermore, women appear to experience higher levels of dyspnoea (Wijnhoven et al, 2003), poorer quality of life and more frequent hospital admission than do men (Weiner et al, 2002c). These observations led Weiner and colleagues to reason that the gender difference might be explained, at least partially, by the fact that women have weaker inspiratory muscles than men (Weiner et al, 2002c). Accordingly, the influence of gender and inspiratory muscle strength (MIP) was examined by comparing the MIP, perception of dyspnoea to threshold loads, and bronchodilator consumption of 22 male and 22 female asthmatic patients with mild-to-moderate bronchoconstriction ($FEV_1 > 60\%$ of predicted) (Weiner et al, 2002c). For the same FEV_1 (% of predicted), the women had significantly weaker inspiratory muscles, whilst dyspnoea during loaded breathing and β_2-agonist consumption was significantly higher than in the men. The women were divided randomly into two groups: half received IMT, and the remainder received sham training. After 20 weeks of IMT, the MIP of the women (+42%) matched that of the men. Accompanying this change was a reduction in the dyspnoea during loaded

breathing and the β_2-agonist consumption of the women in the IMT group, compared with that of the placebo group. Furthermore, after IMT, dyspnoea and β_2-agonist consumption were no longer different to those in the men.

The strong interrelationship between MIP, dyspnoea and β_2-agonist consumption was confirmed in a study designed to examine their interrelationships specifically (Weiner et al, 2002b). There was no correlation between baseline measures of MIP and intensity of dyspnoea during loaded breathing in a sample of 30 patients. However, after IMT both the total medications use and the perception of dyspnoea during loaded breathing showed a direct, quantitative relationship with the increase in MIP. Indeed, 93% of the change in β_2-agonist consumption was explained by the change in MIP. These findings support a role for the absolute strength of the inspiratory muscles in determining the consumption of medication, and dyspnoea.

Critics will argue that changes in dyspnoea during loaded breathing are not the same as exertional dyspnoea, and they would be correct. However, there is evidence that exertional dyspnoea is also attenuated after IMT in people with asthma (12.4% reduction), and after as little as 3 weeks of IMT (McConnell et al, 1998). Most recently, a comprehensive study of IMT using a matched double-blind placebo-controlled design confirmed that exertional dyspnoea was reduced (by 16%) after 6 weeks of IMT (Turner et al, 2011); it also noted further benefits, which included an improvement in exercise tolerance, attenuation of exercise-induced decrease in MIP, and a lower oxygen cost of exercise (reduced by 12% at T_{lim}). The latter was presumed by the authors to derive from improvements in the mechanical efficiency of breathing, which derives some support from their later finding that in healthy people the oxygen cost of voluntary hyperpnoea is reduced by as much 12% after IMT (Turner et al, 2012).

An impressive feature of studies of IMT in patients with asthma is the reduction in β_2-agonist consumption that accompanies IMT. In the three studies in which this has been examined (Weiner et al, 1992; Weiner et al, 2000; Weiner et al, 2002c), this reduction has ranged from 38% to 78%, being greatest in those with the highest baseline consumption. Thus, IMT appears to be particularly helpful for patients with high levels of dyspnoea and β_2-agonist consumption. Furthermore, a double-blind placebo-controlled trial of IMT conducted over 6 months also observed significant improvements in lung function, asthma symptoms, hospitalizations for asthma and absence from school or work (Weiner et al, 1992).

However, a note of caution is warranted at this point, because there are a small group of patients with asthma for whom further reductions in the intensity of dyspnoea sensation may be life threatening. According to one study, around 26% of patients with asthma have abnormally low perceptions of dyspnoea (Magadle et al, 2002); this was associated with low consumption of medication, increased emergency department visits, hospitalizations, near-fatal asthma attacks, and deaths during follow-up (Magadle et al, 2002). A second study confirmed the association between near-fatal asthma and low perceptions of dyspnoea, as well as blunted hypoxic sensitivity (Kikuchi et al, 1994). It would therefore be inappropriate to implement IMT in this subgroup. However, the available evidence suggests that patients with normal or high sensation of dyspnoea *do not* become desensitized to bronchoconstriction following IMT. Weiner et al (2000) noted that IMT did not result in exaggerated ablation of dyspnoea, and concluded that IMT was safe, at least for use in patients with mild asthma.

In summary, the strength of evidence supporting the efficacy of IMT in patients with asthma has not yet achieved that of COPD. This is primarily because of the small number of studies available to date. There is some evidence that dyspnoea and use of medication are greatest in those with the weakest inspiratory muscles (lowest MIP). Preliminary evidence also suggests that, irrespective of MIP, IMT induces improvements in inspiratory muscle strength, exercise capacity, dyspnoea and use of medication. Patients with abnormally low dyspnoea perception are unsuitable candidates for IMT, but there appears to be no evidence that inspiratory muscle weakness is a prerequisite to improvements following IMT. Furthermore, acute bouts of loaded breathing may also facilitate airway clearance. For specific recommendations regarding implementation of IMT see Chapters 5 and 6.

Bronchiectasis

Bronchiectasis is a chronic lung disease that is not normally included within the umbrella of COPD. However, the functional manifestations of bronchiectasis have similarities with those of COPD, including airway obstruction, which leads to detrimental changes in breathing mechanics, attendant exertional dyspnoea and exercise intolerance (Neves et al, 2011). Patients with moderate-to-severe bronchiectasis also have slight respiratory muscle weakness (Moran et al, 2010). It is therefore reasonable to hypothesize that responses to IMT in patients with bronchiectasis would be similar to those of patients with COPD.

To date there have been just two studies in which patients with bronchiectasis have been subjected to IMT. In the first study, moderate-intensity IMT (15 minutes breathing against 30–60% of MIP) was undertaken for 8 weeks in combination with a programme of physical exercise (EX+IMT). The responses of this IMT group were compared with those of a group who received exercise and sham IMT (EX+sham), as well as a control group (Newall et al, 2005). There was a significant increase in MIP in both training groups (18% and 33% for exercise and EX+IMT, respectively), but the increase was not significantly different between the groups. Exercise tolerance

improved significantly in both training groups during a treadmill T_{lim} test and in an incremental shuttle walking test; but the changes were not significantly different between groups. Thus adding IMT to exercise training in these patients did not result in significantly greater improvements in MIP of exercise tolerance. However, a key finding of this study was that, 3 months after cessation of the interventions, exercise tolerance was maintained in the EX+IMT group but not in the EX+sham group. In addition, the EX+IMT group was the only group to show an improved quality of life score, which was also maintained after cessation of training. It is noteworthy that the improvements in all parameters were largest in the EX+IMT group, but it is important to bear in mind that the assessment of IMT was made on an improving baseline of function due to the exercise training, which was implemented in both the IMT and sham groups; the effect of this would be to reduce the effect size of the IMT. Finally, the lack of statistically significant difference between EX+sham and EX+IMT may be due to lack of statistical power, due to the small sample size (~10 participants per group). The failure to distinguish an additional benefit of adding IMT to exercise has also been observed in patients with COPD, but a recent systematic review concluded that '[in COPD] Results showed significant improvements in maximum inspiratory pressure and maximum exercise tidal volume favoring combined IMT and exercise compared with exercise alone' (O'Brien et al, 2008). Conclusions regarding other outcomes await further data.

In a more recent study (Liaw et al, 2011), a low-intensity IMT regimen (30 minutes breathing against 30–38% of MIP) was evaluated in 13 patients, and compared with 13 patients who did no training at all. Both MIP and MEP increased in the IMT group (39% and 44%, respectively), and although there was a significant increase in 6-minute walk distance (14.8%), this just failed to be significantly different from that of the control group. Interpretation of these data is hampered by lack of statistical power, and the absence of a placebo control. Taken together, the two studies provide preliminary evidence that IMT may elicit similar improvements to those shown in patients with COPD. The joint BTS/ACPRC Guidelines make the following recommendation in relation to IMT in bronchiectasis: 'Consider the use of inspiratory muscle training in conjunction with conventional pulmonary rehabilitation to enhance the maintenance of the training effect' (Bott et al, 2009).

Finally, it is worthwhile mentioning that some IMT studies on patients with CF have reported improvements in expectoration immediately after IMT (Asher et al, 1982; Enright et al, 2004); indeed, repeated, deep inhalations against an inspiratory load have been found to be twice as effective (measured by sputum weight) as standardized physiotherapy consisting of postural drainage and the active cycle of breathing technique (Chatham et al,

2004). Thus IMT may also facilitate airway clearance in patients with bronchiectasis.

In summary, interpretation of the evidence relating to the efficacy of IMT in patients with bronchiectasis is hampered by the very small number of studies. Taken together, the two available studies provide preliminary evidence that IMT may elicit similar improvements to those shown in patients with COPD. Further research on IMT as a stand-alone intervention is justified, as the theoretical rationale for IMT in patients with bronchiectasis is very similar to that for patients with COPD. Furthermore, acute bouts of loaded breathing may also facilitate airway clearance. For specific recommendations regarding implementation of IMT see Chapters 5 and 6.

Cystic fibrosis

Although there are a handful of studies of RMT in patients with CF, one of these failed to include a control group (Keens et al, 1977) and one utilized an unreliable method of training (Asher et al, 1982). Of the remaining three, only two studies (de Jong et al, 2001; Enright et al, 2004) met the criteria to be included in a recent systematic review (Reid et al, 2008). Although inevitably limited, this review represents the most up-to-date picture of the influence of IMT upon patients with CF (Reid et al, 2008). Analysis of both studies revealed no significant effects of IMT upon lung function or inspiratory muscle strength (MIP). However, these findings cannot be taken at face value as some important features of the two studies differed. In one study, the training regimen was 20–40% of MIP sustained for 20 minutes (de Jong et al, 2001). This constitutes an endurance training regimen; indeed, endurance increased significantly, but not strength – a finding ascribed by the authors to the low intensity of the training. Accordingly, these data should be interpreted cautiously in respect of the efficacy of IMT. In the other study within the review (Enright et al, 2004), a high-intensity inspiratory muscle-strength-training programme was implemented. This high-intensity training elicited improvements in MIP (18%) and endurance, as well as diaphragm thickness. Furthermore, lung function, incremental cycle performance and psychological status were also improved significantly. Whilst seemingly contradictory, the systematic review of these two studies most likely highlights the differing efficacy of the two types of training implemented.

It is not clear why the fifth study was excluded from the systematic review, but this may be because it was not a randomized trial (Sawyer & Clanton, 1993). However, it was a placebo-controlled trial and therefore merits consideration. After 10 weeks of IMT using a moderate load (50–60% of MIP), there were significant improvements in MIP (13%), lung function and exercise tolerance. The greater training intensity and longer duration of the intervention may explain the discrepancy between this study and that of de Jong et al (2001).

Finally, two IMT studies on patients with CF have reported improvements in expectoration immediately after IMT (Asher et al, 1982; Enright et al, 2004); indeed, repeated deep inhalations against an inspiratory load have been found to be twice as effective (measured by sputum weight) as standardized physiotherapy consisting of postural drainage and the active cycle of breathing technique (Chatham et al, 2004). It has been suggested that the effect is similar to that seen after exercise. This finding may have implications for other patient groups in which airway clearance is problematic.

In summary, interpretation of the evidence relating to the efficacy of IMT in patients with CF is hampered by the very small number of studies. When viewed collectively, the data from placebo-controlled trials suggest that, when moderate- to high-intensity loading is used, MIP improves by 13–18% and is accompanied by a range of clinically significant benefits. Further research on IMT as a stand-alone intervention is justified as there is a good theoretical rationale for IMT in patients with CF (see Ch. 3). Furthermore, acute bouts of loaded breathing may also facilitate airway clearance. For specific recommendations regarding implementation of IMT see Chapters 5 and 6.

Restrictive chest wall disorders

Conditions such as kyphoscoliosis, fibrothorax, thoracoplasty, flail chest and ankylosing spondylitis create a restrictive pulmonary defect in which total respiratory system elastance and resistance are elevated (Donath & Miller, 2009). Furthermore, inspiratory muscle function also tends to be impaired (Lisboa et al, 1985; Cejudo et al, 2009) owing to changes in chest wall and diaphragm configuration.

Given the obvious imbalance in the demand/capacity relationship of the respiratory pump, it is surprising that there has been only one randomized controlled trial of IMT in patients with restrictive chest wall disease (Budweiser et al, 2006). Thirty patients with restrictive lung disorders who were receiving intermittent non-invasive positive-pressure ventilation (NPPV) took part. Half underwent 3 months of endurance RMT (a minimum of 10 minutes of hyperpnoea training), and half sham RMT (incentive spirometry). Surprisingly, endurance RMT induced significant improvements in MIP (27%), which may be because the sample had such low baseline function (42 ± 14.6 cmH$_2$O). Peak $\dot{V}$O$_2$, peak cycle power and health-related quality of life also improved significantly compared with the sham group. Pulmonary function, 6-minute walk distance and blood gases remained unchanged. Most recently there has been an uncontrolled study of 'breathing exercises' in 22 patients with ankylosing spondylitis. These exercises consisted of diaphragmatic breathing, pursed lip breathing, and thoracic expansion exercises. The patients also used an incentive spirometer equipped with a volume-oriented sustained inhalation (Ortancil et al, 2009). There were significant increases in chest expansion (16%), MIP (9%), MEP (16%) and Bath Ankylosing Spondylitis Functional Index scores after 6 weeks of breathing exercise, but the 6-minute walking distance did not change. The absence of a control group and the unusual nature of the intervention make these data difficult to interpret. The data hint that it may be possible to improve chest wall mobility – which merits further exploration using IMT, which has been shown to increase vital capacity in other conditions. The potential role in improving exertional dyspnoea and exercise tolerance remains unclear as neither study showed a change in 6-minute walking distance. Notwithstanding this, the joint BTS/ACPRC Guidelines make the following recommendation in relation to RMT in patients with kyphoscoliosis: 'Consider the use of respiratory muscle training' (Bott et al, 2009).

Finally, it is worthwhile mentioning that repeated, deep inhalations against an inspiratory load have been found to be twice as effective (measured by sputum weight) as standardized physiotherapy consisting of postural drainage and the active cycle of breathing technique (Chatham et al, 2004). Thus, IMT may also facilitate airway clearance.

In summary, interpretation of the evidence relating to the efficacy of RMT in patients with restrictive chest wall disorders is hampered by the very small number of studies. The single placebo-controlled trial suggests that endurance RMT in patients receiving intermittent NPPV may improve peak exercise capacity and health-related quality of life, but not 6-minute walking distance. Further research on strength IMT as a stand-alone intervention is justified, since there is a good theoretical rationale for IMT in patients with restrictive chest wall disorders (see Ch. 3). Furthermore, acute bouts of loaded breathing may also facilitate airway clearance. For specific recommendations regarding implementation of IMT see Chapters 5 and 6.

Chronic heart failure

The literature relating to RMT in patients with chronic heart failure (CHF) has been growing steadily over the past decade. The first study to examine RMT in patients with CHF appeared in the literature in 1995 (Mancini et al, 1995). The 3-month intervention combined isocapnic hyperpnoea, maximum static inspiratory efforts and pressure threshold loading. Training produced improvements in the MIP (37%) and endurance of the respiratory muscles (57%), as well as alleviating dyspnoea during activities of daily living. Exercise performance during submaximal and maximal exercise tests was also enhanced. The authors suggest that RMT may provide 'a simple and useful adjunct to medical therapy' for patients with CHF. These early findings were replicated either fully or in part over the course of the following decade using pressure threshold IMT (Cahalin et al, 1997; Johnson et al, 1998; Weiner et al, 1999; Martinez et al, 2001). Typically, MIP improves 25–30% over an 8- to 12-week period, whereas the magnitude of changes in exercise tolerance and dyspnoea varies

according to the tests used; typically 6-minute walk distance improves by around 20–30% (Mancini et al, 1995; Weiner et al, 1999).

More recently, further studies have consolidated and extended the earlier findings (Laoutaris et al, 2004; Dall'Ago et al, 2006; Padula et al, 2009; Bosnak-Guclu et al, 2011; Mello et al, 2012). Typically, IMT improves MIP and inspiratory muscle endurance, reduces exertional dyspnoea, increases exercise tolerance and improves quality of life. Four systematic reviews have examined the influence of IMT, one focussing upon its effect upon quality of life (Sbruzzi et al, 2012) whereas the other three also examined exercise tolerance (Lin et al, 2012; Plentz et al, 2012; Smart et al, 2012). Sbruzzi and colleagues included four studies in their analysis, concluding that, on balance, these did not support a significant effect of IMT upon quality of life; however, they suggested that further research is required. In contrast, Smart and colleagues included 11 studies (148 IMT participants and 139 placebo or non-training participants). Significant effects were identified for MIP, peak oxygen uptake (1.8 ml·min^{-1}.kg^{-1}, 9.2%), 6-minute walk distance (34 metres), quality of life (12.2 units) and $\dot{V}_E$–$\dot{V}CO_2$ gradient (an index of ventilatory efficiency). Based upon comparison of effect sizes with previous meta-analyses of exercise training in patients with CHF, the authors concluded that: 'IMT improves cardiorespiratory fitness and quality of life to a similar magnitude to conventional exercise training and may provide an initial alternative to the more severely deconditioned CHF patients who may then transition to conventional [exercise training]'. Similar findings for outcomes relating to MIP, exercise tolerance and dyspnoea were also reported in the systematic reviews by Lin et al (2012) and Plentz et al (2012).

Recent studies have also shed light on the potential mechanisms underlying improvements in exercise tolerance following IMT (Chiappa et al, 2008b; Stein et al, 2009). The first study is an elegant experiment that examined whether IMT influenced activation of the inspiratory muscle metaboreflex (Chiappa et al, 2008b). Before IMT, breathing against an inspiratory load activated the inspiratory muscle metaboreflex, inducing vasoconstriction in both resting and exercising limbs. In contrast, after 4 weeks of IMT the metaboreflex response to the same loaded breathing task was delayed, and the time to fatigue during subsequent forearm exercise task was extended. The study also documented a 54% increase in contracted diaphragm thickness, which explained 77% of the change in MIP. The finding of a change in the work threshold for activation of the inspiratory muscle metaboreflex after IMT is similar to that in healthy people described above (McConnell & Lomax, 2006; Witt et al, 2007; Bailey et al, 2010), and suggests that this mechanism plays an important role in mediating improvements in exercise tolerance.

The role of improved oxygen delivery in the improvements in exercise tolerance observed after IMT is supported by Stein and colleagues' retrospective analysis (2009) of the data published by Dall'Ago et al (2006). Stein and colleagues used the oxygen uptake efficiency slope (OUES, or gradient of $\dot{V}O_2$ vs $\log\dot{V}_E$) (Baba et al, 1996) during submaximal treadmill exercise as an index of the 'cardiorespiratory functional reserve' and demonstrated that this was not only improved post-IMT, but that the increase in MIP accounted for 69% of the increase in OUES. The OUES is essentially an index of the rate of increase of $\dot{V}O_2$ in response to a given $\dot{V}_E$; thus it provides an index of the efficiency with which oxygen is being taken up at the lungs, which is in turn affected by the pulmonary diffusion area and alveolar ventilation ($\dot{V}_A$). The OUES also provides an index of systemic perfusion (Baba et al, 1996). Both diffusion area and $\dot{V}_A$ are impaired in patients with CHF, and both have the potential to be improved by IMT. In the case of the diffusion area, the influence of IMT upon the threshold for activation of the inspiratory muscle metaboreflex may enhance pulmonary perfusion (see the section 'Improvements in hypoxic conditions', above). Furthermore, data from healthy people suggest that IMT increases V_T (Romer et al, 2002a), which theoretically improves $\dot{V}_A$, by reducing V_D/V_T. Similar changes in patients with CHF after IMT might also contribute to the improved OUES observed by Stein and colleagues (2009). These mechanistic studies provide good evidence that IMT improves exercise tolerance in patients via credible and important physiological mechanisms.

The influence of IMT upon autonomic balance has also received attention both in patients with CHF and in those with hypertension. Mello et al (2012) found that 12 weeks of IMT not only yielded significant improvements in MIP (47%), peak oxygen uptake (31%) and quality of life, but also these changes were accompanied by an increase in cardiac vagal tone (increase in the ratio of low-frequency to high-frequency components of heart rate variability (LF/HF) and a decrease in muscle sympathetic nerve activity (27%; assessed using microneurography). The influence of IMT upon sympathetic activity and arterial blood pressure (ABP) has also been examined in hypertensive patients (Ferreira et al, 2011); this randomized, placebo-controlled trial lasted 8 weeks, at the end of which the IMT group exhibited a 46% increase in MIP, which was accompanied by a significant reduction in 24-hour systolic and diastolic blood pressures of 8 mmHg and 5 mmHg, respectively. These changes appeared to be underpinned by improvements in autonomic balance as sympathetic activity was reduced significantly (increase in LF/HF). The authors speculated that this might be due to a reduction in the sympathoexcitatory input from the inspiratory muscle metaboreflex. An alternative explanation is that IMT prompted a slower, deeper breathing pattern, which has also been shown to reduce ABP in hypertensive patients, especially when combined with a small inspiratory load (Jones et al, 2010). Breathing exercises have also been shown to increase cardiac vagal tone in healthy people (Hepburn et al, 2005), which is suggestive of an ability to influence autonomic balance. The magnitude of improvements in ABP after

breathing training is comparable to, or better than, those observed following exercise training (2–3 mmHg) (NICE, 2011) and pharmacotherapy ($\sim$13–17 mmHg) (Wright & Musini, 2009).

A recent double-blind, randomized placebo-controlled study has examined the influence of IMT upon functional balance in patients with CHF, as well as the more traditional indices of function such as exercise tolerance and dyspnoea (Bosnak-Guclu et al, 2011). The beneficial effects upon exercise, dyspnoea and quality of life were confirmed, but the study also identified a significant improvement in the Berg Balance Scale score of 1.36 units. This is consistent with the role of the respiratory muscles in postural control (Hodges & Gandevia, 2000).

A recent consensus statement from the Heart Failure Association and the European Association for Cardiovascular Prevention and Rehabilitation concluded that IMT 'can improve exercise capacity and quality of life, particularly in those who present with inspiratory muscle weakness (IMW). Hence, routine screening for IMW is advisable and specific inspiratory muscle training in addition to standard endurance training might be beneficial' (Piepoli et al, 2011). This recommendation is echoed by Ribeiro and colleagues in a recent review of the contribution of inspiratory muscles to exercise limitation in patients with CHF (Ribeiro et al, 2012). Perhaps the only contention in respect of current advice regarding implementation of IMT is the restriction to patients with overt inspiratory muscle weakness. The reasons for this are: (1) inspiratory muscle strength needs to be considered in the broader context of the demand/capacity relationship of the respiratory pump (see Ch. 3), and (2) if one accepts that changes to the threshold for activation of the inspiratory muscle metaboreflex contribute to functional improvements after IMT, the similarity of the changes in metaboreflex activation in patients with CHF and in healthy people (McConnell & Lomax, 2006; Chiappa et al, 2008b) supports the notion that similar mechanisms underlie functional improvements. Accordingly, since healthy people have normal inspiratory muscle function and show functional improvements following IMT, it is reasonable to suggest that IMT should also be considered for patients without overt inspiratory muscle weakness.

In summary, the strength of evidence supporting the efficacy of RMT, and in particular IMT, in patients with CHF is growing, and has now achieved a level where it is possible to recommend IMT as a stand-alone treatment. Improvements in inspiratory muscle strength, exercise capacity and dyspnoea can be expected but improvements in quality of life are less consistent. Studies examining limb blood flow and the OUES response to exercise suggest that changes to the inspiratory muscle metaboreflex response may contribute to enhancement of exercise capacity after IMT. Some studies have included only patients with inspiratory muscle weakness, giving rise to the recommendation that this be a prerequisite for IMT. However, there is no direct evidence indicating that patients with normal MIP cannot also benefit. Further research is required to build critical mass within the evidence base, as well as to evaluate the combined benefits of IMT and exercise. The influence of IMT upon autonomic nervous system balance is also worthy of further exploration. For specific recommendations regarding implementation of IMT see Chapters 5 and 6.

Neurological and neuromuscular disease

Neurological and neuromuscular diseases include conditions that affect the brain, spinal cord, nerves and muscles. Impairment can be the result of intrinsic muscle dysfunction, or arise indirectly via neurological/nerve dysfunction. The functional consequences are broadly divided into spasticity and paralysis. For simplicity, these conditions are considered collectively in this section under the terminology of neuromuscular disease (NMD), beginning with spinal cord injury.

Spinal cord injury

Spinal cord injury (SCI) induces profound changes to pulmonary and respiratory muscle function, as well as breathing mechanics, creating imbalance in the demand/capacity relationship of the respiratory pump. Respiratory symptoms are common in patients with SCI, and breathlessness is present in 73% of people with a lesion at C5 but only 29% of those with a lesion below T8 (Spungen et al, 1997). Around two-thirds of the prevalence of dyspnoea has been attributed to inspiratory muscle paralysis (Spungen et al, 1997). Furthermore, respiratory complications remain a major cause of morbidity and mortality in people with SCI (Schilero et al, 2009), the underlying cause of which is poor cough function. Interestingly, MIP shows a higher correlation with cough function than does MEP (Kang et al, 2006).

As poor respiratory muscle function is linked to dyspnoea and cough function, it is reasonable to suppose that specific RMT may have a beneficial influence. There have been three systematic reviews on the topic (Brooks et al, 2005; Van Houtte et al, 2006; Sheel et al, 2008). The first of these reviews examined IMT and addressed the following outcomes: inspiratory muscle strength and endurance, exercise capacity, dyspnoea, pulmonary function and quality of life. Only three studies satisfied the inclusion criteria and were randomized (Loveridge et al, 1989; Derrickson et al, 1992; Liaw et al, 2000); two included a control group (Loveridge et al, 1989; Liaw et al, 2000) whereas the third compared RMT with abdominal muscle training in which the diaphragm was used to lift weights placed on the abdomen (Derrickson et al, 1992). Two studies were undertaken in the acute phase post-injury, whereas the third was undertaken 1 year post-injury (Loveridge et al, 1989). Thus the literature could be described as a 'mixed bag'. It is perhaps no surprise that the analyses revealed no consistent changes in the outcome variables analysed; even MIP failed to

achieve statistical significance between groups, though the difference was significant within groups in all three studies (MIP increased by 29–61%). The latter stems from two factors: first, one study compared IMT with a different form of diaphragm training (Derrickson et al, 1992); secondly, another observed a 30% improvement in MIP in the control group.

A second systematic review was broader, evaluating all forms of RMT (Van Houtte et al, 2006). Only six of 106 studies met the inclusion criteria, and addressed the following outcomes: inspiratory muscle strength and endurance, pulmonary function, respiratory complications, quality of life and exercise performance. Unfortunately, the authors were forced to conclude that due to 'a limited number of randomized controlled trials, unreported data and heterogeneity ... it was impossible to calculate effect sizes and to perform a meta-analysis'. However, they were able to conclude that the data suggested 'tendencies' for improved expiratory muscle strength, vital capacity and residual volume after RMT.

The most recent systematic review examined the influence of both IMT and general exercise training upon respiratory muscle and lung function in patients with all levels of SCI (Sheel et al, 2008). Thirteen studies were included in the analysis of IMT but, as with previous systematic reviews, heterogeneity of participants and training methods hampered analysis. The authors concluded that there was insufficient evidence to support IMT as a method of improving inspiratory muscle function, lung function or dyspnoea in people with SCI.

The results of these systematic reviews highlight the difficulties of evaluating any intervention in a highly heterogeneous population, especially when the intervention itself lacks standardization. Since the 2009 review, there have been a handful of further studies published, one of which was a randomized, placebo-controlled trial examining the effects of RMT (hyperpnoea) in the acute phase following SCI (Van Houtte et al, 2008). After 8 weeks of training the RMT group exhibited significant improvements in respiratory muscle strength (25%) and endurance (121%) as well a reduction in respiratory complications. Since the 2008 systematic review, a further three studies using controlled designs have examined the influence of IMT upon the exercise performance of wheelchair athletes (Litchke et al, 2008; West et al, 2009; Goosey-Tolfrey et al, 2010). This subgroup of SCI people are more homogeneous, and also more stable in terms of their underlying physiology. In wheelchair athletes, improvements in MIP ranged from 17% to 44%. In one study, similar changes were seen in MIP and MEP in both the IMT and placebo groups, which suggests either that the baseline measures of function were unreliable or that the placebo training intensity (15% MIP) was sufficient to induce changes in function (Goosey-Tolfrey et al, 2010). This study also had poor training compliance (63%), and found no change in lung function or in repeated wheelchair sprint performance. The results of the study that did not implement any placebo training (Litchke et al, 2008) tend to support the suggestion that placebo IMT may be sufficient to increase MIP; in this study, MIP increased significantly (44%) only in the IMT group. These authors also observed no change in $\dot{V}O_{2peak}$ post-IMT. The latter is not surprising, as $\dot{V}O_{2peak}$ represented $\dot{V}O_{2max}$ in these athletes, and IMT does not increase $\dot{V}O_{2max}$ in able-bodied athletes (Romer et al, 2002c). The study by West and colleagues (2009) used a clever placebo, which consisted of using a placebo metered dose inhaler; this study also measured diaphragm thickness. Both MIP and diaphragm thickness improved significantly, and these changes were significantly different from control (23% and 11% respectively). This study also observed a significant increase in arm-cranking power output and V_T, as well as a decrease in $\dot{V}_E/\dot{V}O_2$ at peak power during incremental arm-cranking exercise. Similar changes in breathing pattern have been observed in able-bodied athletes (Romer et al, 2002c).

The joint BTS/ACPRC Guidelines make the following recommendations in relation to IMT in patients SCI: (1) '[IMT] may be considered for patients with upper spinal cord injury to improve respiratory muscle strength', and (2) '[IMT] may be considered for patients with upper spinal cord injury to improve vital capacity and residual volume' (Bott et al, 2009).

Finally, it is worthwhile mentioning that repeated, deep inhalations against an inspiratory load have been found to be twice as effective (as measured by sputum weight) as standardized physiotherapy consisting of postural drainage and the active cycle of breathing technique (Chatham et al, 2004). Thus, IMT may also facilitate airway clearance.

In summary, the role of RMT in patients with SCI remains unclear, and further, careful, systematic research is required before conclusions can be drawn. Issues that demand investigation include: (1) optimal training methods to enhance respiratory muscle function, (2) optimal timing of training (acute, chronic, or both), and (3) the influence of RMT upon relevant clinical outcomes such as lung function, cough, exercise tolerance and quality of life. For specific recommendations regarding implementation of IMT see Chapters 5 and 6.

Other NMDs

Despite the fact that respiratory muscle weakness is a common finding, and respiratory complications are a frequent cause of morbidity and mortality in patients with neuromuscular disease (NMD), RMT has been studied comparatively little in this group of patients. This may stem from misconceptions regarding the ability of diseased muscle to respond to a training stimulus, and potentially harmful effects of exercise (Aboussouan, 2009). Generally, the more severe a patient's disease, the less likely they are to respond to any form of training. Similarly, the more rapid the progress of their disease, the less likely they are to show a training effect. However, the reverse is also true, and large training gains may be possible in patients with mild disease that is progressing slowly.

The umbrella term 'NMD' encompasses a wide range of conditions including amyotrophic lateral sclerosis (ALS), stroke, Parkinson's disease, multiple sclerosis, muscular dystrophy, myasthenia gravis, cerebral palsy, Guillain–Barré syndrome and post-polio syndrome. For many of these conditions, there is a lack of critical mass with respect to studies on the effects of RMT, as well as contradictory evidence. A case in point is Duchenne muscular dystrophy (DMD), where the results have been somewhat contradictory (DiMarco et al, 1985; Martin et al, 1986; Smith et al, 1988; Stern et al, 1989; Vilozni et al, 1994; Wanke et al, 1994; Winkler et al, 2000; Koessler et al, 2001; Topin et al, 2002) and the quality of research design variable, e.g., some lack control groups or randomization. For example, studies fail to agree on fundamental outcomes such as whether respiratory muscle strength and/or endurance improve. However, these discrepancies are most likely methodological in origin, as well as being due to variations in the type of training used. The latter is important, as endurance training does not improve strength, and if strength is the outcome measure of training efficacy then a type II error (falsely accepting the null hypothesis) is the result. Furthermore, some studies contain a diversity of patients with differing conditions and stages of disease progression, making for heterogeneous and diluted outcomes.

In studies in which the patients are either exclusively DMD (Topin et al, 2002), or make up the majority of the sample (Winkler et al, 2000; Koessler et al, 2001), a clearer picture emerges with respect to the influence of IMT. However, this needs to be viewed in the context of the research designs employed. For example, although Topin et al (2002) used a randomized placebo-controlled design, neither Winkler et al (2000) nor Koessler et al (2001) included any control group. The most important observation is that functional improvements appear to be dose dependent, being greatest in those patients who complete the most training sessions. Furthermore, responses are specific to the training stimulus, e.g., where this is endurance biased, improvements in endurance result (46%) with no change in strength (Topin et al, 2002), where a combined protocol is used then both properties improve (Winkler et al, 2000), and where a strength protocol is used then both strength (43%) and endurance (15%) improve (Koessler et al, 2001). The latter arises because of the 'dual conditioning' response to strength training (see Chapter 5). Accompanying the increases in inspiratory muscle strength (MIP) are improvements in or maintenance of lung function (Koessler et al, 2001). So far as functional outcomes such as breathing effort perception are concerned, the only study to examine this utilized a randomized placebo-controlled design and a protocol of discrete pressure threshold IMT and EMT (Gozal & Thiriet, 1999). Improvements in both inspiratory and expiratory muscle strength (30% and 47%, respectively) were observed, but without improvement in lung function. However, there was a significant decline in the perception of effort when breathing against an inspiratory load. This study also noted that improvements in respiratory muscle strength were lost 3 months after cessation of training, but that perception of breathing effort remained attenuated. The most recent British Thoracic Society Guideline on management of children with neuromuscular weakness concludes that 'respiratory muscle training can improve respiratory muscle strength and endurance in children with DMD' (Hull et al, 2012). Collectively, these data provide preliminary support for the use of RMT in patients with DMD, and specifically inspiratory resistance training, which elicits the widest range of benefits; improvements include lung function and dyspnoea.

Post-polio syndrome is often associated with inspiratory muscle dysfunction. Exercise is limited to some extent by ventilatory insufficiency, as indicated by abnormal blood gas values during exercise (Weinberg et al, 1999). The only study of IMT in post-polio included only seven patients in the training group and three control patients. The study found that an endurance biased programme of IMT improved inspiratory muscle endurance (56%) significantly, and some activities of daily living, but did not change inspiratory muscle strength or lung function (Klefbeck et al, 2000). The latter is to be expected if the training is biased towards endurance. It is also noteworthy that these patients used assisted ventilation at night, and half relied upon an electric wheelchair for mobility. Accordingly, these preliminary data suggest that, even in patients with severely compromised physical function, IMT may provide some benefit to activities of daily living, but further research is required.

Myasthenia gravis (MG) is associated with generalized weakness and fatigue, which includes weakness of the inspiratory muscles, which induces dyspnoea at rest and during exercise (Weiner et al, 1998a). To date, there have been a handful of studies employing respiratory muscle resistance training (Weiner et al, 1998a; Fregonezi et al, 2005) or hyperpnoea endurance training (Rassler et al, 2007, 2011). Methodological quality varied, with most studies failing to include control groups (Weiner et al, 1998a; Rassler et al, 2007; Rassler et al, 2011), and just one employing a randomized placebo-controlled design (Fregonezi et al, 2005). In these studies, strength training resulted in significant improvements in the strength of both inspiratory (35%) and expiratory muscles, and an improvement in endurance (53%) (Weiner et al, 1998a; Fregonezi et al, 2005). Significant improvements in lung function and dyspnoea accompanied these changes in strength and endurance (Weiner et al, 1998a); the former may be the result of the increased thoracic mobility observed post-IMT (Fregonezi et al, 2005). Finally, there were also improvements in health-related quality of life post-IMT (Fregonezi et al, 2005). Predictably, endurance RMT resulted in improvements in respiratory muscle endurance ($\sim$101–230%), but no significant change in lung function or inspiratory muscle strength (Rassler et al, 2007,

2011). In addition, the Besinger Score of MG symptoms improved after 4 months of training, but not after 4 weeks (Rassler et al, 2007; Rassler et al, 2011). Thus, these preliminary data suggest that RMT may provide some benefit to patients with MG, but further research is required.

Multiple sclerosis (MS) is a progressively debilitating disease in which respiratory muscle weakness is inevitable (Klefbeck & Hamrah Nedjad, 2003). Both IMT (Klefbeck & Hamrah Nedjad, 2003; Fry et al, 2007) and EMT (Smeltzer et al, 1996; Gosselink et al, 2000; Chiara et al, 2007) have been investigated in patients with MS, as well as a combination of IMT and EMT (Olgiati et al, 1989). Methodological quality varied, with some studies failing to include control groups (Olgiati et al, 1989; Chiara et al, 2007), but others using randomized placebo-controlled designs (Klefbeck & Hamrah Nedjad, 2003), placebo-controlled designs (Smeltzer et al, 1996), or randomized controlled designs (Gosselink et al, 2000; Fry et al, 2007). Both IMT and EMT were found to result in improvements in respiratory muscle strength ($\sim$30–80%), although changes are not always significant (Gosselink et al, 2000), and do not always result in improvements in lung, or other aspects of function (Olgiati et al, 1989; Klefbeck & Hamrah Nedjad, 2003; Chiara et al, 2007). However, the degree of physical disability appears to play a role in activities of daily living, such that improvements are difficult to achieve in patients who are wheelchair or bed bound (Klefbeck & Hamrah Nedjad, 2003). In addition, it may be necessary to increase inspiratory muscle strength considerably ($\sim$80%) in order to enhance lung function (Fry et al, 2007). In the most recent randomized controlled trial of IMT, patients with moderate disability showed impressive improvements in MIP after IMT (81%) that were accompanied by improvements in lung function (Fry et al, 2007). The data led the authors to speculate that 'Enhanced pulmonary function in persons with MS may increase effectiveness of cough, improve speech, reduce bouts of pneumonia, improve performance of ADL, increase tolerance for exercise training, and improve quality of life' (Fry et al, 2007), but this awaits empirical confirmation.

Following stroke, respiratory muscle paralysis may be present on the affected side, resulting in impaired breathing mechanics and dyspnoea (Lanini et al, 2002) as well as impaired lung function (Roth & Noll, 1994). To date, there have been two randomized controlled trials examining the influence of RMT (hyperpnoea) or IMT upon patients following a stroke (Sutbeyaz et al, 2010; Britto et al, 2011). In the study of Sutbeyaz and colleagues (2010), inspiratory muscle strength (MIP) and FVC (forced vital capacity) improved significantly in the IMT group (16% and 7–9%, respectively), but only MIP and MEP improved significantly in the endurance RMT group (14% and 9%, respectively). There were also small, but significant, improvements in MIP (5%) and MEP (5%) in the control group. Furthermore, the IMT group was the only group to exhibit a significant improvement in both exertional dyspnoea and exercise performance during arm cranking, post-intervention (peak $\dot{V}O_2$, heart rate and $\dot{V}_E$). In addition, the Barthel Index and Functional Ambulation Categories scores increased significantly in the IMT group, but not in the other two groups. Finally, health-related quality of life scores also improved significantly in the IMT and RMT groups. In their study of IMT, Britto and colleagues (2011) found that both MIP (52%) and inspiratory muscle endurance (53%) improved post-intervention, and changes were significantly different from the placebo group. However, there were no significant changes in exercise tolerance or quality of life. A Cochrane review of these two studies concluded that 'Further well-designed [randomized controlled trials] are required' (Xiao et al, 2012), but these data provide some preliminary indications that IMT might be of benefit to patients following a stroke.

Parkinson's disease (PD) patients have a number of pulmonary abnormalities including a reduction in respiratory muscle strength, endurance and mechanical efficiency (Tzelepis et al, 1988; Weiner et al, 2002a), accompanied by a restrictive pattern of lung dysfunction (Sabate et al, 1996). Surprisingly, exertional dyspnoea is uncommon, but this is most likely because of the sedentary lifestyles of most PD patients (Inzelberg et al, 2005). This supposition is supported by the fact that, during loaded breathing, dyspnoea is greater in patients with PD than in control participants (Weiner et al, 2002a). A placebo-controlled trial found that, after IMT, inspiratory muscle strength and endurance improve (26% and 45%, respectively), but without any change in lung function (Inzelberg et al, 2005). These improvements in respiratory muscle function were accompanied by, and correlated with, a reduction in the perception of dyspnoea during a loaded breathing test (22%). To date, no study has evaluated whether the improvements in respiratory muscle function and dyspnoea translate into improved exercise tolerance and quality of life.

Amyotrophic lateral sclerosis (or motor neuron disease; ALS/MND) is a neurodegenerative disease involving progressive weakness of voluntary muscles, including respiratory muscles (Just et al, 2010). A decline in lung function accompanies the inspiratory muscle weakness, which contributes to the development of hypoventilation (Pinto et al, 2009) and ultimately to respiratory failure (Cheah et al, 2009). Indeed, both FVC and respiratory muscle strength correlate with prognosis in ALS (Stambler et al, 1998). To date, two randomized controlled studies have evaluated the influence of IMT upon the function of patients with ALS (Cheah et al, 2009; Pinto et al, 2012). One studied 26 patients in the early stages of the disease (Pinto et al, 2012), whereas the other studied 37 consecutive patients (Cheah et al, 2009). In neither study did IMT induce any statistically significant improvements in respiratory muscle or lung function. However, both sets of data exhibited trends towards improving MIP and lung function (Cheah et al, 2009) or offsetting ongoing deterioration of function (Pinto et al, 2012). In both studies, the statistical power was hampered by sample size, and by the shifting baseline of deteriorating function. It is also noteworthy that both studies implemented a training regimen that would be considered an endurance protocol, i.e., a low relative load sustained for 10 minutes. It is possible that briefer bouts of higher-intensity training might yield improvements in MIP and lung function. The data are therefore inconclusive with respect to the effect of IMT upon patients with ALS.

Finally, it is worthwhile mentioning that repeated, deep inhalations against an inspiratory load have been found to be twice as effective (as measured by sputum weight) as standardized physiotherapy consisting of postural drainage and the active cycle of breathing technique (Chatham et al, 2004). Thus, IMT may also facilitate airway clearance in patients with NMD.

In summary, it is clear from the preceding section that the evidence base for RMT in people with NMD is heterogeneous. There are clear differences between disease conditions in both the quality of the evidence and the ease with which it can be interpreted. Since no evidence-based guidelines exist for exercise prescription in general or RMT in particular for patients with NMD, Aboussouan (2009) offers some pragmatic advice in a review on exercise limitation and pulmonary rehabilitation for patients with NMD, suggesting that the selection of any training modality should be based upon the patients' limitations. For example, for RMT it is suggested: '[RMT] should be considered in patients in whom respiratory muscle weakness or fatigue is contributing to the impairment'. An application that awaits empirical assessment is the prophylactic use of RMT as a means of providing a functional 'cushion' against respiratory failure.

Obesity

To date, three studies have examined the influence of RMT in patients with obesity, two of which used hyperpnoea RMT (Frank et al, 2011; Villiot-Danger et al, 2011) and one IMT (Edwards et al, 2012). The premise for the study by Frank and colleagues (2011) was that the attenuating influence of hyperpnoea RMT upon exertional dyspnoea would make exercise 'more enjoyable', thereby increasing spontaneous physical activity. The study had a randomized controlled design in which one group undertook just exercise plus nutrition counselling (E+N) whilst the other undertook RMT (30 minutes hyperventilation five times per week) in addition to E+N. There was a 1-month run-in period during which the RMT group trained and the control group received no intervention. This was followed by a 3-month block of supervised RMT and/or E+N, and a second 3-month block of unsupervised RMT and/or E+N. Both groups improved their 12-minute treadmill walk/run distance, but the improvement was significantly greater in the group who also received RMT (8.7% vs 3.6%). Using a case–control design, Villiot-Danger and colleagues (2011) also implemented hyperpnoea RMT (30 minutes of hyperventilation, 3–4 times per week); 10 participants underwent 26 days of inpatient dietary control and exercise plus RMT, whilst the control group received only dietary control and exercise. There were significantly larger improvements in 6-minute walk distance (54 metres, ~10%), dyspnoea and quality of life in the group who also received RMT. Furthermore, improvements in 6-minute walk distance were correlated significantly with improvements in respiratory muscle endurance. Finally, Edwards and colleagues (2012) examined the influence of IMT in 15 obese and overweight individuals using a randomized placebo-controlled design. The 4-week training intervention consisted of 30 breaths, twice daily at 55% of MIP. There were no changes in lung function, but the 6-minute walk distance increased significantly (62 metres ~20%) in the IMT group, but not in the placebo group. Interestingly, the improvement in 6-minute walk distance correlated positively both with change in MIP and with baseline body mass index.

In summary, specific recommendations regarding the use of RMT and IMT to reduce dyspnoea and improve exercise tolerance in obese people await further research. However, there is preliminary evidence that both RMT and IMT enhance exercise tolerance and reduce dyspnoea in obese individuals, a finding that is supported by a strong theoretical rationale. Accordingly, this is an area worthy of future exploration, particularly in light of the potential of RMT and IMT to enhance the ability to tolerate exercise training for weight loss.

Ageing

Normal ageing is associated with a number of changes that affect breathing, and the senescent changes to the pulmonary system have been dubbed 'senile emphysema' (Janssens et al, 1999). These changes impact upon the demand/capacity relationship of the respiratory muscles, which may contribute to exercise limitation via dyspnoea. Indeed, respiratory muscle strength is independently related to decline in mobility in older people (Buchman et al, 2008). Whether mobility is the chicken or the egg is unclear, but a randomized double-blind placebo-controlled trial has shown that improving inspiratory muscle function through IMT significantly increases participation in moderate-to-vigorous physical activity (Aznar-Lain et al, 2007). The latter may arise because exertional dyspnoea is lower, rendering exercise less uncomfortable.

To date, there have been only a handful of studies of resistance RMT in healthy elderly people (Copestake & McConnell, 1995; Aznar-Lain et al, 2007; Watsford & Murphy, 2008). Collectively, these studies indicate that 6–8 weeks of IMT induce consistent increases in MIP (~20–46%), treadmill exercise capacity (peak performance and T_{lim} duration) and spontaneous physical activity (measured by accelerometry), as well as reducing exertional dyspnoea. One randomized controlled trial implemented IMT+EMT (within the same breath cycle) and demonstrated significant increases in both MIP (20%) and MEP

(30%) (Watsford & Murphy, 2008). In addition, the same study demonstrated that, when walking at 5.5 km·h^{-1}, the heart rate, breathing effort and oxygen uptake were significantly lower in the training group. Similar reductions have also been observed in healthy young people (see the section 'Responses to RMT in healthy people'). Finally, one randomized controlled trial has examined the effect of 8 weeks of hyperpnoea RMT (Belman & Gaesser, 1988); it observed a significant increase in maximum sustained ventilatory capacity (17%), but no significant improvement in incremental or single-stage treadmill performance, or in breathing effort during exercise.

In summary, specific recommendations regarding the use of RMT to reduce dyspnoea and improve exercise tolerance in older people await further research. However, the small number of studies to date suggest that both IMT and IMT+EMT improve a range of exercise-related outcomes in healthy elderly people, although hyperpnoea RMT does not appear to generate any benefits. The strong theoretical rationale for [strength] RMT in older people, combined with the finding of an apparent relationship between improvement in MIP and participation in moderate-to-vigorous physical activity, also supports its use as a potential means of enhancing physical functioning. The demographic shift towards an increasingly older population makes this a potentially impactful area for future research. For specific recommendations regarding implementation of IMT see Chapters 5 and 6.

Miscellaneous conditions

Diabetes

Type 1 and 2 diabetes are associated with inspiratory muscle weakness (Heimer et al, 1990; Kaminski et al, 2011) and in type 1 there is also impairment of inspiratory muscle endurance (Heimer et al, 1990), as well as of vital capacity and FEV$_1$ (Innocenti et al, 1994). These factors may contribute to exercise intolerance via their influence on the demand/capacity relationship of the respiratory pump.

To date, there is only one study of IMT in patients with diabetes, and this was undertaken in patients with type 2, who were selected for their inspiratory muscle weakness (Correa et al, 2011). In this randomized placebo-controlled trial, low-intensity IMT (30 minutes breathing against 30% of MIP) was undertaken for 8 weeks. Inspiratory muscle strength and endurance increased significantly over that of the placebo group; indeed, MIP doubled and endurance tripled. Lung function was normal at baseline and did not improve, and incremental treadmill performance ($\dot{V}O_{2peak}$) also did not improve. The study also evaluated a number of indices of autonomic function, which showed no change. The use of an incremental exercise test is questionable in this study, as peak heart rate data suggest that the patients attained a cardiovascular limited peak at baseline (peak $f_c = 150$ beats · min^{-1}). This being the case, an increase in $\dot{V}O_{2peak}$ post-IMT was extremely unlikely as maximal $\dot{V}O_2$ does not increase after IMT. Submaximal constant intensity tests such as the 6-minute walk test are typically most sensitive to the physiological changes elicited by IMT, and might have revealed a change in exercise tolerance in these patients.

There is one further relevant, and intriguing, controlled trial that is applicable to patients with diabetes. The premise for the study was the observation that 3 weeks of IMT increased the expression of the glucose transporter GLUT-4 in the diaphragm of sheep (Bhandari et al, 2000). Seven of 14 elderly insulin-resistant patients received 12 weeks of low-intensity IMT (30 minutes breathing against 40% of MIP) (Silva Mdos et al, 2012); IMT increased MIP significantly (25%), and this was accompanied by a decrease in insulin resistance, as indicated by a decrease in the 'Homeostatic model assessment for insulin resistance' (HOMA-IR) from 2.9 to 0.9 units. The authors suggested that IMT might offer an important intervention for insulin-insensitive patients who are unable to exercise.

In summary, specific recommendations regarding the use of RMT to reduce dyspnoea and improve exercise tolerance in patients with diabetes await further research. These studies should use tests such as the 6-minute walk test to evaluate functional changes elicited by IMT. Preliminary evidence suggests RMT may reduce insulin resistance, which is also worthy of further research. For specific recommendations regarding implementation of IMT see Chapters 5 and 6.

Renal failure

Respiratory system involvement in renal failure is extremely complex (Prezant, 1990), deriving from both the disease and its treatment. It has been known for many years that uraemic patients possess impaired inspiratory muscle strength and a restrictive pulmonary defect (Gomez-Fernandez et al, 1984). To date, there have been just three studies of IMT in patients receiving haemodialysis (Weiner et al, 1996; Silva et al, 2011; Pellizzaro et al, 2013). The first (available in English only as an abstract) reported improvements in inspiratory muscle function and functional capacity that were not seen in the sham-training control group (Weiner et al, 1996). Unfortunately, the second study had no control group, and although MIP increased by around 70% after low-intensity IMT (15 minutes breathing against 40% of MIP) this was not statistically significant (Silva et al, 2011). There were no changes in lung function, but the 6-minute walk distance increased significantly (20%) and exertional dyspnoea was reduced significantly (27%). The most recent study (Pellizzaro et al, 2013) was a randomized controlled trial in which RMT was compared with peripheral muscle training (PMT) in 39 patients undergoing haemodialysis (11 RMT, 14 PMT, 14 control). The MIP, MEP and 6-minute walk distance increased significantly in both exercise groups, compared with control, with changes in the RMT group being larger than those in the PMT group.

In summary, specific recommendations regarding the use of RMT to reduce dyspnoea and improve exercise tolerance in patients with renal failure await further research, but are supported by preliminary findings of improved exercise capacity after IMT in two studies. For specific recommendations regarding implementation of IMT see Chapters 5 and 6.

Myopathic pharmacological agents

Steroid-induced myopathy is a well-established phenomenon in patients receiving high doses of corticosteroids (Perkoff et al, 1959), and the inspiratory muscles are amongst those affected (Weiner et al, 1995). Other agents, e.g., colchicine and statins, have also been linked with iatrogenic myopathy in case studies.

Patients with COPD are routinely prescribed high doses of corticosteroids during exacerbations to control lung inflammation, but their myopathic effects may have unwanted side effects. Weiner and colleagues hypothesized that the inspiratory muscle weakness induced by the corticosteroids might impair lung function (Weiner et al, 1995). They tested this hypothesis by assessing the influence of acute administration of oral corticosteroids upon the inspiratory muscle and lung function of 12 patients (with conditions other than respiratory disease). The spontaneous response to corticosteroid treatment was compared with the response when treatment was accompanied by a programme of IMT. By the end of the 8-week course of corticosteroid treatment, significant reductions in inspiratory muscle strength ($\sim$30%), endurance ($\sim$50%) and lung function (forced vital capacity reduced by almost 15%) were observed in the group who did not receive IMT; in contrast, in the group who received IMT during treatment, inspiratory muscle and lung function remained stable. The authors concluded that, in order to prevent the detrimental influence of corticosteroids, particularly in respiratory patients in whom inspiratory muscle weakness is already present, IMT might be implemented.

In summary, where myopathic agents are necessary or desirable modes of treatment, Weiner and colleagues' study (1995) suggests that their myopathic influence might be minimized by prophylactic IMT. For specific recommendations regarding implementation of IMT see Chapters 5 and 6.

Surgery

Physical fitness is utilized increasingly as a tool for the risk stratification of patients prior to surgery, with fitter patients showing a lower risk of adverse outcomes (Hennis et al, 2011). The benefit of higher levels of physical fitness prior to surgery has led to the assessment of pre- and post-operative physical training, including IMT (Jack et al, 2011), as tools to enhance outcomes. A recent Cochrane review of preoperative physical therapy for elective cardiac surgery patients concluded that, 'preoperative physical therapy, especially inspiratory muscle training, prevents some postoperative complications, including atelectasis, pneumonia, and length of hospital stay' (Hulzebos et al, 2012).

Inspiratory muscle training has been conducted pre-operatively, post-operatively and both pre- and post-operatively. Pre-operative IMT has been undertaken prior to coronary artery by-pass graft surgery (CABG) (Weiner et al, 1998b; Hulzebos et al, 2006a; Hulzebos et al, 2006b), abdominal surgery (Dronkers et al, 2008, 2010; Kulkarni et al, 2010), oesophagectomy (Dettling et al, 2012), open bariatric surgery (Barbalho-Moulim et al, 2011) and thoracic orthopaedic surgery (Takaso et al, 2010). Post-operative treatment has followed open bariatric surgery (Casali et al, 2011) and cardiac sugery (Kodric et al, 2012), whilst pre- and post-operative treatment has been undertaken in patients undergoing CABG surgery (Savci et al, 2011) and pneumonectomy (Weiner et al, 1997). In most cases, these studies have been randomized controlled trials (Weiner et al, 1997; Weiner et al, 1998b; Hulzebos et al, 2006a; Hulzebos et al, 2006b; Dronkers et al, 2008; Dronkers et al, 2010; Kulkarni et al, 2010; Barbalho-Moulim et al, 2011; Casali et al, 2011; Kodric et al, 2012).

Pre-operative treatment duration has typically ranged from 2 to 4 weeks, using a training regimen with a low intensity (15–30 minutes breathing against 10–60% of MIP). Typically, relative to usual care, pre-operative IMT is associated with improvement or maintenance of MIP and lung function. In addition, there is a reduction in the incidence of atelectasis (Hulzebos et al, 2006b; Dronkers et al, 2008), reduction in the number and severity of post-operative pulmonary complications (Hulzebos et al, 2006a) and a reduction in the number of patients requiring mechanical ventilation (Weiner et al, 1998b). In the largest study to date, Hulzebos and colleagues (2006a) planned to recruit 584 patients. However, the study was stopped after 292 patients following interim analysis revealing that the incidence of pneumonia and length of hospital stay were significantly lower in the IMT group, compared with the usual care–control group. The study was halted because the institutional review board 'thought it was no longer ethical to withhold IMT from the patients in the usual care group' (Hulzebos et al, 2006a). Post-operative IMT has been associated with a more rapid recovery of lung function following bariatric surgery (Casali et al, 2011). However, Dettling and colleagues found no change in the incidence of pneumonia or length of hospital stay following at least 2 weeks of pre-operative IMT in patients subjected to oesophagectomy, despite a significant increase in MIP (Dettling et al, 2012). However, it is noteworthy that MIP declined by around two-thirds post-operatively in the IMT group (to $\sim$37 cmH$_2$O), and by around half in the control group (to $\sim$25 cmH$_2$O), but remained significantly higher in the IMT group. This marked decline may be because of the involvement of the diaphragm during oesophageal resection, and it is possible that the superior MIP post-operatively in the IMT group was insufficient, in absolute terms, to provide any influence upon susceptibility to

pneumonia. Surgically induced diaphragm dysfunction is also a complication of cardiac surgery. A 1-year randomized, placebo-controlled trial of IMT in patients with post-operative diaphragm paralysis found that 78% of patients receiving IMT ($n = 36$) showed improved diaphragm mobility, compared with just 12% of placebo patients ($n = 16$) (Kodric et al, 2012).

In the most recent study to evaluate pre- and post-surgery IMT, functional capacity (6-minute walk test), anxiety score and length of stay in intensive care were all found to improve significantly relative to a group who received usual care in patients who underwent CABG surgery (Savci et al, 2011).

In summary, in patients undergoing surgery to the thorax or abdomen, prophylactic IMT for as little as 2 weeks may provide a functional 'cushion' that enhances recovery and minimizes the risk of post-operative complications. The fact that the largest study of pre-operative IMT to date was halted prematurely because it was considered unethical to withhold the treatment from the control group is a strong recommendation for its routine implementation. Similarly, post-operative IMT may speed recovery and enhance exercise capacity. For specific recommendations regarding implementation of IMT see Chapters 5 and 6.

Mechanical ventilation

Mechanical ventilation can lead to rapid atrophy and loss of respiratory muscle function (Fitting, 1994; Bissett et al, 2012b), precipitating prolongation of mechanical ventilation and difficulty weaning patients from the ventilator (Callahan, 2009; Bissett et al, 2012b). Patients who are weaned successfully from mechanical ventilation have higher MIP than those who do not (20–40 cmH$_2$O vs 40–60 cmH$_2$O) (Epstein et al, 2002; Carlucci et al, 2009). Indeed, MIP has been found to be an independent predictor of delayed weaning (De Jonghe et al, 2007), suggesting that improving MIP might be a therapeutic target in such patients during the weaning process, as well as prophylactically. However, the apparent link between inspiratory muscle weakness and weaning failure is by no means clear-cut, and some studies have failed to find any influence of MIP upon weaning outcome (Meade et al, 2001; Conti et al, 2004). Furthermore, despite the apparent logic of improving MIP, it is far from certain that the inspiratory muscles are 'trainable' under conditions of mechanical ventilation, or that improving strength addresses the complex impediments to weaning sufficiently directly (Bissett et al, 2012b).

The majority of studies examining the influence of IMT upon weaning success have been case reports, or uncontrolled trials in small groups of patients (Aldrich & Uhrlass, 1987; Lerman & Weiss, 1987; Aldrich et al, 1989; Martin et al, 2002; Sprague & Hopkins, 2003; Bissett & Leditschke, 2007), including infants (Brunherotti et al, 2012; Smith et al, 2012). In all such trials, patients who had previously failed to wean from a ventilator have been given brief periods of IMT and periods of spontaneous breathing off the ventilator, with the result that MIP improved and successful weaning was achieved.

A handful of randomized controlled trials have examined the influence of IMT upon weaning (Caruso et al, 2005; Cader et al, 2010; Martin et al, 2011; Cader et al, 2012), and a systematic review was published in 2011 (Moodie et al, 2011). The review included 150 patients and demonstrated a significant effect of training upon MIP and a trend in favour of IMT for weaning success and duration, as well as for survival. It is noteworthy that the study by Cader and colleagues (Cader et al, 2010) included ventilated patients who were intubated and in the early phase of mechanical ventilation (Cader et al, 2010), whilst that of Martin and colleagues included tracheostomized patients with weaning failure (Martin et al, 2011). The studies also differed in the training regimen implemented. Cader and colleagues (2010) employed an IMT regimen consisting of 5 minutes at a load equivalent to 30% MIP, twice daily. In contrast, Martin and colleagues employed a regimen of four sets of 6–10 breaths at the highest tolerable load, with mechanical ventilation between each set. Cader and colleagues (2010) found that, in those who did not die or receive a tracheostomy, the time to weaning was significantly shorter in the experimental group than in the control group (1.7 days), whereas Martin and colleagues (2011) found that 71% of their IMT group weaned successfully compared with 47% of the placebo group. In contrast, the study by Caruso et al (2005) found no change in MIP across the intervention; however, training consisted of imposing an inspiratory load by adjusting the pressure trigger of the mechanical ventilator (ranging from 20% of MIP to 40% of MIP). It is therefore possible that the discrepancy with other studies may be explained by the nature of the training stimulus, which would have consisted of a brief threshold load at the very onset of the breath. This is a very different, and inferior, training stimulus compared with inhaling continuously against an inspiratory threshold load. This is emphasized by a recent randomized controlled trial of pressure threshold IMT in intubated, elderly intensive care patients ($n = 28$) (Cader et al, 2012). The patients in the IMT group ($n = 14$) showed a significant increase in MIP (67%) and a significant decrease in Tobin Index, compared with controls ($n = 14$). The IMT group also had a shorter weaning time (3.64 vs 5.36 days), but this was not significant. However, the time spent in non-invasive positive pressure ventilation was significantly shorter for the IMT group (7.5 vs 23 hours).

In a recent review of IMT in ventilated patents, Bissett and colleagues (2012b) suggested that the benefits of IMT may be wider reaching than simply improving the power of the respiratory pump. For example, they hypothesized that a reduction in inspiratory metaboreflex activation might enhance perfusion, thereby accelerating recovery; this awaits further research.

Finally, it is pertinent to stress that the available evidence suggests that IMT is safe, even for patients undergoing continuous invasive ventilation (Bissett et al, 2012a), and is well tolerated, even in infants (Brunherotti et al, 2012; Smith et al, 2012). Bissett and colleagues used a prospective cohort study to assess the influence of IMT, without supplemental oxygen, in 10 medically stable ventilator-dependent adult patients. They observed no adverse responses during the 195 IMT sessions assessed. Furthermore, IMT provoked no significant changes in heart rate, mean arterial pressure, oxygen saturation or respiratory rate. Training consisted of three to six sets of six breaths at a training threshold that generated a Borg CR-10 rating of between 6 and 8. Furthermore, no adverse events were reported in the studies of Martin et al (2011) or Cader et al (2010).

In summary, the strong theoretical rationale for IMT appears to be supported by positive case study data and emerging data from randomized controlled trials. When IMT is implemented using a resistance-training device, weaning from mechanical ventilation is enhanced. This conclusion is also supported by the outcomes of the systematic review by Bissett and colleagues (2012b), which suggested that IMT is a useful treatment for patients subjected to mechanical ventilation and those experiencing weaning failure. Importantly, they also highlighted the importance of careful selection of patients for IMT, suggesting they must be 'stable, alert and co-operative patients who are able to psychologically tolerate the temporary high inspiratory workload of IMT'. Furthermore they recommended that patients should be 'medically stable and they must not be heavily reliant on high levels of ventilatory support (e.g., PEEP < 10, $FiO_2 < 60\%$). Not all critically ill patients will be suitable for IMT, particularly in the most acute phase of their management. However, any patient who is at risk of ventilator-induced respiratory dysfunction, particularly those whose MV has exceeded seven days, should be screened for suitability for IMT.' Bissett and colleagues have also provided evidence to support the safety of IMT in this vulnerable patient group (Bissett et al, 2012a). The importance of the potential clinical outcomes of IMT in the critical care setting promises to make this a burgeoning area of research.

Obstructive sleep apnoea

There are two mechanical mechanisms by which the collapsibility of the upper airway could be modified: first by improving active neuromuscular tone of the upper airway, and secondly by reducing the passive compliance of the upper airway. The former has two subcomponents, the first being reflex coordination of airway dilator muscles, and the second being the functional properties of these muscles (e.g., strength, fatigue resistance, rate of shortening).

Short-term repetition of motor tasks has been shown to induce cortical reorganization in a range of activities, including the practice of diaphragm breathing (Demoule et al, 2008). These changes are consistent with the ability of task repetition to enhance neuromuscular functioning, thereby optimizing reflex coordination of muscles. Furthermore the hyperpnoea of exercise training has been shown to elicit structural adaptions in both the diaphragm and upper airway muscles of rats (Vincent et al, 2002). The structural changes induced by training also influence the compliance of muscle tissue; e.g., the passive stiffness of locomotor muscles increases in a manner that is independent of increases in either mass or strength (Lindstedt et al, 2002).

It may not be immediately apparent why IMT would influence the physiology of the upper airway musculature, but the negative pressure generated within the airways during inhalation tends to collapse the extrathoracic airways. Thus IMT induces activation of upper-airway-stabilizing muscles in order to maintain upper airway patency (How et al, 2007; Cheng et al, 2011). Because these muscles are activated during IMT, it is reasonable to presume that the upper airway muscles are also trained during IMT.

To date, there have been no randomized controlled trials of RMT in patients with OSA; however, there are some data that hint at potential benefits. For example, one study has shown an improvement in nocturnal saturation in patients with COPD following IMT (Heijdra et al, 1996). In addition, RMT using hyperpnoea training has been shown to reduce the incidence of snoring and daytime sleepiness (Furrer et al, 1998; Frank et al, 2011), but did not improve the apnoea–hypopnoea index in obese patients (Frank et al, 2011). Interestingly, a randomized controlled trial of didgeridoo playing showed it to have a beneficial effect upon daytime sleepiness, apnoea–hypopnoea index and partner-reported sleep disturbance (Puhan et al, 2006). In addition, a cross-sectional study of 906 musicians found that musicians who played double-reed instruments had a significantly lower OSA risk than non-wind musicians, and that risk was predicted by the number of hours spent playing (Ward et al, 2012). Further research is needed, but these data provide an impetus for further exploration of RMT in patients with OSA.

In summary, specific recommendations regarding the use of RMT to reduce the severity of OSA awaits further research. However, implementation is supported by preliminary case study evidence and a theoretical rationale. Accordingly, this is an area worthy of future exploration, particularly in light of the growing prevalence of OSA as a co-morbidity of many chronic conditions. In the mean time, IMT could be considered as a safe, simple and inexpensive adjunctive treatment in patients with OSA. For specific recommendations regarding implementation of IMT see Chapters 5 and 6.

Vocal cord dysfunction and inspiratory stridor

Inspiratory stridor (IS) is an external sign of vocal cord dysfunction (VCD) during exercise; it arises when the vocal cords collapse across that laryngeal opening causing an increase in upper airway flow resistance, increased breathing effort, dyspnoea and sudden exercise intolerance. As was mentioned in the section on OSA, the activation of upper airway muscles during IMT means that it is highly likely that these muscles are also trained during IMT.

Traditional treatments for inspiratory stridor are based on speech therapy techniques, and in extreme cases surgery is used to stabilize the upper airway mechanically (Maat et al, 2007). However, two case studies have shown that exercise-induced symptoms of stridor subside after a short period of IMT (30 breaths breathing against 50–60% of MIP for 4 to 11 weeks), without recurrence (Ruddy et al, 2004; Dickinson et al, 2007). In addition, dyspnoea and exercise intolerance due to vocal fold paralysis have also been treated successfully using IMT (Baker et al, 2003a; Baker et al, 2003b).

In summary, specific recommendations regarding the use of RMT to ameliorate IS and VCD await further research. However, implementation is supported by preliminary evidence from case studies and a theoretical rationale. Accordingly, this is an area worthy of future exploration using randomized controlled designs. In the meantime, IMT could be considered as a safe, simple and inexpensive first-line intervention in patients with VCD. For specific recommendations regarding implementation of IMT see Chapters 5 and 6.

General conclusions

The range of conditions in which RMT has been implemented to date spans the obvious (e.g., COPD) to the unexpected (e.g., diabetes). In conditions where RMT has been implemented, the strength of evidence also varies widely, from conditions where IMT is supported by systematic reviews and meta-analyses (e.g., COPD) to those where there is currently only a theoretical rationale for assessing potential benefits (e.g., OSA). A better understanding of the load/capacity relationship of the respiratory muscles is emerging, and this is providing impetus for research to characterize and address imbalance. Furthermore, the development of a greater understanding of RMT and its potential benefits, combined with greater knowledge regarding implementation, as well as advances in training equipment, should amalgamate to stimulate further advances in RMT research and applications.

REFERENCES

Aboussouan, L.S., 2009. Mechanisms of exercise limitation and pulmonary rehabilitation for patients with neuromuscular disease. Chron. Respir. Dis. 6, 231–249.

Aldrich, T.K., Uhrlass, R.M., 1987. Weaning from mechanical ventilation: successful use of modified inspiratory resistive training in muscular dystrophy. Crit. Care Med. 15, 247–249.

Aldrich, T.K., Karpel, J.P., Uhrlass, R.M., et al., 1989. Weaning from mechanical ventilation: adjunctive use of inspiratory muscle resistive training. Crit. Care Med. 17, 143–147.

Amann, M., Proctor, L.T., Sebranek, J.J., et al., 2009. Opioid-mediated muscle afferents inhibit central motor drive and limit peripheral muscle fatigue development in humans. J. Physiol. 587, 271–283.

Amann, M., Blain, G.M., Proctor, L.T., et al., 2010. Group III and IV muscle afferents contribute to ventilatory and cardiovascular response to rhythmic exercise in humans. J. Appl. Physiol. 109, 966–976.

Asher, M.I., Pardy, R.L., Coates, A.L., et al., 1982. The effects of inspiratory muscle training in patients with cystic fibrosis. Am. Rev. Respir. Dis. 126, 855–859.

Aznar-Lain, S., Webster, A.L., Canete, S., et al., 2007. Effects of inspiratory muscle training on exercise capacity and spontaneous physical activity in elderly subjects: a randomized controlled pilot trial. Int. J. Sports Med. 28, 1025–1029.

Baba, R., Nagashima, M., Goto, M., et al., 1996. Oxygen uptake efficiency slope: a new index of cardiorespiratory functional reserve derived from the relation between oxygen uptake and minute ventilation during incremental exercise. J. Am. Coll. Cardiol. 28, 1567–1572.

Bailey, S.J., Romer, L.M., Kelly, J., et al., 2010. Inspiratory muscle training enhances pulmonary O(2) uptake kinetics and high-intensity exercise tolerance in humans. J. Appl. Physiol. 109, 457–468.

Baker, S.E., Sapienza, C.M., Collins, S., 2003a. Inspiratory pressure threshold training in a case of congenital bilateral abductor vocal fold paralysis. Int. J. Pediatr. Otorhinolaryngol. 67, 413–416.

Baker, S.E., Sapienza, C.M., Martin, D., et al., 2003b. Inspiratory pressure threshold training for upper airway limitation: a case of bilateral abductor vocal fold paralysis. J. Voice 17, 384–394.

Baker, S., Davenport, P., Sapienza, C., 2005. Examination of strength training and detraining effects in expiratory muscles. J. Speech Lang. Hear. Res. 48, 1325–1333.

Bangsbo, J., Iaia, F.M., Krustrup, P., 2008. The Yo-Yo intermittent recovery test : a useful tool for evaluation of physical performance in intermittent sports. Sports Med. 38, 37–51.

Barbalho-Moulim, M.C., Miguel, G.P., Forti, E.M., et al., 2011. Effects of preoperative inspiratory muscle training in obese women undergoing open bariatric surgery: respiratory muscle strength, lung volumes, and diaphragmatic excursion. Clinics 66, 1721–1727.

Beckerman, M., Magadle, R., Weiner, M., et al., 2005. The effects of 1 year of specific inspiratory muscle training in patients with COPD. Chest 128, 3177–3182.

Belman, M.J., Gaesser, G.A., 1988. Ventilatory muscle training in the elderly. J. Appl. Physiol. 64, 899–905.

Bhandari, A., Xia, Y., Cortright, R., et al., 2000. Effect of respiratory muscle training on GLUT-4 in the sheep diaphragm. Med. Sci. Sports Exerc. 32, 1406–1411.

Bissett, B., Leditschke, I.A., 2007. Inspiratory muscle training to enhance weaning from mechanical ventilation. Anaesth. Intensive Care 35, 776–779.

Bissett, B., Leditschke, I.A., Green, M., 2012a. Specific inspiratory muscle training is safe in selected patients who are ventilator-dependent: a case series. Intensive Crit. Care Nurs. 28, 98–104.

Bissett, B., Leditschke, I.A., Paratz, J.D., et al., 2012b. Respiratory dysfunction in ventilated patients: can inspiratory muscle training help? Anaesth. Intensive Care 40, 236–246.

Bosnak-Guclu, M., Arikan, H., Savci, S., et al., 2011. Effects of inspiratory muscle training in patients with heart failure. Respir. Med. 105, 1671–1681.

Bott, J., Blumenthal, S., Buxton, M., et al., 2009. Guidelines for the physiotherapy management of the adult, medical, spontaneously breathing patient. Thorax 64 (Suppl. 1), i1–i51.

Britto, R.R., Rezende, N.R., Marinho, K.C., et al., 2011. Inspiratory muscular training in chronic stroke survivors: a randomized controlled trial. Arch. Phys. Med. Rehabil. 92, 184–190.

Brooks, D., O'Brien, K., Geddes, E.L., et al., 2005. Is inspiratory muscle training effective for individuals with cervical spinal cord injury? A qualitative systematic review. Clin. Rehabil. 19, 237–246.

Brown, P.I., Sharpe, G.R., Johnson, M.A., 2011. Inspiratory muscle training abolishes the blood lactate increase associated with volitional hyperpnoea superimposed on exercise and accelerates lactate and oxygen uptake kinetics at the onset of exercise. Eur. J. Appl. Physiol. 12 (6), 2117–2129.

Brunherotti, M.A., Bezerra, P.P., Bachur, C.K., et al., 2012. Inspiratory muscle training in a newborn with anoxia who was chronically ventilated. Phys. Ther. 92, 865–871.

Buchman, A.S., Boyle, P.A., Wilson, R.S., et al., 2008. Respiratory muscle strength predicts decline in mobility in older persons. Neuroepidemiology 31, 174–180.

Budweiser, S., Moertl, M., Jorres, R.A., et al., 2006. Respiratory muscle training in restrictive thoracic disease: a randomized controlled trial. Arch. Phys. Med. Rehabil. 87, 1559–1565.

Cader, S.A., Vale, R.G., Castro, J.C., et al., 2010. Inspiratory muscle training improves maximal inspiratory pressure and may assist weaning in older intubated patients: a randomised trial. Journal of Physiotherapy 56, 171–177.

Cader, S.A., de Souza Vale, R.G., Zamora, V.E., et al., 2012. Extubation process in bed-ridden elderly intensive care patients receiving inspiratory muscle training: a randomized clinical trial. Clinical Interventions in Aging 7, 437–443.

Cahalin, L.P., Semigran, M.J., Dec, G.W., 1997. Inspiratory muscle training in patients with chronic heart failure awaiting cardiac transplantation: results of a pilot clinical trial. Phys. Ther. 77, 830–838.

Caine, M.P., McConnell, A.K., 1998a. The inspiratory muscles can be trained differentially to increase strength or endurance using a pressure threshold, inspiratory muscle training device. Eur. Respir. J. 12, 58–59.

Caine, M.P., McConnell, A.K., 1998b. Pressure threshold inspiratory muscle training improves submaximal cycling performance. In: Sargeant, A.J., Siddons, H. (Eds.), Third Annual Conference of the European College of Sport Science. Centre for Health Care Development, Manchester, p. 101.

Callahan, L.A., 2009. Invited editorial on 'acquired respiratory muscle weakness in critically ill patients: what is the role of mechanical ventilation-induced diaphragm dysfunction?' J. Appl. Physiol. 106, 360–361.

Carlucci, A., Ceriana, P., Prinianakis, G., et al., 2009. Determinants of weaning success in patients with prolonged mechanical ventilation. Crit. Care 13, R97.

Caruso, P., Denari, S.D., Ruiz, S.A., et al., 2005. Inspiratory muscle training is ineffective in mechanically ventilated critically ill patients. Clinics 60, 479–484.

Casali, C.C., Pereira, A.P., Martinez, J.A., et al., 2011. Effects of inspiratory muscle training on muscular and pulmonary function after bariatric surgery in obese patients. Obes. Surg. 21, 1389–1394.

Cejudo, P., Lopez-Marquez, I., Lopez-Campos, J.L., et al., 2009. Factors associated with quality of life in patients with chronic respiratory failure due to kyphoscoliosis. Disabil. Rehabil. 31, 928–934.

Chatham, K., Ionescu, A.A., Nixon, L.S., et al., 2004. A short-term comparison of two methods of sputum expectoration in cystic fibrosis. Eur. Respir. J. 23, 435–439.

Cheah, B.C., Boland, R.A., Brodaty, N.E., et al., 2009. INSPIRATIonAL – INSPIRAtory muscle training in amyotrophic lateral sclerosis. Amyotroph. Lateral Scler. 10, 1–9.

Cheng, S., Butler, J.E., Gandevia, S.C., et al., 2011. Movement of the human upper airway during inspiration with and without inspiratory resistive loading. J. Appl. Physiol. 110, 69–75.

Chiappa, G.R., Borghi-Silva, A., Ferreira, L.F., et al., 2008a. Kinetics of muscle deoxygenation are accelerated at the onset of heavy-intensity exercise in patients with COPD: relationship to central cardiovascular dynamics. J. Appl. Physiol. 104, 1341–1350.

Chiappa, G.R., Roseguini, B.T., Vieira, P.J., et al., 2008b. Inspiratory muscle training improves blood flow to resting and exercising limbs in patients with chronic heart failure. J. Am. Coll. Cardiol. 51, 1663–1671.

Chiappa, G.R., Queiroga Jr., F., Meda, E., et al., 2009. Heliox improves oxygen delivery and utilization during dynamic exercise in patients with

chronic obstructive pulmonary disease. Am. J. Respir. Crit. Care Med. 179, 1004–1010.

Chiara, T., Martin, D., Sapienza, C., 2007. Expiratory muscle strength training: speech production outcomes in patients with multiple sclerosis. Neurorehabil. Neural Repair 21, 239–249.

Conti, G., Montini, L., Pennisi, M.A., et al., 2004. A prospective, blinded evaluation of indexes proposed to predict weaning from mechanical ventilation. Intensive Care Med. 30, 830–836.

Copestake, A.J., McConnell, A.K., 1995. Inspiratory muscle training reduces exertional breathlessness in healthy elderly men and women. In: International Conference on Physical Activity and Health in the Elderly. University of Sterling, Scotland, p. 150.

Correa, A.P., Ribeiro, J.P., Balzan, F.M., et al., 2011. Inspiratory muscle training in type 2 diabetes with inspiratory muscle weakness. Med. Sci. Sports Exerc. 43, 1135–1141.

Currell, K., Jeukendrup, A.E., 2008. Validity, reliability and sensitivity of measures of sporting performance. Sports Med. 38, 297–316.

Dall'Ago, P., Chiappa, G.R., Guths, H., et al., 2006. Inspiratory muscle training in patients with heart failure and inspiratory muscle weakness: a randomized trial. J. Am. Coll. Cardiol. 47, 757–763.

de Jong, W., van Aalderen, W.M., Kraan, J., et al., 2001. Inspiratory muscle training in patients with cystic fibrosis. Respir. Med. 95, 31–36.

De Jonghe, B., Bastuji-Garin, S., Durand, M.C., et al., 2007. Respiratory weakness is associated with limb weakness and delayed weaning in critical illness. Crit. Care Med. 35, 2007–2015.

Demoule, A., Verin, E., Montcel, S.T., et al., 2008. Short-term training-dependent plasticity of the corticospinal diaphragm control in normal humans. Respir. Physiol. Neurobiol. 160, 172–180.

DePalo, V.A., Parker, A.L., Al-Bilbeisi, F., et al., 2004. Respiratory muscle strength training with nonrespiratory maneuvers. J. Appl. Physiol. 96, 731–734.

Derrickson, J., Ciesla, N., Simpson, N., et al., 1992. A comparison of two breathing exercise programs for patients with quadriplegia. Phys. Ther. 72, 763–769.

Dettling, D.S., van der Schaaf, M., Blom, R.L., et al., 2012. Feasibility and effectiveness of pre-operative inspiratory muscle training in patients undergoing oesophagectomy: a pilot study. Physiother. Res. Int. Apr 10. [Epub ahead of print]. Available at: http://dx.doi.org/10.1002/pri.1524.

Dickinson, J., Whyte, G., McConnell, A., 2007. Inspiratory muscle training: a simple cost-effective treatment for inspiratory stridor. Br. J. Sports Med 41, 694–695; discussion 695.

DiMarco, A.F., Kelling, J.S., DiMarco, M.S., et al., 1985. The effects of inspiratory resistive training on respiratory muscle function in patients with muscular dystrophy. Muscle Nerve 8, 284–290.

Donath, J., Miller, A., 2009. Restrictive chest wall disorders. Semin. Respir. Crit. Care Med. 30, 275–292.

Downey, A.E., Chenoweth, L.M., Townsend, D.K., et al., 2007. Effects of inspiratory muscle training on exercise responses in normoxia and hypoxia. Respir. Physiol. Neurobiol. 156, 137–146.

Dronkers, J., Veldman, A., Hoberg, E., et al., 2008. Prevention of pulmonary complications after upper abdominal surgery by preoperative intensive inspiratory muscle training: a randomized controlled pilot study. Clin. Rehabil. 22, 134–142.

Dronkers, J.J., Lamberts, H., Reutelingsperger, I.M., et al., 2010. Preoperative therapeutic programme for elderly patients scheduled for elective abdominal oncological surgery: a randomized controlled pilot study. Clin. Rehabil. 24, 614–622.

Edwards, A.M., Cooke, C.B., 2004. Oxygen uptake kinetics and maximal aerobic power are unaffected by inspiratory muscle training in healthy subjects where time to exhaustion is extended. Eur. J. Appl. Physiol. 93, 139–144.

Edwards, A.M., Wells, C., Butterly, R., 2008. Concurrent inspiratory muscle and cardiovascular training differentially improves both perceptions of effort and 5000 m running performance compared with cardiovascular training alone. Br. J. Sports Med. 42, 523–527.

Edwards, A.M., Maguire, G.P., Graham, D., et al., 2012. Four weeks of inspiratory muscle training improves self-paced walking performance in overweight and obese adults: a randomised controlled trial. Journal of Obesity 2012, 918202.

Enright, S., Chatham, K., Ionescu, A.A., et al., 2004. Inspiratory muscle training improves lung function and exercise capacity in adults with cystic fibrosis. Chest 126, 405–411.

Enright, S.J., Unnithan, V.B., Heward, C., et al., 2006. Effect of high-intensity inspiratory muscle training on lung volumes, diaphragm thickness, and exercise capacity in subjects who are healthy. Phys. Ther. 86, 345–354.

Epstein, C.D., El-Mokadem, N., Peerless, J.R., 2002. Weaning older patients from long-term mechanical ventilation: a pilot study. Am. J. Respir. Crit. Care Med. 11, 369–377.

Ferreira, J.B., Plentz, R.D., Stein, C., et al., 2011. Inspiratory muscle training reduces blood pressure and sympathetic activity in hypertensive patients: A randomized controlled trial. Int. J. Cardiol Oct 8. [Epub ahead of print].

Fitting, J.W., 1994. Respiratory muscles during ventilatory support. Eur. Respir. J. 7, 2223–2225.

Frank, I., Briggs, R., Spengler, C.M., 2011. Respiratory muscles, exercise performance, and health in overweight and obese subjects. Med. Sci. Sports Exerc. 43, 714–727.

Fregonezi, G.A., Resqueti, V.R., Guell, R., et al., 2005. Effects of 8-week, interval-based inspiratory muscle training and breathing retraining in patients with generalized myasthenia gravis. Chest 128, 1524–1530.

Fry, D.K., Pfalzer, L.A., Chokshi, A.R., et al., 2007. Randomized control trial of effects of a 10-week inspiratory muscle training program on measures of pulmonary function in persons with multiple sclerosis. J. Neurol. Phys. Ther. 31, 162–172.

Furrer, E., Baur, S., Boutellier, U., 1998. Treatment of snoring by training of the upper airway muscles. Am. J. Respir. Crit. Care Med. 157, A284.

Gandevia, S.C., 2001. Spinal and supraspinal factors in human muscle fatigue. Physiol. Rev. 81, 1725–1789.

Geddes, E.L., O'Brien, K., Reid, W.D., et al., 2008. Inspiratory muscle training in adults with chronic obstructive pulmonary disease: An update of a systematic review. Respir. Med. 102, 1715–1729.

Gething, A.D., Williams, M., Davies, B., 2004. Inspiratory resistive loading improves cycling capacity: a placebo controlled trial. Br. J. Sports Med. 38, 730–736.

Gomez-Fernandez, P., Sanchez Agudo, L., Calatrava, J.M., et al., 1984. Respiratory muscle weakness in uremic patients under continuous ambulatory peritoneal dialysis. Nephron 36, 219–223.

Goosey-Tolfrey, V., Foden, E., Perret, C., et al., 2010. Effects of inspiratory muscle training on respiratory function and repetitive sprint performance in wheelchair basketball players. Br. J. Sports Med. 44, 665–668.

Gosselink, R., Kovacs, L., Ketelaer, P., et al., 2000. Respiratory muscle weakness and respiratory muscle training in severely disabled multiple sclerosis patients. Arch. Phys. Med. Rehabil. 81, 747–751.

Gosselink, R., De Vos, J., van den Heuvel, S.P., et al., 2011. Impact of inspiratory muscle training in patients with COPD: what is the evidence? Eur. Respir. J. 37, 416–425.

Gozal, D., Thiriet, P., 1999. Respiratory muscle training in neuromuscular disease: long-term effects on strength and load perception. Med. Sci. Sports Exerc. 31, 1522–1527.

Griffiths, L.A., McConnell, A.K., 2007. The influence of inspiratory and expiratory muscle training upon rowing performance. Eur. J. Appl. Physiol. 99, 457–466.

Hajghanbari, B., Yamabayashi, C., Buna, T., et al., 2012. Effects of respiratory muscle training on performance in athletes: a systematic review with meta-analyses. J. Strength Cond. Res. [Epub ahead of print]. Available at: http://dx.doi.org/10.1519/JSC.0b013e318269f73f.

Heijdra, Y.F., Dekhuijzen, P.N., van Herwaarden, C.L., et al., 1996. Nocturnal saturation improves by target-flow inspiratory muscle training in patients with COPD. Am. J. Respir. Crit. Care Med. 153, 260–265.

Heimer, D., Brami, J., Lieberman, D., et al., 1990. Respiratory muscle performance in patients with type 1 diabetes. Diabet. Med. 7, 434–437.

Hennis, P.J., Meale, P.M., Grocott, M.P., 2011. Cardiopulmonary exercise testing for the evaluation of perioperative risk in non-cardiopulmonary surgery. Postgrad. Med. J. 87, 550–557.

Hepburn, H., Fletcher, J., Rosengarten, T.H., et al., 2005. Cardiac vagal tone, exercise performance and the effect of respiratory training. Eur. J. Appl. Physiol. 94, 681–689.

Hodges, P.W., Gandevia, S.C., 2000. Activation of the human diaphragm during a repetitive postural task. J. Physiol. 522 (pt 1), 165–175.

Holm, P., Sattler, A., Fregosi, R.F., 2004. Endurance training of respiratory muscles improves cycling performance in fit young cyclists. BMC Physiol. 4, 9.

How, S.C., McConnell, A.K., Taylor, B.J., et al., 2007. Acute and chronic responses of the upper airway to inspiratory loading in healthy awake humans: an MRI study. Respir. Physiol. Neurobiol. 157, 270–280.

Hull, J., Aniapravan, R., Chan, E., et al., 2012. British Thoracic Society guideline for respiratory management of children with neuromuscular weakness. Thorax 67 (Suppl. 1), i1–40.

Hulzebos, E.H., Helders, P.J., Favie, N.J., et al., 2006a. Preoperative intensive inspiratory muscle training to prevent postoperative pulmonary complications in high-risk patients undergoing CABG surgery: a randomized clinical trial. J. Am. Med. Assoc. 296, 1851–1857.

Hulzebos, E.H., van Meeteren, N.L., van den Buijs, B.J., et al., 2006b. Feasibility of preoperative inspiratory muscle training in patients undergoing coronary artery bypass surgery with a high risk of postoperative pulmonary complications: a randomized controlled pilot study. Clin. Rehabil. 20, 949–959.

Hulzebos, E.H., Smit, Y., Helders, P.P., van Meeteren, N.L., 2012. Preoperative physical therapy for elective cardiac surgery patients. Cochrane Database Syst, Rev 11.

Illi, S.K., Held, U., Frank, I., et al., 2012. Effect of respiratory muscle training on exercise performance in healthy individuals: a systematic review and meta-analysis. Sports Med. 42, 707–724.

Innocenti, F., Fabbri, A., Anichini, R., et al., 1994. Indications of reduced pulmonary function in type 1 (insulin-dependent) diabetes mellitus. Diabetes Res. Clin. Pract. 25, 161–168.

Inzelberg, R., Peleg, N., Nisipeanu, P., et al., 2005. Inspiratory muscle training and the perception of dyspnea in Parkinson's disease. Can. J. Neurol. Sci. 32, 213–217.

Jack, S., West, M., Grocott, M.P., 2011. Perioperative exercise training in elderly subjects. Best Pract. Res. Clin. Anaesthesiol. 25, 461–472.

Janssens, J.P., Pache, J.C., Nicod, L.P., 1999. Physiological changes in respiratory function associated with ageing. Eur. Respir. J. 13, 197–205.

Johnson, P.H., Cowley, A.J., Kinnear, W.J., 1998. A randomized controlled trial of inspiratory muscle training in stable chronic heart failure. Eur. Heart. J. 19, 1249–1253.

Johnson, M.A., Sharpe, G.R., Brown, P.I., 2007. Inspiratory muscle training improves cycling time-trial performance and anaerobic work capacity but not critical power. Eur. J. Appl. Physiol. 101, 761–770.

Jones, C.U., Sangthong, B., Pachirat, O., 2010. An inspiratory load enhances the antihypertensive effects of home-based training with slow deep breathing: a randomised trial. Journal of Physiotherapy 56, 179–186.

Just, N., Bautin, N., Danel-Brunaud, V., et al., 2010. The Borg dyspnoea score: a relevant clinical marker of inspiratory muscle weakness in amyotrophic lateral sclerosis. Eur. Respir. J. 35, 353–360.

Kaminski, D.M., Schaan, B.D., da Silva, A.M., et al., 2011. Inspiratory muscle weakness is associated with autonomic cardiovascular dysfunction in patients with type 2 diabetes mellitus. Clin. Auton. Res. 21, 29–35.

Kang, S.W., Shin, J.C., Park, C.I., et al., 2006. Relationship between inspiratory muscle strength and cough capacity in cervical spinal cord injured patients. Spinal Cord 44, 242–248.

Keens, T.G., Krastins, I.R., Wannamaker, E.M., et al., 1977. Ventilatory muscle endurance training in normal subjects and patients with cystic fibrosis. Am. Rev. Respir. Dis. 116, 853–860.

Kikuchi, Y., Okabe, S., Tamura, G., et al., 1994. Chemosensitivity and perception of dyspnea in patients with a history of near-fatal asthma. N. Engl. J. Med. 330, 1329–1334.

Kilding, A.E., Brown, S., McConnell, A.K., 2010. Inspiratory muscle training improves 100 and 200 m swimming performance. Eur. J. Appl. Physiol. 108, 505–511.

Kim, J., Davenport, P., Sapienza, C., 2008. Effect of expiratory muscle strength training on elderly cough function. Arch. Gerontol. Geriatr. 48 (3), 361–366.

Klefbeck, B., Lagerstrand, L., Mattsson, E., 2000. Inspiratory muscle training in patients with prior polio who use part-time assisted ventilation. Arch. Phys. Med. Rehabil. 81, 1065–1071.

Klefbeck, B., Hamrah Nedjad, J., 2003. Effect of inspiratory muscle training in patients with multiple sclerosis. Arch. Phys. Med. Rehabil. 84, 994–999.

Kodric, M., Trevisan, R., Torregiani, C., et al., 2012. Inspiratory muscle training for diaphragm dysfunction after cardiac surgery. J. Thorac. Cardiovasc. Surg. (in press).

Koessler, W., Wanke, T., Winkler, G., et al., 2001. 2 years' experience with inspiratory muscle training in patients with neuromuscular disorders. Chest 120, 765–769.

Kulkarni, S.R., Fletcher, E., McConnell, A.K., et al., 2010. Pre-operative inspiratory muscle training preserves postoperative inspiratory muscle strength following major abdominal surgery – a randomised pilot study. Ann. R. Coll. Surg. Engl. 92, 700–707.

Lanini, B., Gigliotti, F., Coli, C., et al., 2002. Dissociation between respiratory effort and dyspnoea in a subset of patients with stroke. Clin. Sci. (Lond.) 103, 467–473.

Laoutaris, I., Dritsas, A., Brown, M.D., et al., 2004. Inspiratory muscle training using an incremental endurance test alleviates dyspnea and improves functional status in patients with chronic heart failure. Eur. J. Cardiovasc. Prev. Rehabil. 11, 489–496.

Leddy, J.J., Limprasertkul, A., Patel, S., et al., 2007. Isocapnic hyperpnea training improves performance in competitive male runners. Eur. J. Appl. Physiol. 99, 665–676.

Lerman, R.M., Weiss, M.S., 1987. Progressive resistive exercise in weaning high quadriplegics from the ventilator. Paraplegia 25, 130–135.

Liaw, M.Y., Lin, M.C., Cheng, P.T., et al., 2000. Resistive inspiratory muscle training: its effectiveness in patients with acute complete cervical cord injury. Arch. Phys. Med. Rehabil. 81, 752–756.

Liaw, M.Y., Wang, Y.H., Tsai, Y.C., et al., 2011. Inspiratory muscle training in bronchiectasis patients: a prospective randomized controlled study. Clin. Rehabil. 25, 524–536.

Lin, S.J., McElfresh, J., Hall, B., et al., 2012. Inspiratory muscle training in patients with heart failure: a systematic review. Cardiopulm. Phys. Ther. J. 23, 29–36.

Lindstedt, S.L., Reich, T.E., Keim, P., et al., 2002. Do muscles function as adaptable locomotor springs? J. Exp. Biol. 205, 2211–2216.

Lisboa, C., Moreno, R., Fava, M., et al., 1985. Inspiratory muscle function in patients with severe kyphoscoliosis. Am. Rev. Respir. Dis. 132, 48–52.

Litchke, L.G., Russian, C.J., Lloyd, L.K., et al., 2008. Effects of respiratory resistance training with a concurrent flow device on wheelchair athletes. J. Spinal Cord Med. 31, 65–71.

Lomax, M., 2010. Inspiratory muscle training, altitude, and arterial oxygen desaturation: a preliminary investigation. Aviat. Space Environ. Med. 81, 498–501.

Lomax, M., Grant, I., Corbett, J., 2011. Inspiratory muscle warm-up and inspiratory muscle training: separate and combined effects on intermittent running to exhaustion. J. Sports Sci. Med. 29, 563–569.

Lötters, F., van Tol, B., Kwakkel, G., et al., 2002. Effects of controlled inspiratory muscle training in patients with COPD: a meta-analysis. Eur. Respir. J. 20 (3), 570–576.

Lougheed, M.D., Lam, M., Forkert, L., et al., 1993. Breathlessness during acute bronchoconstriction in asthma. Pathophysiologic mechanisms. Am. Rev. Respir. Dis. 148, 1452–1459.

Loveridge, B., Badour, M., Dubo, H., 1989. Ventilatory muscle endurance training in quadriplegia: effects on breathing pattern. Paraplegia 27, 329–339.

Lykidis, C.K., White, M.J., Balanos, G.M., 2008. The pulmonary vascular response to the sustained activation of the muscle metaboreflex in man. Exp. Physiol. 93, 247–253.

Maat, R.C., Roksund, O.D., Olofsson, J., et al., 2007. Surgical treatment of exercise-induced laryngeal dysfunction. Eur. Arch. Otorhinolaryngol. 264, 401–407.

Mador, M.J., Krawza, M., Alhajhusian, A., et al., 2009. Interval training versus continuous training in patients with chronic obstructive pulmonary disease. Journal of Cardiopulmonary Rehabilitation and Prevention 29, 126–132.

Magadle, R., Berar-Yanay, N., Weiner, P., 2002. The risk of hospitalization and near-fatal and fatal asthma in relation to the perception of dyspnea. Chest 121, 329–333.

Mancini, D.M., Henson, D., La Manca, J., et al., 1995. Benefit of selective respiratory muscle training on exercise capacity in patients with chronic congestive heart failure. Circulation 91, 320–329.

Markov, G., Spengler, C.M., Knopfli-Lenzin, C., et al., 2001. Respiratory muscle training increases cycling endurance without affecting cardiovascular responses to exercise. Eur. J. Appl. Physiol. 85, 233–239.

Martin, A.J., Stern, L., Yeates, J., et al., 1986. Respiratory muscle training in Duchenne muscular dystrophy. Dev. Med. Child Neurol. 28, 314–318.

Martin, A.D., Davenport, P.D., Franceschi, A.C., et al., 2002. Use of inspiratory muscle strength training to facilitate ventilator weaning: a series of 10 consecutive patients. Chest 122, 192–196.

Martin, A.D., Smith, B.K., Davenport, P.D., et al., 2011. Inspiratory muscle strength training improves weaning outcome in failure to wean patients: a randomized trial. Crit. Care 15, R84.

Martinez, A., Lisboa, C., Jalil, J., et al., 2001. Selective training of respiratory muscles in patients with chronic heart failure. Rev. Med. Chil. 129, 133–139.

McConnell, A.K., 2011. Breathe strong, perform better. Human Kinetics Publishers, Champaign, IL.

McConnell, A.K., Lomax, M., 2006. The influence of inspiratory muscle work history and specific inspiratory muscle training upon human limb muscle fatigue. J. Physiol. 577, 445–457.

McConnell, A.K., Caine, M.P., Donovan, K.J., et al., 1998. Inspiratory muscle training improves lung function and reduces exertional dyspnoea in mild/moderate asthmatics. Clin. Sci. 95, 4P.

McMahon, M.E., Boutellier, U., Smith, R.M., et al., 2002. Hyperpnea training attenuates peripheral chemosensitivity and improves cycling endurance. J. Exp. Biol. 205, 3937–3943.

Meade, M., Guyatt, G., Cook, D., et al., 2001. Predicting success in weaning from mechanical ventilation. Chest 120, 400S–424S.

Mello, P.R., Guerra, G.M., Borile, S., et al., 2012. Inspiratory muscle training reduces sympathetic nervous activity and improves inspiratory muscle weakness and quality of life in patients with chronic heart failure: a clinical trial. Journal of Cardiopulmonary Rehabilitation and Prevention 32 (5), 255–261.

Moodie, L., Reeve, J., Elkins, M., 2011. Inspiratory muscle training increases inspiratory muscle strength in patients weaning from mechanical ventilation: a systematic review. Journal of Physiotherapy 57, 213–221.

Moran, F., Piper, A., Elborn, J.S., et al., 2010. Respiratory muscle pressures in non-CF bronchiectasis: repeatability and reliability. Chron. Respir. Dis. 7, 165–171.

Mota, S., Guell, R., Barreiro, E., et al., 2007. Clinical outcomes of expiratory muscle training in severe COPD patients. Respir. Med. 101, 516–524.

Neves, P.C., Guerra, M., Ponce, P., et al., 2011. Non-cystic fibrosis bronchiectasis. Interactive Cardiovascular and Thoracic Surgery 13 (6), 619–625.

Newall, C., Stockley, R.A., Hill, S.L., 2005. Exercise training and inspiratory muscle training in patients with bronchiectasis. Thorax 60, 943–948.

NICE: National Clinical Guideline Centre, 2011. Hypertension: The clinical management of primary hypertension in adults. Royal College of Physicians, London.www.nice.org.uk/nicemedia/live/13561/56007/56007.pdf.

Nicks, C.R., Morgan, D.W., Fuller, D.K., et al., 2009. The influence of respiratory muscle training upon intermittent exercise performance. Int. J. Sports Med. 30 (1), 16–21.

O'Brien, K., Geddes, E.L., Reid, W.D., et al., 2008. Inspiratory muscle training compared with other rehabilitation interventions in chronic obstructive pulmonary disease: a systematic review update. Journal of Cardiopulmonary Rehabilitation and Prevention 28, 128–141.

Olgiati, R., Girr, A., Hugi, L., et al., 1989. Respiratory muscle training in multiple sclerosis: a pilot study. Schweiz. Arch. Neurol. Psychiatr. 140, 46–50.

Ortancil, O., Sarikaya, S., Sapmaz, P., et al., 2009. The effect(s) of a six-week home-based exercise program on the respiratory muscle and functional status in ankylosing spondylitis. J. Clin. Rheumatol. 15, 68–70.

Padula, C.A., Yeaw, E., Mistry, S., 2009. A home-based nurse-coached inspiratory muscle training intervention in heart failure. Appl. Nurs. Res. 22, 18–25.

Pellizzaro, C.O., Thome, F.S., Veronese, F.V., 2013. Effect of peripheral and respiratory muscle training on the functional capacity of hemodialysis patients. Ren. Fail. 35, 189–197.

Perkoff, G.T., Silber, R., Tyler, F.H., et al., 1959. Studies in disorders of muscle. XII. Myopathy due to the administration of therapeutic amounts of 17-hydroxycorticosteroids. Am. J. Med. 26, 891–898.

Piepoli, M.F., Conraads, V., Corra, U., et al., 2011. Exercise training in heart failure: from theory to practice. A consensus document of the Heart Failure Association and the European Association for Cardiovascular Prevention and Rehabilitation. Eur. J. Heart Fail. 13, 347–357.

Pinto, S., Turkman, A., Pinto, A., et al., 2009. Predicting respiratory insufficiency in amyotrophic lateral sclerosis: the role of phrenic nerve studies. Clin. Neurophysiol. 120, 941–946.

Pinto, S., Swash, M., de Carvalho, M., 2012. Respiratory exercise in amyotrophic lateral sclerosis. Amyotroph. Lateral Scler. 13, 33–43.

Plentz, R.D., Sbruzzi, G., Ribeiro, R.A., et al., 2012. Inspiratory muscle training in patients with heart failure:

meta-analysis of randomized trials. Arq. Bras. Cardiol. 99, 762–771.

Prezant, D.J., 1990. Effect of uremia and its treatment on pulmonary function. Lung 168, 1–14.

Puhan, M.A., Suarez, A., Lo Cascio, C., et al., 2006. Didgeridoo playing as alternative treatment for obstructive sleep apnoea syndrome: randomised controlled trial. BMJ 332, 266–270.

Ram, F.S., Wellington, S.R., Barnes, N.C., 2003. Inspiratory muscle training for asthma. Cochrane Database Syst. Rev. CD003792.

Ramirez-Sarmiento, A., Orozco-Levi, M., Guell, R., et al., 2002. Inspiratory muscle training in patients with chronic obstructive pulmonary disease: structural adaptation and physiologic outcomes. Am. J. Respir. Crit. Care Med. 166, 1491–1497.

Rassler, B., Hallebach, G., Kalischewski, P., et al., 2007. The effect of respiratory muscle endurance training in patients with myasthenia gravis. Neuromuscul. Disord. 17, 385–391.

Rassler, B., Marx, G., Hallebach, S., et al., 2011. Long-term respiratory muscle endurance training in patients with myasthenia gravis: first results after four months of training. Autoimmune Diseases 2011, 808607.

Reid, W.D., Geddes, E.L., O'Brien, K., et al., 2008. Effects of inspiratory muscle training in cystic fibrosis: a systematic review. Clin. Rehabil. 22, 1003–1013.

Ribeiro, J.P., Chiappa, G.R., Callegaro, C.C., 2012. The contribution of inspiratory muscles function to exercise limitation in heart failure: pathophysiological mechanisms. Revista Brasileira de Fisioterapia 16 (4), 261–267.

Romer, L.M., McConnell, A.K., 2003. Specificity and reversibility of inspiratory muscle training. Med. Sci. Sports Exerc. 35, 237–244.

Romer, L.M., McConnell, A.K., Jones, D.A., 2002a. Effects of inspiratory muscle training on time-trial performance in trained cyclists. J. Sports Sci. Med. 20, 547–562.

Romer, L.M., McConnell, A.K., Jones, D.A., 2002b. Effects of inspiratory muscle training upon recovery time during high intensity, repetitive sprint activity. Int. J. Sports Med. 23, 353–360.

Romer, L.M., McConnell, A.K., Jones, D.A., 2002c. Effects of inspiratory muscle training upon time trial performance in trained cyclists. J. Sports Sci. Med. 20, 547–562.

Romer, L.M., McConnell, A.K., Jones, D.A., 2002d. Inspiratory muscle fatigue in trained cyclists: effects of inspiratory muscle training. Med. Sci. Sports Exerc. 34, 785–792.

Romer, L.M., Lovering, A.T., Haverkamp, H.C., et al., 2006. Effect of inspiratory muscle work on peripheral fatigue of locomotor muscles in healthy humans. J. Physiol. 571, 425–439.

Roth, E.J., Noll, S.F., 1994. Stroke rehabilitation. 2. Comorbidities and complications. Arch. Phys. Med. Rehabil. 75, S42–S46.

Roth, E.J., Stenson, K.W., Powley, S., et al., 2010. Expiratory muscle training in spinal cord injury: a randomized controlled trial. Arch. Phys. Med. Rehabil. 91, 857–861.

Ruddy, B.H., Davenport, P., Baylor, J., et al., 2004. Inspiratory muscle strength training with behavioral therapy in a case of a rower with presumed exercise-induced paradoxical vocal-fold dysfunction. Int. J. Pediatr. Otorhinolaryngol. 68, 1327–1332.

Rutchik, A., Weissman, A.R., Almenoff, P.L., et al., 1998. Resistive inspiratory muscle training in subjects with chronic cervical spinal cord injury. Arch. Phys. Med. Rehabil. 79, 293–297.

Sabate, M., Rodriguez, M., Mendez, E., et al., 1996. Obstructive and restrictive pulmonary dysfunction increases disability in Parkinson disease. Arch. Phys. Med. Rehabil. 77, 29–34.

Sadowsky, S., Dwyer, J., Fischer, A., 1995. Failure of hyperoxic gas to alter the arterial lactate anaerobic threshold. J. Cardiopulm. Rehabil. 15, 114–121.

Sapienza, C.M., Davenport, P.W., Martin, A.D., 2002. Expiratory muscle training increases pressure support in high school band students. J. Voice 16, 495–501.

Savci, S., Degirmenci, B., Saglam, M., et al., 2011. Short-term effects of inspiratory muscle training in coronary artery bypass graft surgery: A randomized controlled trial. Scand. Cardiovasc. J. 45, 286–293.

Sawyer, E.H., Clanton, T.L., 1993. Improved pulmonary function and exercise tolerance with inspiratory muscle conditioning in children with cystic fibrosis. Chest 104, 1490–1497.

Sbruzzi, G., Dal Lago, P., Ribeiro, R.A., et al., 2012. Inspiratory muscle training and quality of life in patients with heart failure: systematic review of randomized trials. Int. J. Cardiol. 156, 120–121.

Scherer, T.A., Spengler, C.M., Owassapian, D., et al., 2000. Respiratory muscle endurance training in chronic obstructive pulmonary disease: impact on exercise capacity, dyspnea, and quality of life. Am. J. Respir. Crit. Care Med. 162, 1709–1714.

Schilero, G.J., Spungen, A.M., Bauman, W.A., et al., 2009. Pulmonary function and spinal cord injury. Respir. Physiol. Neurobiol. 166, 129–141.

Sheel, A.W., Reid, W.D., Townson, A.F., et al., 2008. Effects of exercise training and inspiratory muscle training in spinal cord injury: a systematic review. J. Spinal Cord Med. 31, 500–508.

Shoemaker, M.J., Donker, S., Lapoe, A., 2009. Inspiratory muscle training in patients with chronic obstructive pulmonary disease: the state of the evidence. Cardiopulmonary Physical Therapy Journal 20, 5–15.

Silva, V.G., Amaral, C., Monteiro, M.B., et al., 2011. Effects of inspiratory muscle training in hemodialysis patients. Jornal Brasileiro de Nefrologia 33, 62–68.

Silva Mdos, S., Martins, A.C., Cipriano Jr., G., et al., 2012. Inspiratory training increases insulin sensitivity in elderly patients. Geriatrics and Gerontology International 12, 345–351.

Smart, N.A., Giallauria, F., Dieberg, G., 2012. Efficacy of inspiratory muscle training in chronic heart failure patients: A systematic review and meta-analysis. Int. J. Cardiol. May 3. [Epub ahead of print].

Smeltzer, S.C., Lavietes, M.H., Cook, S.D., 1996. Expiratory training in multiple sclerosis. Arch. Phys. Med. Rehabil. 77, 909–912.

Smith, P.E., Coakley, J.H., Edwards, R.H., 1988. Respiratory muscle training in Duchenne muscular dystrophy. Muscle Nerve 11, 784–785.

Smith, B.K., Bleiweis, M.S., Neel, C.R., et al., 2012. Inspiratory muscle strength training in infants with congenital heart disease and prolonged mechanical ventilation: a case report. Phys. Ther. Mar 30. [Epub ahead of print].

Sprague, S.S., Hopkins, P.D., 2003. Use of inspiratory strength training to wean six patients who were ventilator-dependent. Phys. Ther. 83, 171–181.

Spungen, A.M., Grimm, D.R., Lesser, M., et al., 1997. Self-reported prevalence of pulmonary symptoms in subjects with spinal cord injury. Spinal Cord 35, 652–657.

Stambler, N., Charatan, M., Cedarbaum, J.M., 1998. Prognostic indicators of survival in ALS. ALS CNTF Treatment Study Group. Neurology 50, 66–72.

Stein, R., Chiappa, G.R., Guths, H., et al., 2009. Inspiratory muscle training improves oxygen uptake efficiency slope in patients with chronic heart failure. Journal of Cardiopulmonary Rehabilitation and Prevention 29, 392–395.

Stern, L.M., Martin, A.J., Jones, N., et al., 1989. Training inspiratory resistance in Duchenne dystrophy using adapted computer games. Dev. Med. Child Neurol. 31, 494–500.

Stuessi, C., Spengler, C.M., Knopfli-Lenzin, C., et al., 2001. Respiratory muscle endurance training in humans increases cycling endurance without affecting blood gas concentrations. Eur. J. Appl. Physiol. 84, 582–586.

Summerhill, E.M., Angov, N., Garber, C., et al., 2007. Respiratory muscle strength in the physically active elderly. Lung 185, 315–320.

Sutbeyaz, S.T., Koseoglu, F., Inan, L., et al., 2010. Respiratory muscle training improves cardiopulmonary function and exercise tolerance in subjects with subacute stroke: a randomized controlled trial. Clin. Rehabil. 24, 240–250.

Takaso, M., Nakazawa, T., Imura, T., et al., 2010. Surgical correction of spinal deformity in patients with congenital muscular dystrophy. J. Orthop. Sci. 15, 493–501.

Taylor, B.J., Romer, L.M., 2009. Effect of expiratory resistive loading on inspiratory and expiratory muscle fatigue. Respir. Physiol. Neurobiol. 16, 164–174.

Thomas, M.J., Simpson, J., Riley, R., et al., 2010. The impact of home-based physiotherapy interventions on breathlessness during activities of daily living in severe COPD: a systematic review. Physiotherapy 96, 108–119.

Tong, T.K., Fu, F.H., 2006. Effect of specific inspiratory muscle warm-up on intense intermittent run to exhaustion. Eur. J. Appl. Physiol. 97, 673–680.

Tong, T.K., Fu, F.H., Eston, R., et al., 2010. Chronic and acute inspiratory muscle loading augment the effect of a 6-week interval program on tolerance of high-intensity intermittent bouts of running. J. Strength Cond. Res. 24 (11), 3041–3048.

Tong, T.K., Lin, H., McConnell, A., et al., 2012. Respiratory and locomotor muscle blood-volume and oxygenation kinetics during intense intermittent exercise. Eur. J. Sport Sci. 12, 321–330.

Topin, N., Matecki, S., Le Bris, S., et al., 2002. Dose-dependent effect of individualized respiratory muscle training in children with Duchenne muscular dystrophy. Neuromuscul. Disord. 12, 576–583.

Turner, L.A., Mickleborough, T.D., McConnell, A.K., et al., 2011. Effect of inspiratory muscle training on exercise tolerance in asthmatic individuals. Med. Sci. Sports Exerc. 43, 2031–2038.

Turner, L.A., Tecklenburg-Lund, S.L., Chapman, R.F., et al., 2012. Inspiratory muscle training lowers the oxygen cost of voluntary hyperpnea. J. Appl. Physiol. 112, 127–134.

Tzelepis, G.E., McCool, F.D., Friedman, J.H., et al., 1988. Respiratory muscle dysfunction in Parkinson's disease. Am. Rev. Respir. Dis. 138, 266–271.

Tzelepis, G.E., Vega, D.L., Cohen, M.E., et al., 1994. Pressure–flow specificity of inspiratory muscle training. J. Appl. Physiol. 77, 795–801.

Tzelepis, G.E., Kasas, V., McCool, F.D., 1999. Inspiratory muscle adaptations following pressure or flow training in humans. Eur. J. Appl. Physiol. Occup. Physiol. 79, 467–471.

Van Houtte, S., Vanlandewijck, Y., Gosselink, R., 2006. Respiratory muscle training in persons with spinal cord injury: a systematic review. Respir. Med. 100, 1886–1895.

Van Houtte, S., Vanlandewijck, Y., Kiekens, C., et al., 2008. Patients with acute spinal cord injury benefit from normocapnic hyperpnoea training. J. Rehabil. Med. 40, 119–125.

Verges, S., Boutellier, U., Spengler, C.M., 2008. Effect of respiratory muscle endurance training on respiratory sensations, respiratory control and exercise performance: a 15-year experience. Respir. Physiol. Neurobiol. 161, 16–22.

Villiot-Danger, J.C., Villiot-Danger, E., Borel, J.C., et al., 2011. Respiratory muscle endurance training in obese patients. Int. J. Obes. (Lond). 35, 692–699.

Vilozni, D., Bar-Yishay, E., Gur, I., et al., 1994. Computerized respiratory muscle training in children with Duchenne muscular dystrophy. Neuromuscul. Disord. 4, 249–255.

Vincent, K.R., Braith, R.W., Feldman, R.A., et al., 2002. Improved cardiorespiratory endurance following 6 months of resistance exercise in elderly men and women. Arch. Intern. Med. 162, 673–678.

Volianitis, S., McConnell, A.K., Koutedakis, Y., et al., 2001. Inspiratory muscle training improves rowing performance. Med. Sci. Sports Exerc. 33, 803–809.

Wanke, T., Toifl, K., Merkle, M., et al., 1994. Inspiratory muscle training in patients with Duchenne muscular dystrophy. Chest 105, 475–482.

Ward, C.P., York, K.M., McCoy, J.G., 2012. Risk of obstructive sleep apnea lower in double reed wind musicians. Journal of Clinical Sleep Medicine 8, 251–255.

Watsford, M., Murphy, A., 2008. The effects of respiratory-muscle training on exercise in older women. J. Aging Phys. Act. 16, 245–260.

Weinberg, J., Borg, J., Bevegard, S., et al., 1999. Respiratory response to exercise in postpolio patients with severe inspiratory muscle dysfunction. Arch. Phys. Med. Rehabil. 80, 1095–1100.

Weiner, P., Weiner, M., 2006. Inspiratory muscle training may increase peak inspiratory flow in chronic obstructive pulmonary disease. Respiration 73, 151–156.

Weiner, P., Azgad, Y., Ganam, R., et al., 1992. Inspiratory muscle training in patients with bronchial asthma. Chest 102, 1357–1361.

Weiner, P., Azgad, Y., Weiner, M., et al., 1995. Inspiratory muscle training during treatment with corticosteroids in humans. Chest 107, 1041–1044.

Weiner, P., Ganem, R., Zamir, D., et al., 1996. Specific inspiratory muscle training in chronic hemodialysis. Harefuah 130 (73–76), 144.

Weiner, P., Man, A., Weiner, M., et al., 1997. The effect of incentive spirometry and inspiratory muscle training on pulmonary function after lung resection. J. Thorac. Cardiovasc. Surg. 113, 552–557.

Weiner, P., Gross, D., Meiner, Z., et al., 1998a. Respiratory muscle training in patients with moderate to severe myasthenia gravis. Can. J. Neurol. Sci. 25, 236–241.

Weiner, P., Zeidan, F., Zamir, D., et al., 1998b. Prophylactic inspiratory muscle training in patients undergoing coronary artery bypass graft. World J. Surg. 22, 427–431.

Weiner, P., Waizman, J., Magadle, R., et al., 1999. The effect of specific inspiratory muscle training on the sensation of dyspnea and exercise tolerance in patients with congestive heart failure. Clin. Cardiol. 22, 727–732.

Weiner, P., Berar-Yanay, N., Davidovich, A., et al., 2000. Specific inspiratory muscle training in patients with mild asthma with high consumption of inhaled beta(2)-agonists. Chest 117, 722–727.

Weiner, P., Inzelberg, R., Davidovich, A., et al., 2002a. Respiratory muscle performance and the Perception of dyspnea in Parkinson's disease. Can. J. Neurol. Sci. 29, 68–72.

Weiner, P., Magadle, R., Beckerman, M., et al., 2002b. The relationship among inspiratory muscle strength, the perception of dyspnea and inhaled beta2-agonist use in patients with asthma. Can. Respir. J. 9, 307–312.

Weiner, P., Magadle, R., Massarwa, F., et al., 2002c. Influence of gender and inspiratory muscle training on the perception of dyspnea in patients with asthma. Chest 122, 197–201.

Weiner, P., Magadle, R., Beckerman, M., et al., 2003a. Comparison of specific expiratory, inspiratory, and combined muscle training programs in COPD. Chest 124, 1357–1364.

Weiner, P., Magadle, R., Beckerman, M., et al., 2003b. Specific expiratory muscle training in COPD. Chest 124, 468–473.

Wells, G.D., Plyley, M., Thomas, S., et al., 2005. Effects of concurrent inspiratory and expiratory muscle training on respiratory and exercise performance in competitive swimmers. Eur. J. Appl. Physiol. 94, 527–540.

West, C.R., Taylor, B.J., Campbell, I.G., et al., 2009. Effects of inspiratory muscle training in Paralympic athletes with cervical spinal cord injury. Med. Sci. Sports Exerc. 41, S31–S32.

Wijnhoven, H.A., Kriegsman, D.M., Snoek, F.J., et al., 2003. Gender differences in health-related quality of life among asthma patients. J. Asthma 40, 189–199.

Winkler, G., Zifko, U., Nader, A., et al., 2000. Dose-dependent effects of inspiratory muscle training in neuromuscular disorders. Muscle Nerve 23, 1257–1260.

Witt, J.D., Guenette, J.A., Rupert, J.L., et al., 2007. Inspiratory muscle training attenuates the human respiratory muscle metaboreflex. J. Physiol. 584, 1019–1028.

Wright, J.M., Musini, V.M., 2009. First-line drugs for hypertension. Cochrane Database Sys. Rev. CD001841.

Xiao, Y., Luo, M., Wang, J., et al., 2012. Inspiratory muscle training for the recovery of function after stroke. Cochrane Database Sys. Rev. 5, CD009360.

Part | II |

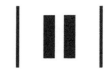

Practical application of respiratory muscle training

Introduction to Part II

In Part I of *Respiratory muscle training: theory and practice* a comprehensive foundation was laid for the practical application of respiratory muscle training (RMT). This included both a review of existing evidence from studies of RMT, and an examination of the theoretical rationale for RMT in a broader range of clinical, and other, conditions. Furthermore, Part I reviewed insights from both healthy people and patients regarding the mechanisms that underlie improvements in exercise tolerance that follow RMT. In Part II, the practical application of RMT, and specifically inspiratory muscle resistance training (IMT), will be described. Chapter 5 describes the different evidence-based methods of RMT, as well as the specific muscle adaptations they elicit, and the pros and cons of the equipment and methods utilized for the implementation of RMT. Chapter 6 considers all aspects of implementation, from

how IMT can be incorporated into a treatment pathway, to optimizing breathing pattern during IMT. This phase of training is referred to as 'Foundation' IMT, and the chapter closes with a case study.

An important issue that was identified in Part I was the 'multi-tasking' role of the trunk muscles, and the conflicts that this creates between breathing, postural control and trunk stabilization. In doing so, a rationale was established for adopting a more functional approach to IMT, and this is expanded in Chapter 7. In addition, this chapter suggests methods that can be used to identifying load/capacity imbalance within the inspiratory muscles, as well as the quantification of the main symptom of inspiratory muscle overload, viz., dyspnoea. Finally, Chapter 7 describes a comprehensive range of over 100 'Functional' IMT exercises, which incorporate a stability and/or postural challenge, including exercises that address specific movements that are known to provoke dyspnoea, e.g. raising the arms above head height.

Chapter 5

Methods of respiratory muscle training

GENERAL TRAINING PRINCIPLES

The respiratory muscles are unique amongst skeletal muscles because of their continuous activity throughout life. For many years it was assumed that this resulted in a state of optimal training adaptation. As was described in Chapter 1, the structural and metabolic properties of the respiratory muscles would seem to support this notion, as they have properties that suit them ideally to their continuous activity. However, it became apparent from research conducted during the 1990s on young athletes that the respiratory muscles, specifically the diaphragm, exhibit fatigue following strenuous exercise (Johnson et al, 1993). The presence of fatigue is an indication that muscles are working at the limits of their capacity. These data therefore provided the first evidence that the respiratory muscles were not immune to fatigue. The data also raised the question of whether the respiratory muscles were capable of responding to training stimuli and displaying improvements in function in the same way that, say, leg muscles respond to running or weight training.

This chapter will describe the generic principles that underpin muscle training, and consider how these can be applied to the respiratory muscles. It will further consider the methods that are available to train the respiratory muscles, and the changes in respiratory muscle function that each method induces. Consideration will also be given to the relative merits of commercially available respiratory muscle training equipment.

There are three training principles that are well established for skeletal muscles – namely 'overload', 'specificity' and 'reversibility' (Pardy & Leith, 1995). The following section provides an overview of the evidence that respiratory muscles respond to these principles in the same manner as other muscles have been shown to (Romer & McConnell, 2003).

Overload

To obtain a training response, muscle fibres must be overloaded. Implicit within this principle is the concept of training *duration, intensity and frequency*. In other words, muscles can be overloaded by requiring them to work for longer, at higher intensity and/or more frequently than they are accustomed to. Most training regimens combine two or three of these factors in order to achieve overload. The overload principle will be considered first for healthy people, and then for patients.

Healthy people

In healthy people, two main forms of overload have been imposed upon the respiratory muscles: (1) external loads at the mouth (*intensity*), and (2) voluntary hyperpnoea (increased breathing volume and flow rate) for extended periods (*intensity and duration*). In both cases, the training takes place daily, or at least three times per week (*frequency*).

Studies employing external loading have typically used load *intensities* in excess of 50% of inspiratory muscle strength (maximal inspiratory pressure: MIP), at a *frequency* of once or twice per day, for 5–7 days per week (McConnell & Romer, 2004). Loading at 50–70% of MIP typically yields task failure (see Ch. 6) within a *duration* of 30 breaths, or 2–3 minutes (*intensity* = 50–70%; *duration* = 30 breaths; *frequency* = twice daily). Statistically significant changes in muscle function have been measured within 3 weeks (Romer & McConnell, 2003), with a plateau in improvement occurring after around 6 weeks of training, despite continuous increases of the training load (Volianitis et al, 2001; Romer & McConnell, 2003). Changes in strength occurring within the first 2 weeks of strength training have traditionally been attributed to a neural adaptation process (Jones et al, 1989), i.e., improving the coordinated activation of synergistic muscles. Although this adaptation undoubtedly makes a contribution to the immediate short-term improvements seen in respiratory muscles, evidence from animal studies suggests that structural adaptation occurs within days of overload (Gea et al, 2000). Furthermore, in human beings, improvements in diaphragm thickness (8–12%) have been reported following just 4 weeks of inspiratory muscle training (IMT) (Downey et al, 2007) confirming the presence of rapid fibre hypertrophy in response to loading. These changes in diaphragm thickness were parallelled by improvements in maximal inspiratory pressure (MIP) (Downey et al, 2007). In placebo-controlled trials of IMT in healthy people, loads of 15% of MIP have been used as the placebo condition. When a 15% load is implemented with 30–60 repetitions it does not provide sufficient overload, as it fails to elicit changes in MIP (see (McConnell & Romer, 2004). Thus research suggests that inspiratory muscle overload in healthy people requires loads of 50–70% of MIP, eliciting muscle adaptations within 3–4 weeks.

Studies using hyperpnoea training have typically induced overload at *intensities* corresponding to 70% of maximum voluntary ventilation (MVV), for a *duration* of 15–40 minutes per day, at a *frequency* of once per day, for 4–5 days per week (Verges et al, 2008a). In the case of hyperpnoea training, overload is achieved by increasing the rate of air flow, with the inspiratory muscles working against the inherent resistance and elastance of the respiratory system (*intensity* = 70%; *duration* = 15–40 minutes; *frequency* = 4–5 days per week). Improvements in muscle function (endurance) are evident within 4 weeks (Verges et al, 2008a). There are currently no data to indicate the point at which functional improvements plateau after commencing of training.

The *intensity* and *frequency* dimensions of overload warrant specific mention, as they need to be balanced carefully so as not to tip the respiratory muscles into a state of 'overtraining'. Most studies have implemented moderate-intensity IMT (50–70%) daily, but the *intensity* and *frequency* balance has yet to be studied systematically, or with consideration for other stimuli that overload the respiratory muscles. In the case of athletes this might be concurrent athletic training, and/or exposure to altitude, but in the case of patients it might be exercise training and/or the effects of an exacerbation. Preliminary unpublished data from healthy young soccer and rugby players (McConnell, unpublished observations) suggests that twice-daily high-intensity IMT (70–80% of MIP) may induce a state of chronic inspiratory muscle fatigue in athletes who are undergoing concurrent whole-body training. These training conditions appear to elicit suboptimal improvements in function. Thus, present evidence suggests that low-to-moderate-intensity loading (30–60% MIP) can be implemented daily, whereas high-intensity loading (>70% MIP) should be implemented no more than once every other day.

Patients

In the majority of reported studies in patients with respiratory disease, training has been undertaken by imposing an external load at the mouth (*intensity*) for 10–30 minutes (*duration*). Typically, training has been undertaken for 2 to 3 months, but structural and biochemical adaptations to the inspiratory muscles are evident within 6 weeks (Ramirez-Sarmiento et al, 2002). A study in patients with chronic obstructive pulmonary disease (COPD) has demonstrated the time course of changes in strength over a 12-month intervention (Weiner et al, 2004). Weiner and colleagues (Weiner et al, 2004) noted the largest improvement in MIP during the first 3 months of their study (32%), followed by smaller increases (∼6%) for the four subsequent 3-month blocks of IMT. Training sessions have typically been conducted in continuous bouts lasting 10–30 minutes, 1–2 times a day, for 5–7 days per week.

The *intensity* dimension has not been studied extensively in patients, but data from seven studies of patients with COPD collated by Pardy & Rochester (1992) suggested a significant positive relationship between the percentage increase in MIP and the relative magnitude of the inspiratory training load. In other words, the higher the load relative to the subject's MIP, the greater was the increase in MIP induced by training. The collated data suggest that, to achieve a 20% increase in MIP, a load of at least 30% of maximum strength is required. This suggestion is also supported by data from a 2002 meta-analysis of IMT (Lotters et al, 2002), and in a study that compared the efficacy of high- (52% MIP) and low-intensity (22%) IMT (Preusser et al, 1994); high-intensity IMT increased MIP by 35% ($p < 0.05$), whereas low-intensity IMT increased MIP by only 10% ($p > 0.05$) (Preusser et al, 1994). Collectively, the literature supports the need for training loads to exceed 30% MIP, but the question of whether more is better when it comes to the magnitude of inspiratory loading has not been examined systematically. A handful of studies have reported the effects of high-intensity training in patients with COPD, and these suggest that when loads are 68% of MIP (Sturdy et al, 2003), 'the highest tolerable inspiratory threshold load' (Hill et al, 2006) or '80% of maximal effort' (Enright et al, 2006), then greater increases in MIP are achieved (29–41%) compared with low-to-moderate intensities (15–23%; Geddes et al, 2008).

However, it is important to note that in all of the studies employing high-intensity IMT the frequency of training has been only 3 days per week, compared with twice daily IMT in the studies using low to moderate loads (i.e., three sessions per week compared with 14). This is potentially very important from a practical point of view, as it suggests that high-intensity training may be far more time efficient, as well as more effective. However, a note of caution should also be expressed, as daily high-intensity IMT may overload the muscles to the extent that chronic inspiratory muscle fatigue and suboptimal adaptations are elicited (see above). Practical suggestions regarding load setting can be found in Chapter 6.

Studies of IMT in patients have typically been of much longer duration than those in healthy young athletes (3 months vs 4–6 weeks). As mentioned previously, Weiner and colleagues noted the largest improvement in MIP during the first 3 months of their study, followed by a gradual plateau of improvement (Weiner et al, 2004). Similar observations were made by Larson et al (1988) after 1 month of training, and by Lisboa et al (1997). This 'plateau' effect is also apparent in studies on healthy people, where MIP increases most rapidly during the first 3 weeks, then rising more slowly to a plateau by around 6 weeks (Volianitis et al, 2001; Romer & McConnell, 2003). The development of a plateau cannot be ascribed to a lack of load progression (increasing the training load to accommodate increases in MIP) as it occurs regardless of this measure. Instead, it is a reflection of a basic property of muscle adaptation to strength-training stimuli (Moritani & deVries, 1979; Hakkinen et al, 1987), which necessitates periodic changes in the nature of the training stimulus in order to maintain the adaptation process; this is one of the reasons why athletes periodize their training.

Specificity

The adaptations elicited by training depend upon the type of stimulus to which the muscle is subjected. This is best illustrated by considering the polar opposites of strength and endurance training: muscles tend to respond to strength-training stimuli (high *intensity* and short *duration*) by improving strength, and to endurance-training stimuli (low *intensity* and long *duration*) by improving endurance.

Training for strength

Generally, respiratory muscles respond to high-load–low-frequency loading with a strength-training response (Pardy & Rochester, 1992; Tzelepis et al, 1994a; Romer & McConnell, 2003). However, as well as load specificity, there is also an element of flow specificity that must be borne in mind as the two are interrelated (Tzelepis et al, 1994a; Romer & McConnell, 2003). This is because of the limitations imposed by the force–velocity relationship of muscles (see Ch. 1); high loads cannot be overcome at high velocities of muscle shortening. Training stimuli with high loads and low velocities (e.g., a Mueller manoeuvre) elicit increases in MIP, but do not elicit increases in maximal shortening velocity (peak inspiratory flow rate) (see Ch. 4, Fig. 4.2). Conversely, training with low loads and high velocities of shortening (e.g., unloaded hyperpnoea) elicit increases in maximal shortening velocity, but not MIP (see Ch. 4, Fig. 4.2) (Tzelepis et al, 1994a; Romer & McConnell, 2003). Interestingly, training stimuli with intermediate loads and shortening velocities elicit

improvements in both qualities (Tzelepis et al, 1994a; Romer & McConnell, 2003), which arguably provides the 'best of both worlds' (see Ch. 4, Fig. 4.2).

A number of studies have now demonstrated in healthy people (Enright et al, 2006; Downey et al, 2007) and patients (Ramirez-Sarmiento et al, 2002; Enright et al, 2004; Chiappa et al, 2008; West et al, 2009) that the increase in MIP that follows strength training of the inspiratory muscles is secondary to hypertrophy.

Training for endurance

An endurance-conditioning response can be elicited with prolonged low-load–high-frequency contractions, which have typically been imposed upon the respiratory muscles using prolonged voluntary hyperpnoea (Boutellier & Piwko, 1992), but endurance can also be improved through strength training (Belman & Shadmehr, 1988; Harver et al, 1989). There is a common misconception that muscle endurance can be improved only using a specific endurance-training stimulus. However, stronger muscles perform a given task at a lower percentage of their maximum capacity than weaker muscles, which has beneficial consequences for fatigue resistance (endurance) (Belman & Shadmehr, 1988). Thus, inspiratory muscle strength training provides a 'dual-conditioning' response. There is no evidence that a specific endurance-training stimulus, such as hyperpnoea, improves MIP (Leith & Bradley, 1976; O'Kroy & Coast, 1993); indeed, this would not be expected as strength improves only when the tension within muscles is increased by the imposition of an external load. Collectively, the data suggest that training regimens with a moderate strength bias have the capacity to improve maximal strength, velocity of shortening and power output (Romer & McConnell, 2003) as well as endurance (Romer & McConnell, unpublished observations). This versatility supports the implementation of training with a bias towards strength at a moderate intensity.

The effect of lung volume (muscle length)

To date, only one study has examined whether the lung volume at which IMT occurs has any influence upon training outcomes (Tzelepis et al, 1994b). The data indicate that improvements in inspiratory muscle strength are specific to the lung volume at which training occurs (Tzelepis et al, 1994b). When three groups of healthy participants performed 6 weeks of repeated static maximum inspiratory manoeuvres at one of three lung volumes (residual volume, functional residual capacity (FRC), or FRC plus one-half of inspiratory capacity), the greatest improvements in strength occurred at the volume at which the participants trained. In addition, the improvements were significantly greater for those who trained at low lung volumes. Furthermore, the range of lung volume over which strength was increased was also greatest for those who trained at low lung volumes.

These data suggest that IMT should be conducted over the greatest range of lung volumes possible, commencing as close as possible to residual volume.

A caveat that must be borne in mind in the context of lung volume specificity is the volume–pressure relationship of the inspiratory muscles (see Ch. 1). The inspiratory muscles become progressively weaker as the lungs inflate, such that under conditions of inspiratory loading the breath may be curtailed before the lungs are completely full. This 'clipping' of inspired volume is influenced by: (1) the magnitude of the load (occurring earlier with heavier loads), and (2) the fatigue state of the inspiratory muscles (occurring earlier in the presence of fatigue) (see also Ch. 6, Fig. 6.2). This means that, for most resistance IMT devices, a compromise must be struck between the magnitude of the load and the volume of the breath, as it is impossible to achieve high loads and high volumes simultaneously. The impact of these issues upon training load selection is considered in Chapter 6. The influence upon the design of IMT products will be considered at the end of this chapter.

Reversibility

The phenomenon of 'use it or lose it' describes the reversibility of training benefits. Despite the continuous activity of the respiratory muscles, even under resting conditions, this is insufficient to protect them against detraining. Sensitivity to prevailing levels of work is illustrated by the dose-response relationship between levels of physical activity and inspiratory muscle function that has been identified in elderly people (Buchman et al, 2008). Furthermore, in circumstances such as mechanical ventilation, where complete inactivity is imposed, inspiratory muscle function deteriorates precipitously;); 18 to 69 hours of complete diaphragmatic inactivity due to mechanical ventilation decreased the cross-sectional areas of diaphragmatic fibres by at least 50% (Tobin et al, 2010).

Detraining

Unfortunately, the extent and time course of inspiratory muscle detraining are not well documented, but two studies of resistance IMT do shed some light on these issues. In healthy young adults, Romer & McConnell (2003) documented regression of IMT-induced changes in inspiratory muscle function (9 weeks of three differing IMT regimens) over an 18-week period of detraining. Decrements were observed at 9 weeks, with no further changes in strength-related measures at 18 weeks post-IMT. In contrast, endurance continued to decline between 9 and 18 weeks of detraining (Romer & McConnell, unpublished observations). Inspiratory muscle function remained significantly above baseline at 18 weeks, with a loss of 32% of the improvement in strength, 65% of the improvement in maximum shortening velocity and 75% of the improvement in inspiratory muscle endurance.

In patients with COPD, Weiner et al (2004) observed the detraining response of a group of COPD patients who had completed a 3-month intensive IMT programme. The detraining group undertook sham training (inspiratory load of 7 cmH$_2$O) for the next 12 months and were reassessed at 3-month intervals. After 3 months of detraining, both MIP and inspiratory muscle endurance remained elevated compared with baseline (MIP 19%, endurance 22%), but after 12 months they were not significantly different from baseline. Collectively, these data suggest that inspiratory muscles respond in a similar manner to other muscles when a training stimulus is removed (Mujika & Padilla, 2000a, b) and that most of the losses of function occur within 2 to 3 months of the cessation of training.

Maintenance

On a more positive note, the two detraining studies described above (Romer & McConnell, 2003; Weiner et al, 2004) also demonstrated that IMT-induced improvements in inspiratory muscle function can be sustained with maintenance training programmes in which training *frequency* is reduced. Training *frequency* can be reduced by as much as two-thirds without loss of function, i.e., to 2 days per week in healthy adults (Romer & McConnell, 2003) and to 3 days per week in patients with COPD (Weiner et al, 2004).

In summary, the literature supports the notion that the general training principles of overload, specificity and reversibility apply as much to the training of respiratory muscles as they do to limb muscles. This means that respiratory training interventions should apply these principles in order to obtain specific functional outcomes (see Ch. 6).

DIFFERENT FORMS OF RMT AND THEIR OUTCOMES

Training methods can be subdivided broadly into two types: (1) resistance training in which the muscles are subjected to external loading that is akin to lifting a weight, and (2) endurance training in which the respiratory muscles are required to work at high shortening velocities for prolonged periods of time. In the case of the latter, the only load imposed upon the respiratory muscles is that of the inherent flow resistance and elastance of the respiratory system.

Resistance training

Conflict of interest statement:

The author is an inventor of two inspiratory muscle training products: (POWERbreathe and POWERbreathe K-Series). In the interests of complete transparency, the author declares a beneficial interest in these products in the form of a share of licence income to the University of Birmingham and Brunel University. The author also acts as a consultant to POWERbreathe International Ltd.

Inspiratory flow resistive loading

Inspiratory flow resistive loading (IFRL) requires inhalation via a variable diameter orifice whereby, for a given flow, the smaller the orifice the greater the resistive load. Studies utilizing IFRL have reported increases in inspiratory muscle strength in the range of 18% to 54% (Leith & Bradley, 1976; Hanel & Secher, 1991). However, an inherent limitation of IFRL is that inspiratory pressure, and thus training load, varies with flow (according to a power function) and not just to orifice size. Therefore, it is vitally important that breathing pattern is monitored during IFRL if a quantifiable training stimulus is to be provided. In a 1992 meta-analysis of respiratory muscle training (RMT) in patients with chronic obstructive pulmonary disease (COPD), it was concluded that studies employing IFRL in which inspiratory flow was not controlled failed to elicit improvements in inspiratory muscle function (Smith et al, 1992). Although modified flow resistive loading devices can be used to control flow (Belman & Shadmehr, 1991), such modifications require complex and expensive hardware making IFRL impractical for routine use.

A novel approach to IFRL, based on the Test of Incremental Respiratory Endurance (TIRE) technique (Chatham et al, 1995), has been used by some investigators to train the inspiratory muscles (Chatham et al, 1996) and to test the effects of this training upon exercise performance (Chatham et al, 1999; Enright et al, 2006; Mickleborough et al, 2008). The TIRE system uses a flow resistive load (2 mm diameter orifice), an electronic manometer attached via a serial interface to a computer, and dedicated software. Initially, several sustained maximal inspiratory efforts through the orifice are performed to provide a baseline pressure–time profile. A target pressure–time profile is then presented, typically set at 80% of the maximal effort. The manoeuvre is then repeated six times with 60 seconds recovery between efforts before the resting time is reduced to 45 seconds. A further six efforts are then completed, whereby the recovery time is reduced to 30 seconds and the user repeats the exercise. There are six different levels in all, with diminishing recovery times down to 5 seconds between breaths (incremental IFRL). The exercise is terminated when the participant either completes the prescribed number of breathing manoeuvres, or the pressure generated falls beneath the reference pressure–time profile.

Incremental IFRL has been shown to increase inspiratory muscle strength in healthy people (Enright et al, 2006; Mickleborough et al, 2008; Mickleborough et al, 2009) and patients with cystic fibrosis (Enright et al, 2004). Although the technique appears to overcome the primary limitations of flow resistive loading, the functional relevance of incremental IFRL is questionable. This type of sustained maximal inspiratory effort bears no relation to the dynamic function of inspiratory muscles during whole-body endurance exercise. The influence of incremental IFRL is therefore likely to be confined to the force (pressure) axis of the force–velocity relationship of the inspiratory muscles (Romer & McConnell, 2003). Furthermore, training sessions are physically demanding and time consuming (a complete training session takes ~30 minutes).

Dynamic inspiratory flow resistive loading

Most recently, an electronic product has been launched with a dynamically adjusting inspiratory flow resistor (dynamic IFRL). The magnitude of the inspiratory load can be manipulated within and between breaths to create an extremely versatile loading system. The device tapers the inspiratory load in such a way that the load is maintained at any pre-set percentage of MIP throughout the breath; in other words, the absolute load declines as the inspiratory muscles weaken during lung inflation. This eliminates the breath 'clipping' that arises with high inspiratory loads and/or inspiratory muscle fatigue. Unlike incremental IFRL, training can be achieved at physiologically relevant inspiratory flow rates. Preliminary data from a pilot study in patients with COPD comparing dynamic IFRL to IPTL (see below) suggests that dynamic IFRL elicits superior improvements in a wide range of functional measures of inspiratory muscle performance (Langer et al, unpublished observations). For example, the patients undertaking dynamic IFRL were able to sustain higher intensity training loads, resulting in superior improvement in MIP after 8 weeks of training (23% vs 15%, $p<0.03$).

Inspiratory pressure threshold loading

Inspiratory pressure threshold loading (IPTL) requires individuals to produce an inspiratory pressure sufficient to overcome a negative pressure load and thereby initiate inhalation. Threshold loading permits loading at a quantifiable, variable intensity by providing near-flow-independent resistance to inspiration. This can be achieved in several ways, e.g., with a weighted plunger (Nickerson & Keens, 1982), a solenoid valve (Bardsley et al, 1993), a constant negative pressure system (Chen et al, 1998), or a spring-loaded poppet valve (Caine & McConnell, 2000) (Fig. 5.1). Threshold loading has been shown to induce improvements in inspiratory muscle strength in healthy young adults (Inbar et al, 2000; Volianitis et al, 2001; Romer et al, 2002b, c; Romer & McConnell, 2003; Edwards & Cooke, 2004; McConnell & Sharpe, 2005; McConnell & Lomax, 2006; Downey et al, 2007; Griffiths & McConnell, 2007; How et al, 2007; Johnson et al, 2007; Witt et al, 2007; Brown et al, 2008, 2010, 2011; Edwards et al, 2008; Klusiewicz et al, 2008; Tong et al, 2008; Kilding et al, 2009; Lomax & McConnell, 2009; Nicks et al, 2009; Verges et al, 2009; Bailey et al, 2010; Lomax,

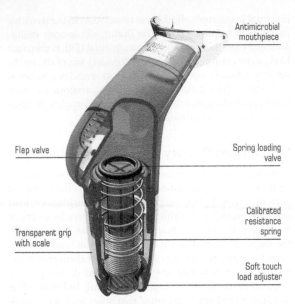

Antimicrobial
mouthpiece

Flap valve

Spring loading
valve

Calibrated
resistance
spring

Transparent grip
with scale

Soft touch
load adjuster

Figure 5.1 A pressure threshold inspiratory muscle trainer illustrating the spring-loaded poppet valve that provides the training load to the inspiratory muscles.
(From POWERbreathe International Ltd, with permission.)

2010; Turner et al, 2012), as well as in patients with COPD (see Gosselink et al, 2011), heart failure (see Smart et al, 2012) and neuromuscular disease (Topin et al, 2002). Maximum rate of muscle shortening (peak inspiratory flow rate) is also improved (Villafranca et al, 1998; Romer et al, 2002a; Romer & McConnell, 2003; Weiner & Weiner, 2006), as are maximal power output (Lisboa et al, 1994; Villafranca et al, 1998; Romer & McConnell, 2003) and inspiratory muscle endurance (Lisboa et al, 1994; Ramirez-Sarmiento et al, 2002; Weiner et al, 2004).

Because of its flow independence, training using IPTL can be undertaken effectively without the need to regulate breathing pattern. In addition, IPTL using a device with a mechanical poppet valve is both portable and easy to use.

Expiratory pressure threshold loading

Expiratory pressure threshold loading (EPTL) requires individuals to produce an expiratory pressure sufficient to overcome a positive pressure load and thereby initiate expiration. As is the case with IPTL, loading can be imposed at a quantifiable intensity by providing near-flow-independent resistance to expiration. This type of training has been far less extensively studied than IPTL, but EPTL has been shown to generate increases in expiratory muscle strength in both healthy people (Suzuki et al, 1995; Baker et al, 2005; Griffiths & McConnell, 2007) and patients with COPD

(Weiner et al, 2003b; Mota et al, 2007) and multiple sclerosis (Smeltzer et al, 1996). Weiner and colleagues also demonstrated an improvement in the endurance performance of the expiratory muscles following EPTL (Weiner et al, 2003a).

Concurrent IPTL and EPTL

The results of studies that have imposed pressure threshold loads upon the inspiratory and expiratory muscles within the same breath cycle suggest that this type of concurrent loading may be counter-productive. For example, when IPTL was added to EPTL after a period of 4 weeks in well-trained rowers, the increase in inspiratory muscle strength over the subsequent 6 weeks of concurrent training was just 13%, which is less than half the value typically attainable when IPTL is implemented without concurrent EPTL (Griffiths & McConnell, 2007). Similar findings were made in young swimmers who undertook simultaneous IPTL/EPTL (Wells et al, 2005). After 12 weeks of training with incrementally increasing inspiratory and expiratory loads, inspiratory and expiratory muscle strength improved by only 8%. This was identical to the change shown over the same period in the sham-training control group. However, one study in healthy elderly people demonstrated improvements in both MIP and MEP following concurrent IPTL/EPTL (Watsford & Murphy, 2008). In this study, the selection of the training load was dictated objectively for the inspiratory load, with the expiratory load being adjusted arbitrarily to a level that was 'tolerable'. This may explain the fact that significant improvements in MIP and MEP were observed in this study, but not in the one by Wells et al (2005). Generally, these data suggest that care is required when using concurrent IPTL and EPTL, as loading both phases of the breathing cycle simultaneously can generate suboptimal improvements in respiratory muscle strength.

Endurance training

Voluntary isocapnic hyperpnoea training

Voluntary isocapnic hyperpnoea (VIH) training requires individuals to maintain high target levels of ventilation for up to 30 minutes. To prevent hypocapnia, participants may simply rebreathe through a dead space. However, most studies have used more elaborate apparatus that supplies supplemental oxygen to avoid hypoxaemia while maintaining isocapnia. Training sessions are typically conducted 3 to 5 times per week at ~60–90% of maximum voluntary ventilation (MVV). Using VIH in healthy people, several investigators have shown increases in endurance during sustained isocapnic ventilation (Boutellier et al, 1992; Boutellier & Piwko, 1992; Markov et al, 1996; Spengler et al, 1999; Stuessi et al, 2001; Leddy et al, 2007; Wylegala et al, 2007; Verges et al, 2008b; Verges et al, 2009), maximum sustainable ventilation (MSV) (Leith & Bradley,

1976; Belman & Gaesser, 1988) and MVV (Leith & Bradley, 1976; Belman & Gaesser, 1988; Spengler et al, 1999; Leddy et al, 2007; Wylegala et al, 2007; Verges et al, 2009). The latter is consistent with improvements in peak velocity of muscle shortening. Typically, pulmonary function indices such as vital capacity and forced expiratory volume in 1 second remain unaffected by VIH (Spengler et al, 1999; Stuessi et al, 2001; Leddy et al, 2007; Wylegala et al, 2007). However, one recent study showed vital capacity increased significantly after VIH (Verges et al, 2009). Studies in patients are less numerous, but VIH appears to elicit similar changes to those observed in healthy people, when implemented in patients with neuromuscular disease (Rassler et al, 2007) and COPD (Mador et al, 2005).

Voluntary isocapnic hyperpnoea is a relatively time-consuming (typically 30 minutes per session) and physically demanding mode of RMT requiring a high degree of motivation. It also requires supplemental carbon dioxide or partial rebreathing in order to prevent hypocapnia (low carbon dioxide levels). Although VIH improves indices of respiratory muscle endurance, it does not improve the maximal pressure-generating capacity of the respiratory muscles (Leith & Bradley, 1976; Verges et al, 2008a). The influence of VIH is thus confined to the velocity (flow) axis of the force–velocity relationship of the inspiratory muscles (Romer & McConnell, 2003).

Summary

The preceding evidence points to resistance training as providing the most versatile training stimulus, as judged by the range of adaptions elicited (strength, power, shortening velocity and endurance). It is also the most time efficient and least arduous method of improving respiratory muscle function. The following section will consider commercially available training equipment, which will provide the final pieces of information required to select a suitable training method i.e., those of portability and relative cost.

PROPRIETARY TRAINING EQUIPMENT

The first part of this section will describe the range of mechanical principles that have been exploited to load the respiratory muscles. This will be followed by a description of the commercial products that utilize these basic principles. However, the latter is limited to those products that have been tested in placebo-controlled trials on patients and/or healthy young people, and shown to generate statistically significant improvements in at least one aspect of respiratory muscle function, as well as being published in peer-reviewed professional journals. The merits and limitations of each device will be summarized in order to assist the selection of the most appropriate device(s) for a given application.

Respiratory training equipment falls into two main categories: devices that impose a resistance-training stimulus and devices that impose an endurance-training stimulus.

Resistance training

These products fall into three main classes on the basis of how the load is generated:

- Passive flow resistance
- Dynamically adjusted flow resistance
- Pressure threshold valve.

Passive flow resistance devices

The mechanical products in this class employ simple dials that allow the user to select inspired airway orifices with differing surface area; the smaller the surface area, the larger is the inspired resistance. However, because these loads are passive, and generated by the inspired air flow (no flow = no load), they are highly sensitive to the influence of inspiratory flow rate, which makes loading unreliable. Because of their simplicity and cheapness of manufacture, the mechanical versions of these products are the most abundant proprietary devices on the market. However, because of their inherent limitations this class contains only one product that meets the requirements for inclusion in this summary, viz., the Pflex® (Respironics Inc. USA; Table 5.1). The main advantages of the Pflex® are its price (less than £15, at the time of writing) and convenience. However, training load and progression are impossible to quantify without providing simultaneous feedback of inspiratory flow rate using another piece of equipment. When used in this way, so-called 'targeted flow resistive training', there is no difference in the quality of the improvement in strength that can be achieved compared with pressure threshold loading products (Hsiao et al, 2003).

The addition of pressure measurement, other electronics and software to a simple flow resistor make load setting reliable and quantifiable, but also adds considerably to the cost and bulk of the equipment. The only product of this type to be supported by published data is the TrainAir® (Project Electronics Ltd., UK), which is based on the Test of Incremental Respiratory Endurance (TIRE) technique (Chatham et al, 1995) described above. The equipment requires interface to a laptop, and its cost (about £500) makes it the preserve of specialist clinics. The training is also very time consuming and strenuous. In its favour are the continuous biofeedback of training intensity, and built-in assessment of inspiratory muscle function.

Dynamically adjusted flow resistance devices

This is a new approach to respiratory training that, at the time of writing, is supported only by unpublished pilot data. However, a description is included here because this

Table 5.1 Comparison of evidence-based proprietary respiratory muscle training equipment*

Training equipment	Strength Power	Shortening velocity	Endurance	Overload range	Overload reliability	Portability	Ease of use	Mouth-piece comfort	Suitability for home use	Participant motivation	Session duration	Ease of load setting	Quantification of function	Contrain-dications	Expense	Overall score	Ranking
Pflex®	2			2	1	5	2	1	5	3	3	1	1	4	5	35	E
TrainAir®	5		3	5	5	2	2	5	1	1	1	5	5	4	1	45	C
POWER-breathe® (Pressure threshold)	5	5	3	5	5	5	5	5	5	5	5	4	1	4	5	72	A
Threshold®	5	5	3	2	5	5	5	1	5	5	5	4	1	4	5	65	B
SpiroTiger®	1		5	5	5	2	3	5	1	1	1	5	5	3	1	43	D

* Please refer to the Author's Conflict of Interest Statement on p. 138.

1 = poor; 5 = excellent. A = top ranked; E = bottom ranked. No score indicates no evidence.

■ Training quality and versatility
■ Participant comfort and convenience

method of loading will become more widely used in the future. As described above, the inherent limitation of a passive flow resistor is that variations in flow rate result in variations in load; this has been overcome in the new generation of flow resistance devices by using continuous, dynamic adjustment of the flow resistor. In essence, the surface area of a variable flow orifice is varied within a breath according to the prevailing respiratory flow rate. The controlled variable can be either the pressure load or the respired flow rate. Currently the only product of this type available is the POWERbreathe® K-Series (POWERbreathe International Ltd.), which was launched in 2010. The product ranges in price from £250 to £450, with the higher-priced products being downloadable and programmable by the user, as well as providing real-time computer-based biofeedback during training. The ability to make within- and between-breath adjustments makes this type of device extremely versatile from the loading perspective. Of the many unique features offered by this method is the ability to taper the load according to the prevailing strength of the muscles. In the case of inspiratory loading, for example, the load can be profiled to maintain it at the same percentage of MIP irrespective of lung volume. This means that the premature curtailment of inspiration (breath 'clipping') that occurs with heavy-pressure threshold loading does not arise; thus, higher loads and higher tidal volumes can be achieved. As with other electronic devices, price makes this method the preserve of specialist clinics.

Pressure threshold devices

There are two products of this type that meet the requirements for inclusion in this summary. One has been applied to both the medical and sports settings (POWERbreathe®, POWERbreathe International Ltd.), the other to just the clinical environment (Threshold®, Respironics Inc.). Both products are supported by extensive, high-quality published research. The principal differences between the products are their loading ranges (see Table 5.1), mouthpiece, separation of inspiratory and expiratory flow paths and price (Threshold about £14 vs POWERbreathe® about £30). The loading range of the Threshold® renders it unusable by anyone whose baseline maximal inspiratory pressure (MIP) exceeds ~ 60 cmH$_2$O. This is because its load-setting range of 9 to 41 cmH$_2$O is unable to accommodate an adequate training load ($\sim 50\%$ MIP) for individuals with a MIP of >80 cmH$_2$O. Thus, someone starting training with a MIP of 60 cmH$_2$O, and improving by 30%, will rapidly reach the limits of the spring to provide an adequate training stimulus. The other product (POWERbreathe®) is supplied in a range of models with load settings spanning 17–98 cmH$_2$O, 23–186 cmH$_2$O and 29–274 cmH$_2$O; there is also a model that is approved for UK National

Health Service prescription (POWERbreathe® Medic). The POWERbreathe® product also separates inspiratory and expiratory flow paths such that the inspiratory valve is protected from expirate. Finally, the Threshold® (like the Pflex®) provides only a hard plastic tube mouthpiece that makes it challenging for some users to maintain an airtight seal, whereas the POWERbreathe® has a flexible flanged mouthpiece that is both comfortable and airtight; it can also be interfaced via a facemask. The low price of these devices make them ideal for use by patients in a domiciliary setting.

Endurance training

There is only one commercial product providing this type of respiratory training (SpiroTiger®, Idag AG, Switzerland). Like the two pressure threshold trainers, the efficacy of the SpiroTiger is supported by an extensive number of published research papers, primarily in a sports setting. As described in the section above, the overloading stimulus is provided by vigorous hyperventilation for periods of around 30 minutes. Because the product requires a rebreathing circuit and a method to monitor the training intensity, it is bulky and expensive (about £500), which renders it primarily a clinic- or sports-based training system. The training is also time consuming and extremely strenuous, requiring a very high level of user commitment in order to achieve and sustain the prescribed training intensity of ~ 60–90% of maximum voluntary ventilation.

MERITS AND LIMITATIONS OF DIFFERENT TRAINING METHODS AND EQUIPMENT

Table 5.1 summarizes the merits and limitations of the various training equipment, taking into consideration factors such as reliability, range of functional outcomes, price, ease of use, training session duration, etc. By referring to this table, it is possible to highlight the factors that are important for a given application, and to select the most appropriate form of apparatus. The table also provides an overall score for each piece of equipment.

Table 5.1 suggests that the most versatile, cost-effective, convenient and time-efficient method of respiratory training is provided by inspiratory pressure threshold loading, which is supported by the overall score received for these products. This method is also the most widely used, and best supported by research evidence. *Accordingly, all subsequent advice and guidance in this book will be provided for pressure threshold IMT.*

For the latest information on equipment and accessories for RMT, visit www.physiobreathe.com.

REFERENCES

Bailey, S.J., Romer, L.M., Kelly, J., et al., 2010. Inspiratory muscle training enhances pulmonary O(2) uptake kinetics and high-intensity exercise tolerance in humans. J. Appl. Physiol. 109, 457–468.

Baker, S., Davenport, P., Sapienza, C., 2005. Examination of strength training and detraining effects in expiratory muscles. J. Speech Lang. Hear. Res. 48, 1325–1333.

Bardsley, P.A., Bentley, S., Hall, H.S., et al., 1993. Measurement of inspiratory muscle performance with incremental threshold loading: a comparison of two techniques. Thorax 48, 354–359.

Belman, M.J., Gaesser, G.A., 1988. Ventilatory muscle training in the elderly. J. Appl. Physiol. 64, 899–905.

Belman, M.J., Shadmehr, R., 1988. Targeted resistive ventilatory muscle training in chronic obstructive pulmonary disease. J. Appl. Physiol. 65, 2726–2735.

Belman, M.J., Shadmehr, R., 1991. A target feedback device for ventilatory muscle training. J. Clin. Monit. 7, 42–48.

Boutellier, U., Piwko, P., 1992. The respiratory system as an exercise limiting factor in normal sedentary subjects. Eur. J. Appl. Physiol. Occup. Physiol. 64, 145–152.

Boutellier, U., Buchel, R., Kundert, A., et al., 1992. The respiratory system as an exercise limiting factor in normal trained subjects. Eur. J. Appl. Physiol. Occup. Physiol. 65, 347–353.

Brown, P.I., Sharpe, G.R., Johnson, M.A., 2008. Inspiratory muscle training reduces blood lactate concentration during volitional hyperpnoea. Eur. J. Appl. Physiol. 104, 111–117.

Brown, P.I., Sharpe, G.R., Johnson, M.A., 2010. Loading of trained inspiratory muscles speeds lactate recovery kinetics. Med. Sci. Sports Exerc. 42, 1103–1112.

Brown, P.I., Sharpe, G.R., Johnson, M.A., 2011. Inspiratory muscle training abolishes the blood lactate increase associated with volitional hyperpnoea superimposed on exercise and accelerates lactate and oxygen uptake kinetics at the onset of exercise.

Eur. J. Appl. Physiol. 112 (6), 2117–2129.

Buchman, A.S., Boyle, P.A., Wilson, R.S., et al., 2008. Respiratory muscle strength predicts decline in mobility in older persons. Neuroepidemiology 31, 174–180.

Caine, M.P., McConnell, A.K., 2000. Development and evaluation of a pressure threshold inspiratory muscle trainer for use in the context of sports performance. Journal of Sports Engineering 3, 149–159.

Chatham, K., Baldwin, J., Oliver, W., et al., 1996. Fixed load incremental respiratory muscle training: A pilot study. Physiotherapy 82, 422–426.

Chatham, K., Baldwin, J., Griffiths, H., et al., 1999. Inspiratory muscle training improves shuttle run performance in healthy subjects. Physiotherapy 85, 676–683.

Chatham, K., Conway, J., Enright, S., et al., 1995. A new test of incremental respiratory endurance (TIRE). Am. J. Respir. Crit. Care Med. 151, A416.

Chen, R.C., Que, C.L., Yan, S., 1998. Introduction to a new inspiratory threshold loading device. Eur. Respir. J. 12, 208–211.

Chiappa, G.R., Roseguini, B.T., Vieira, P.J., et al., 2008. Inspiratory muscle training improves blood flow to resting and exercising limbs in patients with chronic heart failure. J. Am. Coll. Cardiol. 51, 1663–1671.

Downey, A.E., Chenoweth, L.M., Townsend, D.K., et al., 2007. Effects of inspiratory muscle training on exercise responses in normoxia and hypoxia. Respir. Physiol. Neurobiol. 156, 137–146.

Edwards, A.M., Cooke, C.B., 2004. Oxygen uptake kinetics and maximal aerobic power are unaffected by inspiratory muscle training in healthy subjects where time to exhaustion is extended. Eur. J. Appl. Physiol. 93, 139–144.

Edwards, A.M., Wells, C., Butterly, R., 2008. Concurrent inspiratory muscle and cardiovascular training differentially improves both perceptions of effort and 5000 m running performance compared with cardiovascular training alone. Br. J. Sports Med. 42, 523–527.

Enright, S., Chatham, K., Ionescu, A.A., et al., 2004. Inspiratory muscle training improves lung function and exercise capacity in adults with cystic fibrosis. Chest 126, 405–411.

Enright, S.J., Unnithan, V.B., Heward, C., et al., 2006. Effect of high-intensity inspiratory muscle training on lung volumes, diaphragm thickness, and exercise capacity in subjects who are healthy. Phys. Ther. 86, 345–354.

Gea, J., Hamid, Q., Czaika, G., et al., 2000. Expression of myosin heavy-chain isoforms in the respiratory muscles following inspiratory resistive breathing. Am. J. Respir. Crit. Care Med. 161, 1274–1278.

Geddes, E.L., O'Brien, K., Reid, W.D., et al., 2008. Inspiratory muscle training in adults with chronic obstructive pulmonary disease: An update of a systematic review. Respir. Med. 102, 1715–1729.

Gosselink, R., Wagenaar, R.C., Decramer, M., 1996. Reliability of a commercially available threshold loading device in healthy subjects and in patients with chronic obstructive pulmonary disease. Thorax 51, 601–605.

Gosselink, R., De Vos, J., van den Heuvel, S.P., et al., 2011. Impact of inspiratory muscle training in patients with COPD: what is the evidence? Eur. Respir. J. 37, 416–425.

Griffiths, L.A., McConnell, A.K., 2007. The influence of inspiratory and expiratory muscle training upon rowing performance. Eur. J. Appl. Physiol. 99, 457–466.

Hakkinen, K., Komi, P.V., Alen, M., et al., 1987. EMG, muscle fibre and force production characteristics during a 1 year training period in elite weight-lifters. Eur. J. Appl. Physiol. Occup. Physiol. 56, 419–427.

Hanel, B., Secher, N.H., 1991. Maximal oxygen uptake and work capacity after inspiratory muscle training: a controlled study. J. Sports Sci. 9, 43–52.

Harver, A., Mahler, D.A., Daubenspeck, J.A., 1989. Targeted inspiratory muscle training improves respiratory muscle function and reduces dyspnea in patients with chronic obstructive pulmonary disease. Ann. Intern. Med. 111, 117–124.

Hill, K., Jenkins, S.C., Philippe, D.L., et al., 2006. High-intensity inspiratory muscle training in COPD. Eur. Respir. J. 27, 1119–1128.

How, S.C., McConnell, A.K., Taylor, B.J., et al., 2007. Acute and chronic responses of the upper airway to inspiratory loading in healthy awake humans: an MRI study. Respir. Physiol. Neurobiol. 157, 270–280.

Hsiao, S.F., Wu, Y.T., Wu, H.D., et al., 2003. Comparison of effectiveness of pressure threshold and targeted resistance devices for inspiratory muscle training in patients with chronic obstructive pulmonary disease. J. Formos. Med. Assoc. 102, 240–245.

Inbar, O., Weiner, P., Azgad, Y., et al., 2000. Specific inspiratory muscle training in well-trained endurance athletes. Med. Sci. Sports Exerc. 32, 1233–1237.

Johnson, B.D., Babcock, M.A., Suman, O.E., et al., 1993. Exercise-induced diaphragmatic fatigue in healthy humans. J. Physiol. 460, 385–405.

Johnson, M.A., Sharpe, G.R., Brown, P.I., 2007. Inspiratory muscle training improves cycling time-trial performance and anaerobic work capacity but not critical power. Eur. J. Appl. Physiol. 101, 761–770.

Jones, D.A., Rutherford, O.M., Parker, D.F., 1989. Physiological changes in skeletal muscle as a result of strength training. Q. J. Exp. Physiol. 74, 233–256.

Kilding, A.E., Brown, S., McConnell, A.K., 2009. Inspiratory muscle training improves 100 and 200 m swimming performance. Eur. J. Appl. Physiol. 108, 505–511.

Klusiewicz, A., Borkowski, L., Zdanowicz, R., et al., 2008. The inspiratory muscle training in elite rowers. J. Sports Med. Phys. Fitness 48, 279–284.

Larson, J.L., Kim, M.J., Sharp, J.T., et al., 1988. Inspiratory muscle training with a pressure threshold breathing device in patients with chronic obstructive pulmonary disease. Am. Rev. Respir. Dis. 138, 689–696.

Leddy, J.J., Limprasertkul, A., Patel, S., et al., 2007. Isocapnic hyperpnea

training improves performance in competitive male runners. Eur. J. Appl. Physiol. 99, 665–676.

Leith, D.E., Bradley, M., 1976. Ventilatory muscle strength and endurance training. J. Appl. Physiol. 41, 508–516.

Lisboa, C., Munoz, V., Beroiza, T., et al., 1994. Inspiratory muscle training in chronic airflow limitation: comparison of two different training loads with a threshold device. Eur. Respir. J. 7, 1266–1274.

Lisboa, C., Villafranca, C., Leiva, A., et al., 1997. Inspiratory muscle training in chronic airflow limitation: effect on exercise performance. Eur. Respir. J. 10, 537–542.

Lomax, M., 2010. Inspiratory muscle training, altitude, and arterial oxygen desaturation: a preliminary investigation. Aviat. Space Environ. Med. 81, 498–501.

Lomax, M., McConnell, A.K., 2009. Influence of prior activity (warm-up) and inspiratory muscle training upon between- and within-day reliability of maximal inspiratory pressure measurement. Respiration 78, 197–202.

Lotters, F., van Tol, B., Kwakkel, G., et al., 2002. Effects of controlled inspiratory muscle training in patients with COPD: a meta-analysis. Eur. Respir. J. 20, 570–577.

Mador, M.J., Deniz, O., Aggarwal, A., et al., 2005. Effect of respiratory muscle endurance training in patients with COPD undergoing pulmonary rehabilitation. Chest 128, 1216–1224.

Markov, G., Orler, R., Boutellier, U., 1996. Respiratory training, hypoxic ventilatory response and acute mountain sickness. Respir. Physiol. 105, 179–186.

McConnell, A.K., Lomax, M., 2006. The influence of inspiratory muscle work history and specific inspiratory muscle training upon human limb muscle fatigue. J. Physiol. 577, 445–457.

McConnell, A.K., Romer, L.M., 2004. Respiratory muscle training in healthy humans: resolving the controversy. Int. J. Sports Med. 25, 284–293.

McConnell, A.K., Sharpe, G.R., 2005. The effect of inspiratory muscle training upon maximum lactate steady-state

and blood lactate concentration. Eur. J. Appl. Physiol. 94 (3), 277–284.

Mickleborough, T.D., Stager, J.M., Chatham, K., et al., 2008. Pulmonary adaptations to swim and inspiratory muscle training. Eur. J. Appl. Physiol. 103 (6), 635–646.

Mickleborough, T.D., Nichols, T., Lindley, M.R., et al., 2009. Inspiratory flow resistive loading improves respiratory muscle function and endurance capacity in recreational runners. Scand. J. Med. Sci. Sports 20 (3), 458–468.

Moritani, T., deVries, H.A., 1979. Neural factors versus hypertrophy in the time course of muscle strength gain. Am. J. Phys. Med. 58, 115–130.

Mota, S., Guell, R., Barreiro, E., et al., 2007. Clinical outcomes of expiratory muscle training in severe COPD patients. Respir. Med. 101, 516–524.

Mujika, I., Padilla, S., 2000a. Detraining: loss of training-induced physiological and performance adaptations. Part I: short term insufficient training stimulus. Sports Med. 30, 79–87.

Mujika, I., Padilla, S., 2000b. Detraining: loss of training-induced physiological and performance adaptations. Part II: long term insufficient training stimulus. Sports Med. 30, 145–154.

Nickerson, B.G., Keens, T.G., 1982. Measuring ventilatory muscle endurance in humans as sustainable inspiratory pressure. J. Appl. Physiol. 52, 768–772.

Nicks, C.R., Morgan, D.W., Fuller, D.K., et al., 2009. The influence of respiratory muscle training upon intermittent exercise performance. Int. J. Sports Med. 30, 16–21.

O'Kroy, J.A., Coast, J.R., 1993. Effects of flow and resistive training on respiratory muscle endurance and strength. Respiration 60, 279–283.

Pardy, R.L., Leith, D.E., 1995. Ventilatory muscle training. In: Roussos, C., Macklem, P.T. (Eds.), The thorax. Marcel Dekker, New York, pp. 1353–1371.

Pardy, R.L., Rochester, D.F., 1992. Respiratory muscle training. Seminars in Respiratory Medicine 13, 53–62.

Preusser, B.A., Winningham, M.L., Clanton, T.L., 1994. High- vs low-intensity inspiratory muscle interval training in patients with COPD. Chest 106, 110–117.

Ramirez-Sarmiento, A., Orozco-Levi, M., Guell, R., et al., 2002. Inspiratory muscle training in patients with chronic obstructive pulmonary disease: structural adaptation and physiologic outcomes. Am. J. Respir. Crit. Care Med. 166, 1491–1497.

Rassler, B., Hallebach, G., Kalischewski, P., et al., 2007. The effect of respiratory muscle endurance training in patients with myasthenia gravis. Neuromuscul Disord 17, 385–391.

Romer, L.M., McConnell, A.K., 2003. Specificity and reversibility of inspiratory muscle training. Med. Sci. Sports Exerc. 35, 237–244.

Romer, L.M., McConnell, A.K., Jones, D.A., 2002a. Effects of inspiratory muscle training on time-trial performance in trained cyclists. J. Sports Sci. 20, 547–562.

Romer, L.M., McConnell, A.K., Jones, D.A., 2002b. Effects of inspiratory muscle training upon recovery time during high intensity, repetitive sprint activity. Int. J. Sports Med. 23, 353–360.

Romer, L.M., McConnell, A.K., Jones, D.A., 2002c. Inspiratory muscle fatigue in trained cyclists: effects of inspiratory muscle training. Med. Sci. Sports Exerc. 34, 785–792.

Smart, N.A., Giallauria, F., Dieberg, G., 2012. Efficacy of inspiratory muscle training in chronic heart failure patients: A systematic review and meta-analysis. Int. J. Cardiol. (in press).

Smeltzer, S.C., Lavietes, M.H., Cook, S.D., 1996. Expiratory training in multiple sclerosis. Arch. Phys. Med. Rehabil. 77, 909–912.

Smith, K., Cook, D., Guyatt, G.H., et al., 1992. Respiratory muscle training in chronic airflow limitation: a meta-analysis. Am. Rev. Respir. Dis. 145, 533–539.

Spengler, C.M., Roos, M., Laube, S.M., et al., 1999. Decreased exercise blood lactate concentrations after respiratory endurance training in humans. Eur. J. Appl. Physiol. Occup. Physiol. 79, 299–305.

Stuessi, C., Spengler, C.M., Knopfli-Lenzin, C., et al., 2001. Respiratory muscle endurance training in humans increases cycling endurance without affecting blood gas concentrations. Eur. J. Appl. Physiol. 84, 582–586.

Sturdy, G., Hillman, D., Green, D., et al., 2003. Feasibility of high-intensity, interval-based respiratory muscle training in COPD. Chest 123, 142–150.

Suzuki, S., Sato, M., Okubo, T., 1995. Expiratory muscle training and sensation of respiratory effort during exercise in normal subjects. Thorax 50, 366–370.

Tobin, M.J., Laghi, F., Jubran, A., 2010. Narrative review: ventilator-induced respiratory muscle weakness. Ann. Intern. Med. 153, 240–245.

Tong, T.K., Fu, F.H., Chung, P.K., et al., 2008. The effect of inspiratory muscle training on high-intensity, intermittent running performance to exhaustion. Appl. Physiol. Nutr. Metab. 33, 671–681.

Topin, N., Matecki, S., Le Bris, S., et al., 2002. Dose-dependent effect of individualized respiratory muscle training in children with Duchenne muscular dystrophy. Neuromuscul. Disord. 12, 576–583.

Turner, L.A., Tecklenburg-Lund, S.L., Chapman, R.F., et al., 2012. Inspiratory muscle training lowers the oxygen cost of voluntary hyperpnea. J. Appl. Physiol. 112, 127–134.

Tzelepis, G.E., Vega, D.L., Cohen, M.E., et al., 1994a. Pressure-flow specificity of inspiratory muscle training. J. Appl. Physiol. 77, 795–801.

Tzelepis, G.E., Vega, D.L., Cohen, M.E., et al., 1994b. Lung volume specificity of inspiratory muscle training. J. Appl. Physiol. 77, 789–794.

Verges, S., Boutellier, U., Spengler, C.M., 2008a. Effect of respiratory muscle endurance training on respiratory sensations, respiratory control and exercise performance: a 15-year experience. Respir. Physiol. Neurobiol. 161, 16–22.

Verges, S., Kruttli, U., Stahl, B., et al., 2008b. Respiratory control, respiratory sensations and cycling endurance after respiratory muscle endurance training. Adv. Exp. Med. Biol. 605, 239–244.

Verges, S., Renggli, A.S., Notter, D.A., et al., 2009. Effects of different respiratory muscle training regimes on fatigue-related variables during volitional hyperpnoea. Respir. Physiol. Neurobiol. 169, 282–290.

Villafranca, C., Borzone, G., Leiva, A., et al., 1998. Effect of inspiratory muscle training with an intermediate load on inspiratory power output in COPD. Eur. Respir. J. 11, 28–33.

Volianitis, S., McConnell, A.K., Koutedakis, Y., et al., 2001. Inspiratory muscle training improves rowing performance. Med. Sci. Sports Exerc. 33, 803–809.

Watsford, M., Murphy, A., 2008. The effects of respiratory-muscle training on exercise in older women. J. Aging Phys. Act. 16, 245–260.

Weiner, P., Weiner, M., 2006. Inspiratory muscle training may increase peak inspiratory flow in chronic obstructive pulmonary disease. Respiration 73, 151–156.

Weiner, P., Magadle, R., Beckerman, M., et al., 2003a. Comparison of specific expiratory, inspiratory, and combined muscle training programs in COPD. Chest 124, 1357–1364.

Weiner, P., Magadle, R., Beckerman, M., et al., 2003b. Specific expiratory muscle training in COPD. Chest 124, 468–473.

Weiner, P., Magadle, R., Beckerman, M., et al., 2004. Maintenance of inspiratory muscle training in COPD patients: one year follow-up. Eur. Respir. J. 23, 61–65.

Wells, G.D., Plyley, M., Thomas, S., et al., 2005. Effects of concurrent inspiratory and expiratory muscle training on respiratory and exercise performance in competitive swimmers. Eur. J. Appl. Physiol. 94, 527–540.

West, C.R., Taylor, B.J., Campbell, I.G., et al., 2009. Effects of inspiratory muscle training in Paralympic athletes with cervical spinal cord injury. Med. Sci. Sports Exerc. 41, S31–S32.

Witt, J.D., Guenette, J.A., Rupert, J.L., et al., 2007. Inspiratory muscle training attenuates the human respiratory muscle metaboreflex. J. Physiol. 584, 1019–1028.

Wylegala, J.A., Pendergast, D.R., Gosselin, L.E., et al., 2007. Respiratory muscle training improves swimming endurance in divers. Eur. J. Appl. Physiol. 99, 393–404.

Website

www.physiobreathe.com.

Chapter | 6 |

Implementing respiratory muscle training

GENERAL PRINCIPLES OF FOUNDATION IMT

In Chapters 4 and 5, the functional benefits and practical methods of respiratory muscle training (RMT) were reviewed. From the evidence presented there, it was apparent that the most widely used and validated type of RMT is pressure threshold inspiratory muscle training (IMT). Accordingly, the guidance provided in this chapter is for the application of this type of training.

The diversity of potential applications for IMT makes it impossible to provide specific guidance for all potential applications. Accordingly, this chapter provides guidance that is either generic or applies to the most popular and best-supported application of pressure threshold inspiratory muscle training (IMT), viz., the improvement of inspiratory muscle function for the purposes of alleviating dyspnoea and/or improving exercise tolerance. However, in the context of indications for IMT, readers are encouraged to consider the application of the techniques described in this chapter to alternative settings, e.g., weaning from mechanical ventilation. In this respect, a number of non-exercise-related indications are also provided (see also Chs 3 and 4 and Box 6.1).

Context of RMT in the treatment pathway

The evidence presented in Chapters 3 and 4 identified a wide range of patients in whom: (1) disease can create an imbalance in the demand/capacity relationship of the respiratory pump, and/or (2) IMT has been shown to improve one, or multiple, clinically meaningful outcomes. The diversity of patients, and the healthcare systems that care for them, makes prescriptive guidance on the place of IMT in the care pathway inappropriate. However, the vast majority of patients who could benefit from IMT are living with long-term chronic conditions such as respiratory disease, heart failure, obesity and neuromuscular disease. For these patients, the point at which IMT is delivered will be determined by local policies for the management of chronic disease. At the time of writing, the United Kingdom's National Health Service (NHS) is undergoing a major restructuring that is shifting the delivery of services to locations that are closer to its service users (patients). This inevitably means that services hitherto delivered in specialist units within secondary care will in future be delivered by 'up-skilled' primary care providers, or by local subcontractors to primary care providers. Simultaneously, there is likely to be an increase in the diversity of service providers for services such as rehabilitation, which have typically (but not exclusively) been provided in secondary care by NHS employees. These changes within the NHS are likely to bring its structure and delivery framework closer to that of the private healthcare systems that exist in other countries. The implications of such changes are that IMT could be provided in the patient's home as part of, for example, a primary care 'breathing clinic' service delivered by a nurse specialist, or by a specialist rehabilitation service within secondary care – either of which might be delivered by private sector or NHS providers. In practical terms, these changes should make very little difference to the patients' experience, provided that the appropriate expertise exists to assess their needs, and to provide the guidance required to support the optimal implementation of IMT whether in their own homes or within an outpatient setting.

The evidence presented in Chapter 4 supports the use of IMT both as a stand-alone intervention, and as part of a multi-dimensional rehabilitation programme, for a wide range of patients. The benign nature of IMT, and the ability of virtually all patients to meet the demands necessary to elicit improved function, make it a versatile intervention for patients with dyspnoea and exercise intolerance, or indeed for those who avoid activity because of their fear of exertional dyspnoea. Furthermore, co-morbidities that preclude exercise training are no barrier to IMT, making it an ideal intervention for severely compromised patients. A systematic review of home-based physiotherapy interventions for patients with chronic obstructive pulmonary disease (COPD) found that home-based IMT significantly improved dyspnoea (Transitional Dyspnoea Index) by 2.36 units, compared with controls (Thomas et al, 2010). Furthermore, a recent systematic review comparing IMT and rehabilitation concluded that the magnitude of improvement in exercise tolerance (and associated parameters) in response to IMT was indistinguishable statistically from that derived following a period of exercise training '(O'Brien et al, 2008). In other words, IMT yielded the same benefits as exercise training, making it a very cost-effective stand-alone intervention. The ideal setting for the stand-alone implementation of IMT is primary care. The barrier to implementation in this setting is a general lack of specialist expertise relating to IMT, which is not typically part of the curriculum for respiratory clinicians. This book endeavours to facilitate the acquisition of that expertise and the inclusion of IMT within the clinical curricula of specialist nurses, physiotherapists and physicians.

Finally, the context of IMT needs to be defined in terms of its application as either 'Foundation IMT' or 'Functional IMT' (see Ch. 7). In this book, the stand-alone implementation of IMT has been termed 'Foundation IMT', which is also the first phase of a two-phase process that leads to Functional IMT. Respiratory muscles have a number of important non-respiratory roles (see Ch. 3), which is why patients find walking more 'dyspnoegenic' than cycling. A training modality that is applied widely in sport is 'functional' training, i.e., the training of functional movements (e.g., a squat), rather than the training of muscles (e.g., leg extensors). This approach has not yet been applied to IMT in patients. However, for people who already have overloaded respiratory muscles, the competing functions of, say, postural control may be sufficient to render an everyday activity impossible because of intolerable dyspnoea. Accordingly, the rationale for implementing a training modality that addresses these competing demands is very strong. The specialist nature of Functional IMT makes its implementation the preserve of rehabilitation specialists and, therefore, probably unsuitable for implementation outside of the rehabilitation setting.

Indications and contraindications for IMT

Chapters 3 and 4 presented the theoretical and evidence-based rationales for RMT, respectively. The rationale for RMT is based upon ameliorating imbalance within the demand/capacity relationship of the respiratory muscles. This information is summarized in Box 6.1. The following section contains a more detailed overview of these issues.

Indications

Chapter 3 summarized the wide range of conditions in which respiratory muscle dysfunction is present, as well as the disease-specific factors that contribute to an imbalance of the demand/capacity relationship of the inspiratory and expiratory muscles. Chapter 4 summarized the evidence for improvement in clinical outcomes following RMT. For the reasons provided in Chapters 4 and 5, the current chapter deals with training of the inspiratory muscles. The simplistic approach to identifying patients who could benefit from rebalancing of the demand/capacity relationship is to assess maximal inspiratory pressure (MIP) and to apply a diagnostic criterion for 'weakness' based upon reference to population norms (see Ch. 1), e.g., 60% of the predicted normal value.

However, this approach fails to take account of a number of important issues. First, strength (MIP) is a one-dimensional index of muscle function that is difficult to interpret in limb muscles, but is infinitely more difficult for the respiratory muscles. This is primarily because MIP is merely a surrogate measure of strength, and is several steps removed from the true force-generating capacity of the inspiratory muscles (ATS/ERS, 2002). Secondly, in patients with a tendency to hyperinflate, MIP is not a fixed index of function but one that is dependent upon the prevailing degree of hyperinflation. Thirdly, the interpretation of MIP needs to be made in the context of the prevailing loading conditions, and work requirements, of the inspiratory muscles – in other words, whether the demand/capacity relationship of the inspiratory muscles is in a state of imbalance. In the presence of an increased demand for inspiratory muscle work, a muscle that appears 'normal' in absolute terms is rendered weak functionally.

In most chronic conditions, inspiratory muscle dysfunction manifests as dyspnoea and exercise intolerance. Thus, a more pragmatic approach to assessing the extent to which the inspiratory muscles are functionally overloaded is to consider the intensity of dyspnoea that an increased demand for inspiratory muscle work provokes. Any patients who complain of dyspnoea that limits their activities of daily living are therefore candidates for IMT (see also the sections 'Patient selection' below, and 'Assessing patient needs' in Ch. 7).

Notwithstanding the preceding rationale, the absence of exertional dyspnoea should not be a reason to discount IMT as a potential management tool for exercise intolerance. The inspiratory muscle metaboreflex described in Chapters 3 and 4 is probably the reason that a substantial number of patients with respiratory disease stop exercising because of leg discomfort, rather than dyspnoea (Hamilton et al, 1996). In such cases, improving inspiratory muscle function raises the intensity of inspiratory muscle work associated with

Box 6.1 Indications and contraindications summary

Indications

1. Primary indications are dyspnoea and/or exercise intolerance.

2. Main classes of disease, or conditions, where research supports a beneficial influence of IMT upon clinical outcomes in sub-groups of patients (see Ch. 4):

- Respiratory
- Cardiac
- Neuromuscular
- Surgery
- Healthy ageing

3. Specific conditions where either (1) IMT has been shown to produce some clinically significant benefits (see Ch. 4), or (2) there is a theoretical rationale for IMT based upon the presence of inspiratory muscle dysfunction and/or abnormal respiratory mechanics, producing a demand/capacity imbalance within the respiratory pump (see Ch. 3):

- Amyotrophic lateral sclerosis
- Ankylosing spondylitis
- Anorexia nervosa
- Arthritis
- Artificially ventilated patients
- Asthma
- Bronchiectasis
- Cancer
- Cerebral palsy
- Chronic heart failure
- COPD
- Corticosteroid use (oral)
- Cystic fibrosis
- Diabetes (type 1 and 2)
- Diaphragm paralysis
- Hypothyroidism
- Kyphoscoliosis
- Multiple sclerosis
- Muscular dystrophies
- Myasthenia gravis
- Obesity
- Obstructive sleep apnoea
- Parkinson's disease
- Post-polio
- Pregnancy
- Pulmonary arterial hypertension
- Renal failure
- Sarcoidosis and interstitial lung disease
- Senescence
- Spinal cord injury
- Surgical patients (thoracic and abdominal)
- Ventilator-induced myopathy and failure to wean
- Ventilatory failure (vulnerability to)
- Vocal cord dysfunction and stridor

4. Some specific physiological indicators of potential load/capacity imbalance of the respiratory muscles, and/or inadequate respiratory muscle function. The following are not unique to load/capacity imbalance of the respiratory muscles, but can be used as part of a process of differential diagnosis:

- Reduced respiratory muscle strength
- Dyspnoea
- Orthopnoea
- Expiratory flow limitation
- Hyperinflation
- Reduced respiratory system compliance
- Elevated ratio of dead space to tidal volume (V_D / V_T)
- Tachypnoea
- Hypoxaemia
- Hypercapnia
- Poor cough function
- Inability to breathe without the aid of mechanical ventilation

Contraindications

There have been no reports of adverse events following IMT, but there is a *theoretical* risk of barotrauma-related events. Accordingly, caution should be exercised in the following situations:

- A history of spontaneous pneumothorax (i.e., not due to traumatic injury)
- A pneumothorax due to a traumatic injury that has not healed fully
- A burst eardrum that has not healed fully, or any other condition of the eardrum

The sub-group of asthma patients with unstable asthma and abnormally low perception of dyspnoea are also unsuitable candidates for IMT.

---

metaboreflex activation. This can increase the exercise tolerance of non-dyspnoeic patients by improving leg blood flow.

Finally, readers are encouraged to consider the application of the techniques described in this chapter to ameliorating the demand/capacity imbalance of the inspiratory muscles in non-exercise-related contexts. Some indications for these applications are provided in Box 6.1.

Contraindications

Inspiratory muscle training is associated with large negative pressure swings within the chest (intrathoracic

decompression), and this naturally engenders concern regarding barotrauma-related events. For example, clinicians sometimes express concern regarding the risks of IMT for patients with bullae/blebs, especially those with COPD.

Implicitly, the measurement of maximal respiratory pressures is associated with larger pressure changes, so it is perhaps appropriate to consider also the risks associated with these measurements, as they represent a 'worst case scenario' for the risk of barotrauma during IMT. The first published measurements of maximal respiratory pressures were made by Black & Hyatt in the late 1960s (Black & Hyatt, 1969), and the first studies of IMT by Leith & Bradley (1976). Thus, the research base spans over 40 years, but there is no mention of any complications or adverse events in any of the studies within the published literature. In other words, of the hundreds of studies of IMT and/or maximal inspiratory mouth pressure measurement (incorporating many thousands of patients), no study has ever reported a patient withdrawal due to an event precipitated by barotrauma. Similarly, there are no case studies of IMT reporting isolated incidents of adverse events during the treatment, or assessment of any person undertaking measurement of maximal inspiratory pressures (MIP), or IMT. Despite the intrathoracic pressure swings, even patients with heart failure experience no deterioration of their cardiac output during training (McConnell et al, 2005).

Notwithstanding this, there are some *theoretical* risks associated with sub-atmospheric pressures within the chest, throat, inner ear and sinuses. Accordingly, there are some conditions in which IMT may not be appropriate:

- A history of spontaneous pneumothorax (i.e., not due to traumatic injury)
- A pneumothorax due to a traumatic injury that has not healed fully
- A burst eardrum that has not healed fully, or any other condition of the eardrum.

There is also an important subgroup of asthma patients for whom IMT is inappropriate, i.e., those with unstable asthma and abnormally low perception of dyspnoea. In these patients, it is the disruption of the normal relationship between dyspnoea and bronchoconstriction that is thought to contribute to their poor adherence to medication and consequent clinical instability (Magadle et al, 2002). Since IMT may reduce their perception still further, it is inadvisable.

Unlike pharmacological treatments, IMT has no side effects or drug interactions.

Patient selection

There remains a perception that only patients with evidence of inspiratory muscle weakness (see section 'Assessment of respiratory muscle function') or ventilatory limitation during physical activity can benefit from IMT. The logic of this has always been questionable, particularly given that Olympic standard athletes are known to benefit, and they certainly have no compromise to the function of their ventilatory pump. The misconception is perpetuated by the fact that patients with a MIP < 60 cmH$_2$O appear to show larger improvements than those with stronger inspiratory muscles (Lotters et al, 2002; Gosselink et al, 2011). However, even when inspiratory muscle weakness is not an inclusion criterion, improvements in dyspnoea and exercise performance still follow IMT (Lotters et al, 2002). A pragmatic way to view these observations is that weaker individuals have more to gain from IMT.

In addition, it is also worth noting that research has shown repeatedly that there is a close correlation between

the post-IMT decrease in dyspnoea and the improvement in MIP, regardless of MIP at baseline, or whether the participants are patients or healthy young athletes. Thus, it is the extent to which MIP can be improved that dictates the magnitude of improvement in dyspnoea. In this respect also, weaker patients have more to gain, as they appear to show the largest improvements in MIP after IMT (Lotters et al, 2002; Gosselink et al, 2011).

Notwithstanding this, there is nevertheless a dose–response relationship that relates the magnitude of improvement to the number of completed IMT sessions (Winkler et al, 2000), i.e., the more diligently the IMT training regimen is adhered to the better is the outcome. This means that patient motivation is arguably the most important criterion for enrolment. Accordingly, the best candidates for IMT are well-motivated individuals with dyspnoea and/or exercise intolerance.

See Chapter 7 (section 'Assessing patient needs') for guidance on assessing dyspnoea and the functional limitations it imposes.

Precautions

In patients with coronary artery disease, it is prudent to minimize hypocapnia by using slower breathing frequency and/or the rebreathing technique described below in 'Practical issues'. In addition, IMT may induce slight ear discomfort in people who have had a recent head cold, sinusitis, or any condition that leads to difficulty in equalizing pressure between the ear and airway. Accordingly, it is wise to delay IMT until such symptoms have resolved.

In patients who have experienced an acute exacerbation, or chest infection, clinical judgement should be applied regarding the risk of provoking excessive fatigue of the inspiratory muscles. In this situation, reducing the intensity and/or frequency of IMT may be prudent.

Patients should be cautioned against sharing their training equipment, as this presents an infection risk.

PRACTICAL ISSUES

This section provides guidance on some preliminary issues that require consideration prior to embarking upon a programme of Foundation IMT (inspiratory muscle training).

Posture during training

Recumbent and semi-recumbent postures are known to impair respiratory muscle function, which is optimized in upright positions (Koulouris et al, 1989; Griffiths & McConnell, 2012). Accordingly, posture has an influence on the ability to overcome a given load during IMT. This concept will be developed in Chapter 7 in the context of functional IMT, but posture also has a role to play in obtaining optimal results during the Foundation phase, especially in patients who are unable to adopt an upright position. The premise for this is that larger improvements can be achieved in a shorter time frame if training overload is maximized. Since inspiratory muscle function is optimized in upright positions, the highest training loads can be tolerated when seated or standing, and these represent the ideal positions to commence a period of IMT.

However, there are some caveats to the use of seated or standing postures. The respiratory muscles contribute to postural control, which is a confounding influence during IMT. If the inspiratory muscles are relieved of their postural role, they are able to 'focus' upon breathing. Consequently maximal inspiratory pressure (MIP), maximal expiratory pressure (MEP) and maximal voluntary ventilation (MVV) are all higher in a standing, supported, leaning posture (Cavalheri et al, 2010). Thus standing, and leaning forward against the back of a chair, table, window ledge or just by placing the hands on the knees, increases the tolerable training load and the number of repetitions that can be achieved. The logic of this is immediately apparent when one considers what people do when they are breathless: they instinctively lean on something so that their respiratory muscles can be focussed on the act of breathing.

During the early Foundation phase of IMT the objective is to maximize functional adaptations of the inspiratory muscles in their respiratory role. Hence, in the Foundation phase, the ideal posture is standing with postural unloading, i.e., isolation of the respiratory role of the trunk muscles. Only once this foundation has been laid is it appropriate to challenge the respiratory and non-respiratory functions simultaneously, i.e., with functional training. The next stage towards this objective is training in a standing position without postural unloading, and the final stage is Functional IMT. Accordingly, posture during IMT should be progressed from leaning to unsupported standing.

For some patients, standing will not be acceptable, or even possible, so for those unable to undertake IMT in the standing position (at least at the start of the training), sitting is perfectly good. It is also possible to unload the postural role of the inspiratory muscles when sitting, which is achieved by leaning forward against a table or placing the hands on the knees. However, patients should be encouraged to train in a standing position as soon as possible, as this represents progress towards functionality.

For patients who are confined to bed, IMT is also possible, but these patients can tolerate only low training loads, which may limit the rate and magnitude of progress. Furthermore, since the objective is for patients to be restored to normal functioning, it is important that IMT is progressed to an unsupported, upright position as soon as they are able to tolerate this.

Optimizing breathing technique

Maximizing the training stimulus to the inspiratory muscles, as well as the range of adaptations it elicits, is arguably the most important objective in terms of achieving the best possible training results. Choosing the right type of training device is the first step to maximizing results. In the case of the methods described in this book, the focus is on pressure threshold IMT, for which there are two evidence-based products available (see Ch. 5, Table 5.1). Once the training device has been selected, the second step is to optimize the training stimulus that it generates. Unfortunately, simply breathing through a training device will not achieve this. However, the following section explains the optimal approach for pressure threshold IMT and the physiology that underlies this approach. Firstly, the fundamentals of 'good' breathing technique will be considered, i.e., how to develop efficient, comfortable, diaphragm-focussed breathing. Secondly, the optimization of breathing pattern (the combination of respiratory flows, volumes and the timing of breaths) for IMT will be explained.

Diaphragm breathing

Disease-related changes to the mechanics of breathing can lead to a reduction in diaphragm mobility, and, consequently, its contribution to breathing. This phenomenon has been well documented in COPD where it is largely due to hyperinflation (Unal et al, 2000). Diaphragm breathing training programmes have been shown to improve diaphragm mobility and exercise tolerance (Paulin et al, 2007; Yamaguti et al, 2012), as well as breathing pattern and oxygen saturation (Fernandes et al, 2011). However, in patients with COPD who have asynchronous thoracoabdominal motion, diaphragm breathing may exacerbate dyspnoea (Fernandes et al, 2011) and reduce the efficiency of breathing (Gosselink et al, 1995). Consequently, the appropriateness of diaphragm breathing for a specific patient needs to be evaluated on a case-by-case basis. Given that the likely readers of this book are healthcare professionals with an interest, and considerable expertise, in the realm of 'breathing', there is a danger of 'teaching grandmother to suck eggs' in providing advice on diaphragm breathing. However, relearning normal efficient breathing strategies is the 'essential groundwork' that underpins Foundation IMT. Accordingly, expert readers are merely encouraged to ensure that patients receive appropriate diaphragm breathing training as part of their Foundation IMT. For those readers who would welcome some further guidance on teaching diaphragm breathing, please feel free to read on, but also feel free to seek this elsewhere, as the following section is merely included for the sake of completeness.

This first phase of the process of developing efficient breathing can be thought of as 'getting in touch with the diaphragm'. Human babies breathe almost exclusively with their diaphragm, but most human adults have lost touch with their most important respiratory muscle and become 'chest breathers', i.e., they breathe using the accessory muscles of the rib cage. Without re-establishing diaphragm breathing, IMT will neglect the most important inspiratory muscle.

However, this emphasis upon diaphragm breathing should not be confused with the objective of focussing the IMT upon the diaphragm; this is not what is being advocated (the reasons for this are explained below in the section 'Breathing pattern during IMT'). Rather, the objective is to ensure that the complex inspiratory musculature is used holistically, and in concert, during both training and activities of daily living. This section provides guidance on how to reintroduce the diaphragm into the normal, instinctive process of breathing, so that when breathing is challenged, the diaphragm is a subconscious, central part of the response. The mechanism by which isolated, conscious activation of muscles restores their automatic activation is poorly understood, but it has been likened to flipping a rope back into a well-worn groove. Short-term repetition of motor tasks has been shown to induce cortical reorganization in a range of activities including the practice of diaphragm breathing (Demoule et al, 2008). These changes are consistent with the ability of task repetition to enhance neuromuscular functioning. For example, for muscles that are involved in automatic, anticipatory postural adjustments, such as transversus abdominis, it is thought that isolated specific training can normalize previously abnormal patterns of motor activation (Tsao & Hodges, 2007).

As a general rule, diaphragm-breathing practice should be undertaken only when the patient is in a clinically stable condition. The next factor to consider is the posture adopted during diaphragm-breathing practice. Since the postural role of the respiratory muscles can be a confounding influence, a progressive approach that starts with postural unloading can be helpful. A progressive approach is also helpful for patients who are hyperinflated, but in this case it is essential to ensure that progression does not lead to the development of dysfunctional breathing (see above). Using progression, patients advance from seated leaning, to upright seated, to standing.

Visual and tactile feedback both provide very helpful means of coaching diaphragm breathing. To achieve this, the patient should be positioned in front of a mirror (large enough to see their torso), with palms placed lightly on the ribs with the fingers facing forwards and the tips of the fingers almost touching at the end of a normal exhalation (Fig. 6.1). The exercise should commence by describing (to the patient) the movement of the diaphragm during inhalation and the effect this has on the abdominal wall, i.e., the diaphragm flattens and moves downwards like a piston, pushing the abdominal organs downwards and outwards. A demonstration is helpful,

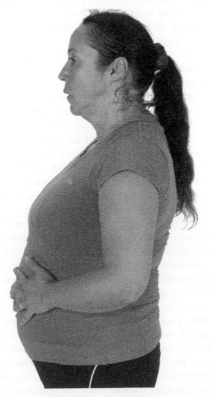 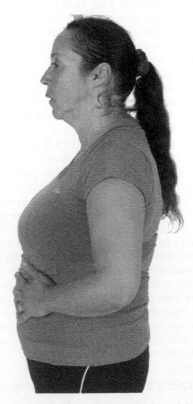

A
B

Figure 6.1 Placing the hands on the abdomen to feel movement of the abdominal wall during diaphragm breathing: (A) inhalation, (B) exhalation.

after which the following instructions can be used to guide the patient's breathing:

- Commence diaphragm breathing at the end of a normal exhalation
- Keep your abdomen, shoulders and chest relaxed, and take a deep, slow inhalation through your nose
- Watch the movement of your abdomen and rib cage in the mirror
- On inhalation, you should see and feel your abdomen bulge forwards and your ribs move sideways and forwards
- Watch your finger tips and try to move them apart using your abdomen as you inhale
- If your chest rises, the diaphragm is not being used properly – relax the shoulders and chest
- Exhalation should be relaxed, with no muscle activity – allow the air to 'fall out' of your chest as your lungs and rib cage 'spring' back
- You may find it helpful to purse your lips as this helps you to breathe out further, and also slows your exhalation, but be careful not to force the air out – relax and let the air fall out
- Be careful not to hold the breath at the end of the inhalation – relax and let the air fall out.

Use of an external breathing pacer that provides an auditory and visual cue (obtainable via www.physiobreathe.com/apps) can be very helpful for supporting the process of developing an efficient breathing pattern, i.e., deep breaths accompanied by a slow exhalation. In addition, a Theraband®, or similar wide elastic resistance band, wrapped around the lower ribs can help to focus effort on this area. The resistance of the band intensifies the sensation of working with the diaphragm (if the patient still finds the exercise too challenging, see below). Diaphragm breathing should be practised until the patient feels confident about how to activate the diaphragm, and what a diaphragm inhalation feels and looks like. Once this technique has been mastered, it should be tried with eyes closed, focussing on the sensation of the air filling the lungs and the sensation of the diaphragm plunging down into the abdomen.

During the diaphragm breathing exercise, breathing rate should be no more than 12 breaths per minute, and preferably 8. With practice it might be possible to reduce this to 6 breaths per minute. The inhalation phase will typically be slightly longer than exhalation because exhalation is passive, i.e., the only phase that is actively controlled is inhalation. However, this will not be the case in obstructed patients, who typically take longer to exhale. Patients can count the breath in and out. For example, for an obstructed patient, if the objective is 10 breaths per minute this means that each breath should take 6 seconds (60/10); count '1–2' during inhalation, and '3–4–5–6' during exhalation. It is vital that the extension of the breath duration is not achieved by breath holding at the

end of inhalation or exhalation; the increase in duration should come about through a slower, deeper, more controlled breath so that each phase starts immediately the other ends. Remind patients that exhalation should be passive, and that the air should 'fall out' of the lungs as quietly as possible. There are some useful biofeedback applications for smartphones and tablet computers that can facilitate the development of slow, deep breathing, which healthcare professionals can use in a clinic setting and that can be suggested to patients as tools to help them to practise at home (see www.physiobreathe.com/apps). These tools set the duration of each phase of breathing and the breathing frequency, count the number of breaths, and time the practice session.

A typical practice session should last around 4 minutes each day (2 minutes with visual feedback and 2 without). Patients should also be encouraged to keep checking periodically throughout the day to make sure that they using diaphragm breathing during everyday activities, including physical activity. The latter can be facilitated by encouraging patients to practise their diaphragm breathing during everyday activities such as walking (e.g., breathe in for 2 steps and out for 3). However, they need to switch from nose to mouth breathing for these sessions. The aim of this process is to use conscious control of breathing to restore the unconscious control of breathing to a more diaphragm-focussed activity.

If the exercises described above are too challenging, patients should lie on their back during diaphragm-breathing practice. This brings about a number of beneficial changes. Firstly, the respiratory muscles are no longer involved in postural activities (holding the trunk upright), which makes it easier to focus on relaxing everything except the diaphragm. The second thing that happens is that the abdominal contents rest against the underside of the diaphragm, giving it something to work against. Finally, it is much easier to be completely relaxed when lying down. The exercise is started with small breaths 'into the abdomen' through the nose. Exhalation is a relaxed process in which the air 'falls out' of the lungs. Patients should increase the size of the breaths progressively until they become slow and deep, being careful not to hold the breath at the end of the inhalation. As described above, the breathing rate should be no more than 12 breaths per minute, but it may be possible to work down to 6. Once diaphragm breathing has been achieved lying down, it should then be practised standing upright in front of a mirror, as described above, and starting over from the beginning.

The restoration of diaphragm in breathing can be undertaken in parallel with the first few weeks of Foundation IMT, and the two activities will reinforce one another.

Developing breath control is a skill that can and should be practised because it maximizes breathing efficiency and minimizes the distracting influence of breathing discomfort. The first stage in achieving this is achieving diaphragm-focussed breathing, which provides the 'groundwork' for good breath control; once this becomes second nature the second phase is much easier. Phase two involves developing breath control to overcome the natural desire to breathe as quickly as possible during periods when breathing demand is high and when breathing discomfort/distress is present. By not allowing breathing to become rapid and shallow, voluntary breathing control imposes a deep, slow, calm and efficient pattern. The only time that this can be practised properly is in situations where breathing demand/distress is high, but only when patients are clinically stable. So they should be encouraged to practice deep, slow breath control during periods when they feel dyspnoeic. Keeping breathing calm and relaxed under stressful conditions can help to minimize stress and anxiety, and build a sense of mastery. See also Chapter 7 (section on 'Breath control') for some exercises that promote deep, slow, controlled breathing.

Breathing pattern during IMT

An important principle for maximizing the benefits of IMT is that training should maximize inspiratory muscle recruitment. This means maximizing both the number of inspiratory muscles involved and the level of activation that is achieved. At the present time, it is not known whether the adaptations resulting in clinical improvements are attributable to the diaphragm, the inspiratory accessory muscles, or both. Accordingly, during IMT, breathing movements should take place over the largest range possible, and maximize recruitment of the inspiratory musculature. The next two sections will consider issues of technique in relation to tidal volume and inspiratory flow rate.

Tidal volume

Although muscle is a very adaptable tissue, training adaptations are also highly specific to the nature of the training stimulus. Adaptations elicited by IMT are specific to a number of characteristics of the training stimulus, including the lung volume at which training takes place (see Ch. 5). The practical implication of this is that IMT should be undertaken across the widest range of lung volume possible, i.e., from as close to residual volume as possible to the point at which it is impossible to inhale any more. Failure to do this will lead to suboptimal adaptation at some lung volumes, which is particularly important in patients who hyperinflate when minute ventilation increases. An important consideration in maximizing tidal volume (V_T) during IMT is the training load; loading too 'heavily' can compromise both the V_T that can be achieved and the amount of work that can be undertaken during training, which will also impair the training response (Box 6.2). This impairment occurs because V_T has a strong influence upon the amount of work done per breath, and the most important determinant of the ability to inhale deeply is the training load (McConnell & Griffiths, 2010). Functional weakening of the inspiratory muscles during inhalation means that, if the load is too high, the inspiratory muscles are not able to overcome the load at higher lung volumes (where the inspiratory muscles are weaker), despite maximal effort. The heavier the load, the more severely the breath is 'clipped'.

This means that the training load must be set with these factors in mind. Figure 6.2 illustrates the interrelationships

---

Box 6.2 Why high pressure threshold training loads produce paradoxical results

Typically, one expects that increasing the magnitude of the weight lifted would increase the magnitude of the training stimulus delivered to a muscle. However, for the inspiratory muscles this appears not to be the case (McConnell & Griffiths, 2010). A recent study in healthy people examined the effects of various inspiratory loads upon a range of training-related variables, including the number of repetitions that could be tolerated, the volume of each breath during the training session, the amount of work completed during the session, and whether the session activated the inspiratory muscle metaboreflex (changing the threshold for activation of this reflex is one of the important mechanisms by which IMT improves performance; see Ch. 4).

As expected, the number of breaths (repetitions) declined as the load increased (e.g., just 4 breaths at 90% of MIP compared with 84 breaths at 60%), and V_T declined with increasing load, as well as during each session (because of the pressure–volume relationship and fatigue, respectively). The most surprising finding was the influence of heavy loads (greater than 70% MIP) upon the amount of work that was undertaken per breath (work = load × V_T). Because V_T was lower with heavy loads, the amount of work done per breath

was reduced markedly. This effect is completely counterintuitive, because, during limb muscle training, heavier loads usually require more work (because the range of movement doesn't change a great deal when moving from moderate to heavy loads). The detrimental effect of the reduction in V_T on the training stimulus delivered to the inspiratory muscles was compounded by the reduction in the number of breaths at heavy loads. In other words, the total amount of work done by the inspiratory muscles is reduced markedly by increasing the load above 70% of MIP.

A further interesting finding was that the only training load to activate the inspiratory muscle metaboreflex was the 60% load, and this also happened to be the load closest to the 30-repetition maximum (RM). What do we conclude from all this? First, heavy loading does not deliver the increase in the intensity of the training stimulus that one might expect it to. Second, to prevent 'work' from being jeopardized, the choice of load must be balanced carefully against the effect that it has on V_T and RM (loading at 50% to 70% appears to tread this line most effectively). Third, if activating the metaboreflex during training is necessary in order to increase its threshold for activation, then the 30RM load delivers this.

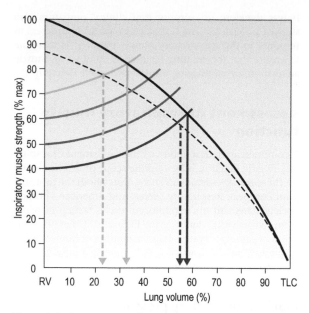

Figure 6.2 The interactions between inspiratory muscle strength (black line), various training loads (40%, 50%, 60% and 70% of maximal inspiratory pressure [faded lines]), and the breath volume that can be achieved during training, as well as the effect of fatigue (dotted lines). For example, at 40% of MIP it is possible to inhale to around 60% of vital capacity, whereas at 70% of MIP it is only possible to inhale to around 35% of vital capacity.
(Adapted from McConnell AK, 2011. Breathe strong, perform better. Human Kinetics, Champaign, IL, with permission.)

of maximal inspiratory pressure (MIP), lung volume and training load, as well as the effect of fatigue on the V_T that can be achieved. Note that the breath volume is clipped progressively earlier in the breath with increasing loads.

Inspiratory flow rate

To understand the advice below, it is necessary to return briefly to the force–velocity relationship of muscle. Essentially, this property dictates that the faster a muscle contracts, the less force it is able to generate, and *vice versa* (see Ch. 4, Fig. 4.1). An example of the force–velocity relationship at work is the difference in force one can exert on the pedals when cycling in a low gear compared with a high gear. This property can be exploited to optimize the training stimulus that the muscle receives. For example, assume that, because of the force–velocity relationship, as the rate of muscle contraction doubles the force it can generate is halved, despite the same [maximal] effort being applied under both conditions. When muscles contract maximally at any speed, the number of muscle fibres that are recruited to the contraction is also maximized, despite the fact that faster contractions result in lower forces. Now consider the effect of doubling the rate of contraction slightly differently: when a muscle is contracting very slowly to move a load that requires, say, half its maximal force-generating

capacity, doubling the rate of contraction against the same load now requires ~100% of the muscle's force-generating capacity (because its ability to generate force has been halved). This means that ~100% of the muscle fibres are recruited for half the force. This can be turned to an advantage during IMT because it means that it is possible to train close to 100% of a muscle's force-generating capacity no matter what load is being applied, provided that the load is moved as fast as possible (i.e., with maximal effort). Under any given loading condition, fast muscle contractions recruit more muscle fibres than slow contractions (Aagaard et al, 2000). Furthermore, recent evidence suggest that training improvements following bench press training are maximized at higher velocities of muscle shortening (Padulo et al, 2012). Therefore, maximal effort ensures maximum velocity, and the recruitment of the greatest number of muscle fibres.

Muscle recruitment has an important impact on the response to training for two reasons. First, fibres that are not recruited will not be trained. So, if the velocity of contraction is slow, a load requiring half of a muscle's force-generating capacity will require recruitment of [and train] only about half of its fibres; however, if the same load is overcome as fast as possible then close to 100% of fibres will be recruited and trained. Secondly, maximizing recruitment is an important part of the neural adaption to training, which also contributes to optimizing training outcomes. Training improves strength through two mechanisms: (1) stimulating muscle fibres to grow, and (2) neural adaptations, which ensure that all available fibres within a muscles are recruited and that all muscles that bring about a given movement are recruited.

In order to stimulate muscle hypertrophy, muscle fibres must be subjected to mechanical stress, which requires the application of at least moderate-intensity loading. This is why high-velocity–low-load training does not improve strength no matter how much effort is applied at low training loads. The practical implications of this for IMT are that strength and speed (power) can be improved only if the training load is at least moderate (50–60% of maximal strength), and the velocity of contraction (inhalation rate) is as fast as possible.

Accordingly, IMT should be conducted with maximum effort; i.e., each inhalation should be executed as fast as possible. This should take around 1–2 seconds and be accompanied by a loud rushing sound as air is sucked through the valve of the training device at high velocity. Encourage patients to make this sound as loud as possible, because this indicates high flow rates. Be aware that the heavier the relative load, the slower will be the maximal flow rate that can be generated (and the smaller the lung volume; see Fig. 6.2). In contrast to the maximal nature of the inspiratory effort, exhalation should be passive, quiet and take 3 to 4 seconds. Use of an external breathing pacer that provides an auditory cue (obtainable via www.physiobreathe.com/apps) can be very helpful for supporting the process.

Because of the higher-than-normal breath volume and breathing frequency, some light-headedness may result from the hyperventilation-induced hypocapnia. This is harmless for the duration of a 30-breath session, and also seems to lessen in severity as training progresses (but see also 'Precautions', above). If it is problematic, ask the patient to pause at the end of exhalation and wait for the urge to breathe in again. For maximal training overload the training breaths should be completed as quickly as possible, but this has to be balanced against the effects of the hypocapnia. A method that can be used to overcome the loss of carbon dioxide is to place the training device inside a bag that has a slit down one side (a supermarket carrier bag is ideal). By rebreathing from the bag, the loss of carbon dioxide is largely abolished and light-headedness is prevented. This allows patients to complete the breaths rapidly, so maximizing the training benefits.

Combining inspiratory and expiratory training

Evidence suggests that loading of the inspiratory and expiratory phases of the same breath produces suboptimal results, and that even healthy young people find this simultaneous loading uncomfortable (Griffiths & McConnell, 2007). Accordingly, this approach is NOT recommended. If expiratory muscle training is to be added to IMT, each should be delivered as a discrete bout of exercise separated by a few minutes of recovery.

Secretions

Repeated, deep inhalations against an inspiratory load have been found to be twice as effective (sputum weight) as standardized physiotherapy consisting of postural drainage and the active cycle of breathing technique (Chatham et al, 2004). These data support anecdotal evidence that patients with conditions such as bronchiectasis or bronchitis experience loosening of secretions following IMT. Accordingly, patients need to be warned of this and given the appropriate advice regarding clearance techniques.

MONITORING PROGRESS

There are two levels at which progress should be assessed: (1) changes in inspiratory muscle function, and (2) changes in clinical outcomes that result from the former. Monitoring inspiratory muscle function has two purposes: first to ensure that the training regimen is stimulating adaptation within the inspiratory muscles, and secondly to ensure that improvements in function are accommodated by increasing training intensity. Early research on IMT was hampered by the fact that deficiencies in training equipment and methods resulted in little or no change in maximal inspiratory pressure (MIP).

It was therefore no surprise that clinical outcomes also showed no change. The first stage in assessing progress in response to IMT (inspiratory muscle training) is therefore to ensure that the training regimen is stimulating muscle adaptation, by monitoring inspiratory muscle function.

Assessment of respiratory muscle function

A comprehensive description of the assessment of respiratory muscle function is beyond the scope of this book, but for those readers wishing to know more about the topic the joint European Respiratory Society and American Thoracic Society statement on respiratory muscles testing provides comprehensive guidance (ATS/ERS, 2002). For the purposes of gaining a practical understanding of how to assess inspiratory muscle function for monitoring purposes, some basic guidance is provided below.

Maximal respiratory pressures

The most widely used index of IMT-induced changes in inspiratory muscle function is the MIP, which provides a surrogate measure of strength. This chapter provides guidance for IMT, and a description of MIP (Mueller manoeuvre) is therefore essential. However, the measurement of maximal expiratory pressure (MEP; Valsalva manoeuvre) is also given here for the sake of completeness, and because measurement of MEP can provide reassurance regarding the absence of any placebo effects of IMT (MEP generally does not increase after IMT).

Respiratory pressures are measured against an occluded airway (incorporating a 1 mm diameter leak to maintain an open glottis) at prescribed lung volumes (see below). Some spirometry equipment incorporates MIP assessment, but there are also hand-held devices that are more convenient for a clinic setting (MicroRPM®, CareFusion Inc.; POWERbreathe® KH1, POWERbreathe International Ltd). The measurement of MIP (and MEP) is subject to the influence of lung volume (Rahn et al, 1946), motivation and skill acquisition (Volianitis et al, 2001a; Hawkes et al, 2007), as well as the effect of repeated measurement upon the excitability of the motor pathway (Hawkes et al, 2007; Ross et al, 2007). Consequently, it is important to control for these confounding factors as far possible by careful coaching, by habituating patients to the measurement, by making repeated measurements until consistency of MIP is achieved (Box 6.3) and by ensuring consistency of lung volume between measurements. In addition, the use of an inspiratory muscle 'warm-up' (see "Inspiratory muscle 'warm-up' and stretching", below) has been shown to reduce variability, to reduce the number of measurements required to achieve consistency and to remove the effects of changes in motor pathway excitability (Volianitis et al, 2001a; Lomax & McConnell, 2009).

Box 6.3 **Conducting a MIP and MEP test**

1. Ensure that your equipment is calibrated and working properly.
2. Ensure that all equipment that will come in to contact with the participant (e.g., mouthpiece), or that s/he will inhale through, is sterile, and/or protected by a disposable viral filter.
3. Complete any necessary consent documentation.
4. Explain to the participant exactly what you wish them to do before starting the test. During the measurement of MIP and MEP the participant will be unable to generate any air flow against the mouth pressure meter, which contains only a small (1 mm) leak; they must be prepared for this.
5. Measurements can be made seated or standing, but ensure that no clothing restricts the thorax, and that a nose-clip is in place.
6. Because of the length–tension relationship of the respiratory muscles, inspiratory pressures (MIP) are measured at residual volume and expiratory pressures (MEP) at total lung capacity.
7. Ideally, MIP measurements should be preceded by a bout of prior loading ('warm-up') to reduce the effect of repeated measurement (Volianitis et al, 2001a). If suitable equipment is not available for this procedure, up to 18 repeated trials may be necessary to establish reliable data (Volianitis et al, 2001a). However, a pragmatic compromise between rigour and time constraints is to record up to 10 efforts.
8. For MIP assessment, ensure that the participant 'squeezes out slowly' to residual volume.
9. Then instruct them to 'breathe in hard … pull, pull, pull' holding the effort for at least 2 seconds and no more than 3 seconds, and maintaining encouragement throughout. Then instruct the participant to 'relax and come off the mouthpiece' (having a piece of tissue ready for saliva).
10. Take the meter from the participant and record the measured value.
11. Leave the nose-clip in place and allow at least 30 to 60 seconds rest before repeating.
12. If there were deficiencies in the quality of the manoeuvre, e.g., s/he did not sustain the effort for long enough, explain what went wrong and what can be done to improve things on the next attempt.
13. For MEP assessment, ensure that the participant breathes in fully to total lung capacity.
14. Then instruct them to 'breathe out hard … push, push, push', holding the effort for no more than 3 seconds (then as in 10–12 above). During the expiratory effort there is a tendency for air to leak around the lips/mouthpiece. Leaks can be prevented if the participant pinches their lips in place around the mouthpiece by encircling them with the thumb and forefinger.
15. Serial measurements of MIP or MEP should not differ by more than 20% (ATS/ERS, 2002), or 10% for research purposes, and should be repeated until three measurements meet the criterion. At least five measurements should be made.
16. Report the largest of the three technically satisfactory measurements (best of three).
17. If 10 manoeuvres are performed without achieving the 20% criterion, then record the highest value measured and note that it is not a 'best of three'.

Common faults include:
- Incomplete inhalation or exhalation (difference in starting lung volume)
- Not maintaining the effort for long enough
- Air leakage during the MEP effort.

Precautions/contraindications include:
- A history of spontaneous pneumothorax (i.e., not due to traumatic injury)
- A pneumothorax due to a traumatic injury that has not healed fully
- A burst eardrum that has not healed fully, or any other condition of the eardrum
- Stress incontinence (MEP only).

Because maximum respiratory pressures are indices of maximal strength, they are highly effort dependent and require well-motivated participants. Efforts must be sustained for at least 1.5 seconds in order that an average pressure over 1 second can be calculated (by the measuring instrument). This averaging enhances the reliability of the measurement. Because of the length–tension relationship of the respiratory muscles, maximal inspiratory pressure (MIP) is measured at residual volume and maximal expiratory pressure (MEP) at total lung capacity.

Care must also be taken to ensure that any task learning and other effects are expressed fully before measured values are recorded. It has been shown that there is a considerable effect of repeated measurement upon MIP, even in experienced participants; in one study (Volianitis et al, 2001a) after 18 repeated trials the MIP was 11.4% higher than the best of the first three measurements made. This effect is large enough to mask changes in MIP due to the effects of inspiratory muscle fatigue and to make detection of training induced improvements statistically difficult. However, this learning effect can be overcome to a large extent by a bout of submaximal inspiratory loading prior to the assessment of MIP (two sets of 30 breaths against an inspiratory threshold load equivalent to 40% of the best MIP measured during the first three efforts; see the section 'Inspiratory muscle 'warm-up' and stretching', below).

Following this prior loading, the difference between the best of the first three efforts and the 18th measurement was only 3%. Thus the time taken to obtain reliable measurements of MIP can be curtailed considerably by implementing a bout of prior loading (see Box 6.3).

The issue of reference values for MIP and MEP is a contentious one. Earlier, it was argued that a diagnosis of 'weakness' cannot be made on the basis of MIP (or MEP) alone because this takes no account of the demand side of the demand/capacity relationship. In addition, respiratory pressures are surrogates of true force-generating capacity, and subject to the influence of chest wall geometry, which may change. Perhaps most importantly, the correlation of respiratory pressures with anthropometric indices is extremely poor (Enright et al, 1994; McConnell & Copestake, 1999). Nevertheless, as there is a compulsion to define 'weakness' objectively in a clinical setting, some form of reference is required. The largest study to generate reference values for healthy older men and women contained 4443 participants aged 65 years or over (Enright et al, 1994). The resulting reference equations are given below, but it is important to note that the equations account for only between 8% (MIP women) and 18% (MEP women) of the variation in measured values. The 'lower limits of normal' for the sample were defined statistically as the fifth percentile of the group.

Equations

The following equations are from the study by Enright et al (1994) (weight is in pounds, age in years):

Inspiratory
Men: MIP $(cmH_2O) = 153 + (-1.27 \, age) + (0.131 \, weight)$
Women: MIP $(cmH_2O) = 96 + (-0.805 \, age) + (0.133 \, weight)$

Expiratory
Men: MEP $(cmH_2O) = 347 + (-2.95 \, age) + (0.25 \, weight)$
Women: MEP $(cmH_2O) = 219 + (-2.12 \, age) + (0.344 \, weight)$

The lower limits of normal (cmH_2O) are the values to be subtracted from the predicted value to define the lower limit:

Men	Women
MIP = −41	MIP = −32
MEP = −71	MEP = −52

Sniff inspiratory pressure

Because of the difficulties and limitations of measuring maximal respiratory pressures, alternative indices of global inspiratory pressure generating capacity have been sought. The maximal sniff inspiratory pressure was developed originally in an invasive form, in which gastric and oesophageal pressures were measured with balloon-tipped catheters. However, the test was modified and validated as a non-invasive variant in which pressure is measured in the nostril (Heritier et al, 1994); as nostril pressure reflects nasopharyngeal pressure, it is a reasonable approximation of intrathoracic pressure. Because sniffing is a familiar manoeuvre, the test is argued to be easier for participants to execute maximally. However, maximal sniffs still require practice.

Pressure is typically measured via a catheter that is wedged in one nostril, occluding it. The participant then sniffs through the unoccluded nostril from functional residual capacity. Limitations of the technique are that it is affected by the patency of the nasopharynx, and is therefore susceptible to the effects of nasal congestion, as well as being unsuitable for people with major septal defects (Heritier et al, 1994).

Typically, 5–10 maximal sniff efforts are made 'until a consistent value' is obtained (Steier et al, 2007). There are no prediction equations based upon a large cohort of healthy people, but weakness has been defined as a pressure of less than 50 cmH_2O for men and 45 cmH_2O for women (Steier et al, 2007).

Peak inspiratory flow rate

A very simple index of inspiratory muscle function that has been shown to improve in response to moderate intensity IMT is the peak inspiratory flow rate (Romer & McConnell, 2003; Weiner & Weiner, 2006). This can be measured during spirometry, using a mechanical peak inspiratory flow meter (In-Check®, Clement Clarke Ltd.), or an electronic IMT device (POWERbreathe KH1®, POWERbreathe International Ltd). The measurement requires patients to exhale to residual volume and to inhale as quickly as possible. The emphasis is upon speed and not volume during the manoeuvre; likening the effort to a 'maximal gasp' can be helpful for eliciting maximal values. However, it is important to note that the peak flow is achieved at around 50% of vital capacity, so although full lung inflation is not essential it is important that the volume excursion is substantial.

There are no normative values for peak inspiratory flow rate, so its utility is as a measure of change due to factors such as exacerbation, fatigue or training.

Inspiratory muscle endurance

Endurance is 'the ability to sustain a specific muscular task over time' (ATS/ERS, 2002) and is by definition task specific. Although no agreed standards exist for the assessment of inspiratory muscle endurance, the tests fall into two main classes: (1) hyperpnoea tests and (2) inspiratory loaded breathing tests. The latter is subdivided further into (i) the time to the limit of tolerance breathing against a fixed load and (ii) the pressure achieved during an incremental loading task.

A hyperpnoea endurance test is typically designed to identify the maximum sustainable ventilation (MSV), which is expressed as a percentage of the maximum voluntary ventilation (MVV) or, in patients, as a percentage of the predicted MVV (MVV%). In healthy people MSV is 60–80% of MVV. The procedure requires 10–25 minutes, and in obstructed patients should be preceded by a bronchodilator (ATS/ERS, 2002). There is no standardized equipment, but the breathing circuit must have a low inherent flow resistance, maintain isocapnia and provide visual feedback of minute ventilation ($\dot{V}_E$). The test commences with a 12 second MVV, after which one of two methods can be used. In the maximum effort technique, participants are required to sustain 70–90% of their MVV using biofeedback of $\dot{V}_E$. Participants continue to try to maintain this $\dot{V}_E$ for 8 minutes, and the average $\dot{V}_E$ sustained for the final minute is taken as the MSV. The maximum incremental technique is analogous to a $\dot{V}O_{2max}$ test, and continues until the limit of tolerance. Participants are required to increment their $\dot{V}_E$ by 10% every 3 minutes, commencing at 20% of their MVV. The MSV is calculated from the last 10 breaths of the final minute of the highest target $\dot{V}_E$. Reassuringly, the two approaches give very similar values for MSV (Thomas et al, 2010).

There are no normative values for MSV, which varies widely. Its utility is therefore limited to providing a measure of change due to factors such as exacerbation, fatigue or training.

Inspiratory loaded breathing tests are designed to identify either the time to the limit of tolerance (T_{lim}) at a given percentage of MIP or the maximum pressure load that can be achieved during an incremental loading test. Typically, during a fixed-load T_{lim} test, a load is selected that results in task failure within 5 to 10 minutes (Goldstein et al, 1989). The correct load can be identified by a 'trial and error' approach, by using a load that corresponds to around 80% of the load achieved during an incremental test (Hill et al, 2007), or by using a load equivalent to 70% of the MIP (Hart et al, 2002). Another disadvantage of the T_{lim} endurance test is that, after an intervention, the T_{lim} may be extended considerably, leading to extremely long post-intervention tests that are typically terminated at 15 minutes by the experimenter (Hill et al, 2007). Incremental inspiratory loading tests typically commence at 10% of MIP, with increases in load of 10% per minute, until task failure (Hill et al, 2007). Performance in the test is expressed as the highest load tolerated for a minimum of 30 seconds.

The problem with both of these tests is the confounding influence of breathing pattern. Participants with the lowest duty cycle (the ratio of inspiratory time to breath duration) tend to have the longest T_{lim} (Hart et al, 2002). An inevitable consequence of a low duty cycle is a smaller V_T, and a lower amount of inspiratory muscle work (McConnell & Griffiths, 2010). Thus, breathing strategy plays a large role in determining performance in both of these tests of inspiratory muscle endurance. Until a method is developed to control the amount of inspiratory muscle work undertaken during inspiratory endurance tests, their results will continue to be a reflection of both behavioural strategies and physiological function.

Evaluating clinical benefits

The parameters selected as clinically significant outcomes will vary enormously between patient populations, or even between individual patients, e.g., in a mechanically ventilated patient the ability to breathe unassisted, or in a patient with COPD the ability to walk continuously for 6 minutes. The outcomes selected therefore need to be specific to the clinical problem being addressed, but selection must also be tempered with realism regarding the clinical factors that are likely to be sensitive to the effects of IMT. For example, IMT will not improve maximal oxygen uptake ($\dot{V}O_{2max}$) in a patient with heart failure in whom oxygen transport is limited by central factors related to cardiac output. However, the same patient may exhibit an improvement in 6-minute walk distance after IMT, though not because $\dot{V}O_{2max}$ has improved (see Ch. 4).

The starting point for all outcome assessment is confirmation that respiratory muscle function has improved (see above). Thereafter, the approach is highly specific to the patient and the disease. Table 6.1 contains a summary of disease-specific factors that have been shown to be sensitive to the effects of IMT in a range of clinical groups (see Ch. 4 for details). The outcomes listed in the table are limited to controlled studies or meta-analyses, but where this level of evidence is lacking for a specific condition some suggested outcomes have been provided, based upon the rationale presented in Chapter 3. The specific methods and instruments employed to assess these factors are well-established, disease-specific and beyond the scope of this book. The exception to this is the assessment of dyspnoea, which is described in Chapter 7 in the section 'Assessing patient needs' (for functional training of the respiratory muscles).

Notwithstanding the disease specificity of outcomes, there are some generic principles for assessing ambulatory patients with dyspnoea and exercise intolerance. In these patients the literature suggests that in most, irrespective of their disease, IMT has the potential to elicit improvements in inspiratory muscle strength and endurance, dyspnoea, exercise tolerance and quality of life. There are well-established, disease-specific techniques for assessing all of these parameters. A notable absentee from the preceding list of outcomes is lung function, since changes appear to be disease specific. For example, there is no evidence that IMT, or indeed exercise training, increases expiratory flow in patients with COPD (Magadle et al, 2007). However, expiratory flow and vital capacity may improve in patients with asthma (Weiner et al, 1992), as well as those in whom inspiratory muscle weakness creates a restrictive defect (Weiner et al, 1998a).

Table 6.1 Summary of main clinically and statistically significant outcomes (compared with control or placebo) following stand-alone use of IMT for a range of clinical conditions*

Clinical condition	Outcomes improved significantly	Supporting references**
Chronic obstructive pulmonary disease	MIP, IME, ExTol, Dysp$_{EX}$, Dysp$_{DL}$, Dysp$_{LB}$, QoL, UHR	Beckerman et al, 2005; Geddes et al, 2008; Shoemaker et al, 2009; Gosselink et al, 2011
Asthma	MIP, IME, ExTol, Dysp$_{EX}$, Dysp$_{LB}$, MedCon	Weiner et al, 1992; McConnell et al, 1998; Weiner et al, 2000a; Weiner et al, 2000b; Weiner et al, 2002a; Weiner et al, 2002b; Turner et al, 2011
Bronchiectasis	§ MIP, IME, ExTol, Dysp$_{EX}$, Dysp$_{DL}$, Dysp$_{LB}$, QoL, UHR, AC	
Chronic heart failure	MIP, IME, ExTol, Dysp$_{EX}$, Dysp$_{DL}$, QoL	Cahalin et al, 1997; Johnson et al, 1998; Weiner et al, 1999; Martinez et al, 2001; Laoutaris et al, 2004; Dall'Ago et al, 2006; Padula et al, 2009; Bosnak-Guclu et al, 2011; Lin et al, 2012; Plentz et al, 2012
Neuromuscular disease	MIP, IME, LF, Dysp$_{EX}$, Dysp$_{DL}$, QoL	Weiner et al, 1998a; Winkler et al, 2000; Koessler et al, 2001; Topin et al, 2002; Fregonezi et al, 2005; Inzelberg et al, 2005; Fry et al, 2007; Sutbeyaz et al, 2010; Hull et al, 2012
Obesity	§ MIP, ExTol	Edwards et al, 2012
Ageing	MIP, ExTol, Dysp$_{EX}$, PA	Copestake & McConnell, 1995; Aznar-Lain et al, 2007
Cystic fibrosis	MIP, IME, LF, ExTol, AC	Sawyer & Clanton, 1993; de Jong et al, 2001; Chatham et al, 2004; Enright et al, 2004
Restrictive chest wall disorders	§ MIP, IME, LF, ExTol, Dysp$_{EX}$, Dysp$_{DL}$, Dysp$_{LB}$, QoL	
Sarcoidosis and interstitial lung disease	§ MIP, IME, LF, ExTol, Dysp$_{EX}$, Dysp$_{DL}$, Dysp$_{LB}$, QoL	
Diabetes	MIP, IME	Correa et al, 2011
Renal failure	MIP, IME, ExTol	Weiner et al, 1996
Cancer	§ MIP, IME, ExTol, Dysp$_{EX}$, Dysp$_{DL}$, QoL	
Anorexia nervosa	§ MIP, IME, LF, ExTol, Dysp$_{EX}$, Dysp$_{DL}$, QoL	
Myopathy (iatrogenic)	MIP, IME, LF (reductions offset by IMT)	Weiner et al, 1995
Surgery	MIP, LF, ExTol, PPC	Weiner et al, 1998b; Hulzebos et al, 2006a; Hulzebos et al, 2006b; Dronkers et al, 2008; Casali et al, 2011; Savci et al, 2011; Hulzebos et al, 2012
Mechanical ventilation	MIP, WS^, S^	Moodie et al, 2011; Cader et al, 2012
Spinal cord injury	MIP, LF^	Van Houtte et al, 2006; West et al, 2009
Pregnancy	§ MIP, IME, ExTol, Dysp$_{EX}$	
Obstructive sleep apnoea	§ MIP, IME, AHI, QoL	
Vocal cord dysfunction	§ MIP, IME, ExTol, Dysp$_{EX}$	

* Where this level of evidence is lacking for a specific condition, some suggested outcomes have been provided, based upon the rationale presented in Chapter 3.
** See Chapter 4 for details.
AC = airway clearance; AHI = apnoea–hypopnoea index; Dysp$_{EX}$ = exertional dyspnoea; Dysp$_{DL}$ = dyspnoea during activities of daily living; Dysp$_{LB}$ = dyspnoea during loaded breathing; ExTol = exercise tolerance; IME = inspiratory muscle endurance; LF = lung function; MedCon = medication consumption; MIP = maximal inspiratory pressure; PA = physical activity; PPC = post-operative pulmonary complications; QoL = quality of life; S = survival; UHR = use of healthcare resources; WS = weaning success; § = statistically significant evidence is lacking, but there is a physiological rationale supporting a beneficial effect of IMT (see Ch. 3); ^ = trend favouring IMT.

GETTING STARTED

This section provides guidance on the practicalities of initiating a programme of IMT (inspiratory muscle training), and describes the Foundation phase of the training process. A summary of the most important guidance from this section can be found in Table 6.2. In addition, Box 6.4 summarizes the key aspects of Foundation IMT.

Protocol selection

Much of the variation between study outcomes can be ascribed to variations in training protocols. For example, one study might report that IMT improves maximal inspiratory pressure (MIP), whereas another reports that MIP remains unchanged, and that inspiratory muscle endurance improves. In the case of the former, the protocol

---

Box 6.4 **Foundation IMT essentials**

- Use a training load of 50–60% of MIP, or set intensity to the 30-repetition maximum (30RM) using a process of trial and error.
- Use stretching and warm-up to prepare for IMT.
- Inhale against the load with maximum effort (as fast as possible).
- Breathe in AND out as far as possible during each breath.
- Train twice per day – morning and evening (not less than 6 hours apart).
- Remember that repetition failure of the inspiratory muscles is an 'inability to achieve a satisfying breath'.
- Increase the training load at least once per week.
- Progress the training by: (1) maintaining it at 50–60% of the new MIP, or (2) keeping the load at the new 30RM to account for improvement.
- Train to 'failure' in a window between 25 and 35 breaths per session.
- Keep in mind that time of day, other activities and health status may affect IMT because of residual fatigue. Accordingly, evening IMT sessions may be more challenging than morning sessions – but don't reduce the training load.
- If you suspect that there is any residual fatigue of the inspiratory muscles, take a day off from IMT.
- Keep an IMT diary.

Table 6.2 Training recommendations summary

Protocol characteristic	Recommendation
Inspiratory load	• At least 30% of maximal inspiratory pressure (MIP) • Typically, 50% to 60% of MIP, or the maximum load that can be sustained for 30 breaths
Repetitions	• 30 breaths, ideally continuous (Foundation IMT) • Short breaks permitted but should be minimized
Frequency	• Daily, one or two times per day (morning and evening)
Duration	• 12 weeks
Load increments	• At least weekly, to maintain required percentage of new MIP, or to maintain 30 breaths to 'failure' (30RM) • Increments can be more frequent using the 30RM principle
Maintenance training	• Can be initiated after 12 weeks of IMT • Reduce frequency to once every other day
Functional training	• Can be initiated after 6 weeks of Foundation IMT • Undertaken at least 3 days per week • Always in tandem with Foundation IMT, which should be undertaken at least 3 days per week

---

might consist of 30 repetitions against a load equivalent to 60% of MIP, whereas the latter might consist of 15 minutes' continuous breathing against a load of 30%. The *specificity* principle of training dictates that you get what you ask for when it comes to training outcomes. The decision regarding the appropriateness of a given protocol for a specific disease condition, or individual patient, is ultimately a pragmatic professional judgement.

Notwithstanding this, there are some considerations that are worthwhile highlighting, as these may facilitate the process of identifying the most appropriate protocol (see also Chs 3, 4 and 5):

- Most patients lack inspiratory muscle strength, and their apparent lack of endurance is secondary to a lack of strength
- Demand/capacity imbalance within the respiratory pump is rebalanced most effectively by increasing the strength and power of the pump
- Strength-biased training protocols generate the widest range of improvements in inspiratory muscle functional properties (strength, shortening velocity, power and endurance)
- Dyspnoea and sense of breathing effort typically improve only if MIP improves, which requires a strength-biased training protocol

- Strength-biased training protocols are more time efficient and may enhance compliance
- Strength-biased training protocols have been shown to produce the widest range of physiological and functional changes in healthy young people.

On the basis of the points summarized above, a protocol that is biased towards improving strength appears to address the widest range of deficits and to elicit the widest range of functional improvements. In practice, this typically means a load that is equivalent to 50–60% of the current MIP, continued to the limit of tolerance (typically 30 continuous breaths).

As well as the load setting, a training protocol needs to define the training frequency. Typically, studies in both patients and healthy individuals have employed a twice-daily regimen for 5–7 days per week.

Setting the training load

The general principles of training overload were described in Chapter 5, which also included a summary of the evidence relating to different types of training and training regimens. The following guidance is based upon these insights.

For people who are already feeling out of breath, the most challenging aspect of embarking on a programme of IMT is learning to tolerate the increased breathing effort that is inevitably associated with the training. This phase needs to be handled with particular sensitivity. A vital step in overcoming the anxiety that breathing through a resistance can provoke is the realization that the increased effort stops as soon as the training stops. So unlike the dyspnoea that one experiences during, say, climbing a flight of stairs, which can takes minutes to subside, the breathing effort of IMT ceases immediately the training device is removed. In addition, the sense of dyspnoea during IMT has a subtly different quality to that experienced during physical activity: the former is a sense of increased effort, whereas the latter also incorporates a sense of 'air hunger' that is akin to suffocation – hence the anxiety that it provokes. Practising breathing through the training device in order to become familiar with the sensation, and its qualities, is a vital part of preparing a patient for IMT.

The next phase is to identify and set an appropriate training load. The approach taken will depend upon whether there is access to equipment for assessing inspiratory muscle strength (maximal inspiratory pressure: MIP). If this is not available then the 'repetition maximum' (RM) principle is used to set the training load. Typically, a moderate load (50–60% of MIP) can be sustained for around 30 or so breaths. Accordingly, the objective is to identify the 30RM and to train at the maximum load that can be sustained for only 30 breaths (this is detailed below). Patients, who are by definition unwell, may find even the lowest setting of the training device very challenging and be unable to complete 30 breaths without stopping. If this is the case, the load should remain at the lowest setting for the first week. Short breaks are allowable (and necessary for patients who need to cough) but should be minimized, as otherwise the training stimulus will be diminished or even lost completely.

Initially, the focus should be on inhaling deeply and forcefully, and exhaling slowly and gently. The objective in the first instance is to develop good breathing technique (see above) and to complete 30 breaths without the need to stop and rest. As soon as 30 breaths can be achieved without stopping, it is time to increase the training load by a quarter turn of the load tensioner (2–3 cmH$_2$O on a typical pressure threshold training device) (see Ch. 5, Fig. 5.1). Note that it may require a number of weeks for some severely compromised patients to achieve this (see the section 'Progressing training', below).

Some patients may find that they can complete more than 30 breaths easily at the lowest setting on day 1. If this is the case, the load should be increased by one-quarter turn each day until a load is reached where 30 breaths is that maximum that can be achieved continuously. Once this load is reached, further increases in the training load should be made according to the guidance on progressing training.

Where there is access to equipment for measuring MIP, the training load can be set using objective criteria. The training should commence at a load equivalent to 30–40% of MIP provided that this is tolerable; this is the lowest intensity that has been shown to elicit improvements in function (Lotters et al, 2002). If this load is not tolerated then commence training as described above until 30 breaths can be completed at the lowest setting. Most training devices do not have a calibrated scale printed on them, but many will provide a conversion chart that enables the level settings printed on the device to be cross-referenced to the corresponding load in cmH$_2$O. Once the starting load of 30–40% can be tolerated, the load should be increased by one-quarter turn each day for the next 7–10 days until up to 50–60% of baseline MIP is reached (see 'Progressing training').

Many patients experience life-changing results very quickly (see 'Case study', below), and this can prompt such enthusiasm that they to want to train more than twice per day. This is definitely inadvisable. Recovery is an important part of the training process, and the inspiratory muscles are already being subjected to a very challenging regimen of twice-daily specific IMT. Patients should therefore be discouraged from training more than twice daily, and they should ensure that the two sessions are separated by at least 6 hours.

In Chapter 7, guidance about the loads to be used during functional training exercises will be divided into 'light' and 'moderate'. These correspond to the following 'repetition maximum' and MIP percentage settings:

- *Light:* equivalent to the 50–100-repetition maximum (20–40% of MIP)
- *Moderate:* equivalent to the 20–40-repetition maximum (50–60% of MIP).

Repetition failure

Repetition failure is a slightly alien concept to people who have never engaged in any form of weight training. Essentially, it refers to the notion that, at some point during repeated lifting of a weight, fatigue will make it impossible to lift the weight, resulting in 'failure'. Most weight training is undertaken to the point of failure, because this optimizes the loading conditions that stimulate muscle adaptation (Toigo & Boutellier, 2006). For most muscles, the weakest point in the movement is at, or close to, the starting point. For example, when performing a bicep curl, the biceps are weakest at the onset of the exercise (when the elbow is extended), which means that failure usually occurs at the start of the movement with the result that the repetition cannot be started. In the case of the inspiratory muscles, the opposite is true: they are strongest at the start of the movement (at residual volume), becoming weaker as one inhales (see Fig. 6.2). This means it may be possible to open the valve, but not possible to take a meaningful breath. So how should failure defined for IMT? A pragmatic approach is to tell the patients that once it is impossible to achieve a 'satisfying breath' then failure has been reached and the session is complete. Some patients may require some encouragement in order to push themselves to this point, but it is the best way to achieve the results they are working towards. Notwithstanding this, it is not disastrous if patients train only until they have completed 30 breaths, provided that the training load is at least 60% of their current MIP and the breathing technique described above is followed (maximizing inspiratory flow and volume).

The influence of daily activities and exacerbations

Acute deteriorations in a patient's clinical condition, as well as other strenuous activities during the day, can affect the ease with which a training session can be completed. It is important that patients understand that there may be temporary setbacks. Some will be short lived (e.g., overdoing it physically on a particular day), but some will take some time to overcome (e.g., an exacerbation of COPD or asthma). In the former case it is not usually necessary to reduce training loads, which should be avoided as much for the impact psychologically as physiologically. In the latter case, however, cessation of IMT is often required during an exacerbation, which means that some training gains are lost and the load must be reduced when training is recommenced. How soon should training recommence after an exacerbation? This is normally dictated by patients' ability and enthusiasm for the training, but IMT should be recommenced as soon as possible, and certainly as soon as they are well enough to recommence the normal (for them) activities of daily living.

Use of training diaries

Keeping a training diary is an excellent way to keep track of the number of sessions completed, the increments in training load, the number of breaths completed and how the session felt. This is an invaluable tool for both patient (e.g., enhancing motivation) and healthcare professional (e.g., monitoring compliance and progress). Some training devices provide a training diary in their user manuals (e.g., POWERbreathe® Medic).

Figure 6.3 provides a template for a training diary that can be reproduced. As well as training load etc., the template provides space for notes on how the training felt and other activities or health-related issues that may impact upon the training, as well as the patient's response to it. This facilitates cross-referencing of circumstances that may be helpful for the patient and healthcare professional in interpreting sudden up- or down-turns in training and/or symptoms.

PROGRESSING TRAINING

Patients should be encouraged to train beyond 30 breaths if they feel able to and can still achieve a 'satisfying breath' (see the section 'Repetition failure', above). In this way, they maximize progress. Once 30 continuous breaths can be completed then further increases in the training load should be made once per week, or as soon as 30 breaths can be exceeded. The increase in load should be sufficient to reduce the number of breaths that can be achieved before failure to between 25 and 30. On most training devices this will be about one-quarter to one-half turn on the spring tensioner. Bringing the number of breaths down to 25 is acceptable because within a few days the maximum number of breaths will be back up to 30. As a rough rule of thumb, the training load should be increased by at least one-quarter turn each week for the first 8 to 12 weeks of training. Alternatively, small increases can be made as soon as the maximum number of breaths exceeds 33 to 35. If patients find that increasing the training load is too challenging then they should be encouraged to focus on optimizing their breathing technique during the training, i.e., maximizing inspiratory flow rate and tidal volume (V_T). These measures can also increase the training stimulus, by increasing the power output achieved during the inhalation (maximizing flow) and the work done (maximizing volume).

If the patient is undertaking the training with the support of a clinician with access to equipment to measure maximum inspiratory pressure (MIP), the load should be increased weekly to maintain the training load at 50–60% of the patient's new MIP.

The duration of the intensive, twice-daily Foundation phase of training varies according to the circumstances in which the IMT is being undertaken, and the objectives.

Week number	Monday		Tuesday		Wednesday		Thursday		Friday		Saturday		Sunday	
	Level	Breaths	Level	Breaths	Level	Breaths	Level	Breaths	Level	Breaths	Level	Breaths	Level	Breaths
Morning														
Evening														

Notes	How did you feel, and did you complete all breaths without stopping?
Monday	
Tuesday	
Wednesday	
Thursday	
Friday	
Saturday	
Sunday	

Please use the following codes to record notes on training

A Trained as expected

B Less than expected (please indicate number of breaths)

C Did not train (forgot)

D Did not train (too busy)

E Did not train (too difficult)

F Did not train (lack of motivation)

G Did not train (too unwell)

H Did not train (too tired)

I Did not train (other reason, please specify)

J Increased training load

K Had to stop during the 30 breaths (please indicate how many and why)

Figure 6.3 Suggested template for a training diary.
(Adapted from McConnell AK, 2011. Breathe strong, perform better. Human Kinetics, Champaign, IL, with permission.)

The first major consideration is whether the Foundation IMT is being undertaken as a stand-alone intervention or as part of a structured rehabilitation programme (see the section 'Rehabilitation component', below). Long-term studies of stand-alone IMT in patients with COPD suggest that improvements in function occur most rapidly over the first 12 weeks, but continue for up to 12 months (Beckerman et al, 2005). These data suggest that the duration of the Foundation phase of IMT should be at least 12 weeks.

Selection of the next phase of training depends upon a number of factors, including patient motivation, but there are essentially four options:

1. Continue Foundation training for as long as the patient is motivated to do so. For some patients, changing a routine may create problems with respect to compliance. Alternatively, they may need more than 12 weeks before they feel ready to change.

2. Enter the Maintenance training phase (see next section). Some patients may find the twice-daily Foundation routine onerous, in which case moving to a Maintenance training regimen may retain their compliance.

3. Enter the Functional training phase, which incorporates activities of daily living (see Ch. 7). Motivated patients who have experienced good results during the Foundation phase may feel motivated to develop their training and to incorporate some functional elements in to their daily regimen.

4. Enter a rehabilitation programme, in which IMT is a component. Having undertaken a period of IMT, patients who were previously unable to benefit from exercise training may have recovered sufficient function to be able to enrol in a rehabilitation programme. In these patients, IMT can be continued in whatever form is most appropriate for the programme and the patient (Foundation, Maintenance or Functional). See also the section 'Incorporating RMT into a rehabilitation programme'.

If the benefits of IMT are to be retained, the intervention must be continued according to one of the options listed above. In circumstances where patients cease IMT completely at the end of the Foundation phase, it is possible to recover the benefits using periodic phases of Foundation IMT. IMT should ideally resume before all of the benefits have regressed, as it is easier to recover post-training gains when starting from an elevated baseline. Data suggest that complete regression of gains in MIP occurs over a period of around 12 months (Weiner et al, 2004). However, it appears that around half of the strength gained is retained for up to 12 weeks. This magnitude of improvement is probably at the threshold of what is required in order to elicit enhancement of exercise tolerance and reduction in dyspnoea. Accordingly, 12 weeks probably represents the maximum period that should be permitted before recommencing IMT. It is also possible, though not proven experimentally, that the duration of the IMT during these periodic bouts of training can be shorter. Thus a design for a periodic training regimen might be 12 weeks of Foundation IMT, followed by repeated cycles of 12 weeks of detraining and 6 weeks of Foundation IMT.

Whether Foundation IMT is being used as a stand-alone intervention or as part of a rehabilitation programme, its duration should ideally be 12 weeks as this represents the period during which the largest improvements in function are gained. However, this does not mean that briefer periods of Foundation training are worthless – far from it.

The duration of many pulmonary rehabilitation programmes is typically 6–12 weeks; thus, there may be logistical issues relating to the duration of the Foundation phase and its relationship to the rehabilitation programme. In an ideal scenario where the Foundation phase has a 12-week duration, this can be dovetailed with the rehabilitation programme in a number of ways (see section 'Incorporating RMT into a structured rehabilitation programme', below).

MAINTENANCE TRAINING

Once the Foundation phase of training has been completed, some patients are perfectly satisfied with the results that they have achieved and are content to enter a phase of Maintenance training. Research has shown that training frequency can be reduced by as much as two-thirds without any loss of functional benefits (Weiner et al, 2004). In other words, training can switch from twice daily to training once every other day. There is, of course, no reason at all that someone cannot switch directly from Maintenance training to Functional training if they so wish.

INCORPORATING RMT INTO A STRUCTURED REHABILITATION PROGRAMME

The strategy used to incorporate IMT into a rehabilitation programme depends upon a range of largely logistical issues including the duration of the rehabilitation programme, whether patients wait for a period of a few weeks before commencing rehabilitation, and the state of readiness of the patient for whole-body exercise. In the last case,

it may be appropriate to consider commencing Foundation IMT during the period that precedes rehabilitation, as a form of Pre-habilitation.

Pre-habilitation

A study on athletes showed that implementing IMT prior to whole-body training improved the outcome of the whole-body training (Tong et al, 2010); thus, it is reasonable to suggest that Foundation IMT might be considered as 'pre-habilitation' for patients awaiting commencement of exercise training. The improvements in dyspnoea and exercise tolerance that accompany IMT should ease the transition of patients into a programme of whole-body physical activity that most patients will find unfamiliar and challenging. By undertaking IMT before commencing a programme, patients should be able to tolerate higher intensities of exercise (as was the case for the athletes studied by Tong et al, 2010), as well as finding exercise less uncomfortable.

Studies on healthy young people suggest that significant improvements in exercise tolerance are measurable after 4–6 weeks of Foundation IMT. Ideally then, any pre-habilitation phase of IMT should be 4–6 weeks in duration, but any duration is likely to be better than none at all. Furthermore, commencing IMT during the period leading up to the rehabilitation programme is also likely to have a number of psychological benefits, e.g., a sense of making progress, a sense of readiness, a sense of empowerment, and building good habits of self-discipline.

In practice, limited resources may dictate that patients are required to manage this phase of IMT largely autonomously. However, following an initial assessment, some coaching regarding breathing technique, load setting and progression, most patients should be capable of undertaking domiciliary IMT. Indeed, this is generally the model employed in research studies of IMT. Notwithstanding this, where resources permit, weekly reviews of progress including a check of MIP and an increment of the training load (where patients have not increased the load themselves) is desirable (Padula et al, 2009).

Rehabilitation component

Inspiratory muscle training can be incorporated very readily into a structured rehabilitation programme. However, the method of achieving synergy between IMT and exercise training will most likely be a pragmatic combination of what is physiologically desirable and the constraints imposed by local logistics. Table 6.3 represents a suggestion of the ideal synergy between IMT and exercise training.

The precise form in which the IMT is incorporated into any given rehabilitation session will also be dictated by local factors. For example, where patients exercise in a group environment using a circuit-based approach, IMT can form one station of the circuit. The exercise performed

Table 6.3 Suggested incorporation of IMT into a rehabilitation programme*

Phase	Weeks	IMT type	Frequency per week
Pre-habilitation	−6–0	Foundation	14 (twice daily)
Rehabilitation	1–6	Foundation	14 (twice daily)
Rehabilitation	7–12	Foundation	10 (twice daily)
Rehabilitation	7–12	Functional	2
Post-rehabilitation	13 onwards	Foundation	4 (twice daily)
Post-rehabilitation	13 onwards	Functional	2

*Assumptions: Patients are enrolled in a 12-week rehabilitation programme, and undergo a pre-enrolment assessment 6 weeks before commencement of a 2 days per week outpatient rehabilitation programme. Immediately after the pre-assessment visit, patients embark upon a pre-habilitation period of Foundation IMT, which is monitored weekly.

at this station can either be a full 30-breath Foundation IMT workout, a proportion of the 30-breath workout (if performed more than once) or one of the Functional IMT exercises described in Chapter 7. Alternatively, a Foundation IMT workout can be undertaken at the start or end of the rehabilitation session (as part of a warm-up or cool-down) or immediately after a bout of aerobic training; the latter has the benefit of providing a degree of specificity, as the inspiratory muscles may already be slightly fatigued by the preceding exercise, which means that they will receive the greatest relative training overload during IMT.

INSPIRATORY MUSCLE 'WARM-UP' AND STRETCHING

'Warm-up'

The concept of 'warm-up' is well established in sport and exercise, and the use of a specific inspiratory muscle 'warm-up' has been shown to enhance performance and reduce breathing effort in healthy young people (Volianitis et al, 2001b). Despite the terminology, these effects are unlikely to be temperature-dependent, and are probably due to neural and blood flow effects. There is every reason to anticipate that patients can experience the same benefits of inspiratory 'warm-up' prior to physical activity as healthy young athletes, i.e., a reduced intensity of dyspnoea during subsequent activities. Accordingly,

the use of a 'warm-up' is recommended prior to any physical activity, but especially those exercises precipitating sudden, large increases in breathing requirement.

To execute the 'warm-up' effectively, it is necessary to find the appropriate loading intensity. This must be sufficiently intense to stimulate the response, but not so intense that it induces fatigue. Research has shown that the correct intensity is around 40% of maximal inspiratory pressure (MIP) (Volianitis et al, 1999). If the patient's MIP is not known, it is possible to set the load based on the 30-repetition maximum load setting and the characteristics of the spring that loads the valve in the training device; assuming that the training load is 50% to 60% (for a 30-breath regimen), the load setting that corresponds to 40% can be estimated. Table 6.4 is a chart that can be used to look up the correct 'warm-up' setting based on the training setting. Once the correct load has been identified, two sets of 30 breaths with 1 minute of rest in between should be completed no more than 10 minutes before a training session.

It is also desirable, but not essential, to undertake the 'warm-up' immediately before IMT. This is because MIP (and presumably blood flow) is enhanced, and it is therefore possible to sustain higher training loads if the IMT session is preceded by an inspiratory muscle 'warm-up'. Of course, if the IMT is undertaken immediately after exercise training then an inspiratory muscle 'warm-up' is redundant because the muscles are already warmed up.

It is worth noting that the influences of IMT and 'warm-up' appear to be additive (Lomax et al, 2011).

Table 6.4 'Warm-up' load settings, based upon the 30-repetition maximum training load

Current training load (level)	Ideal 'warm-up' load (level)
10	8
9	7
8	6.5
7	5.5
6	5
5	4
4	3
3	2.5
2	1.5
1	1
0	0

Note: This method assumes that the training device has 10 load settings and that the training load is the 30-repetition maximum.

Stretching

The trunk and rib cage receive almost no attention when it comes to stretching; however, these areas include numerous muscles, their attachments and associated connective tissue (e.g., the rib cage) that can potentially be a site of great resistance to inhalation. Any resistance to thoracic expansion increases the work of breathing and the associated perception of breathing effort. At least one study has shown that a 4-week programme of thoracic stretching exercises resulted in significant improvements in chest wall expansion (circumferences at three levels) and functional residual capacity (Minoguchi et al, 2002); a number of stretching and mobilization exercises based upon this programme are described in Chapter 7.

INSPIRATORY MUSCLE 'COOL-DOWN'

Just as the warm-up is well established in conditioning science, so too is the notion of an active 'cool-down' or active recovery. The primary objective of an active 'cool-down' is to clear metabolites from the muscles, particularly lactate. Essentially, when muscles work at a low to moderate intensity, the rate at which they consume lactate (for use as a fuel) exceeds the rate at which they produce it, making them net consumers. Therefore, rather than resting when a workout is complete, athletes perform an active 'cool-down' because this is the fastest and most efficient way to clear lactate.

At the end of an exercise training session, clearing metabolites may help with the process of recovery and adaptation. During training that requires repeated high-intensity

efforts, active recovery between efforts hastens lactate clearance and may therefore improve training quality by promoting the ability to tolerate higher-intensity or longer bouts of exercise. There is every reason to believe that patients who exercise above that lactate threshold can derive similar benefits from an active recovery, but the activity need not be confined to the limb muscles.

As we learned in Chapter 1, the inspiratory muscles are highly aerobic, with a large blood supply, making them ideal candidates for lactate consumption during recovery. Recent research suggests that breathing against a small inspiratory load (the lowest setting on most devices) immediately after exercise accelerates the clearance of lactate (Chiappa et al, 2008), though this is not a universal finding (Johnson et al, 2011). A whole-body active recovery takes around 5 minutes to speed up lactate clearance. In contrast, under conditions where inspiratory loading accelerates lactate clearance, it does so immediately exercise stops, and may also clear the lactate much more quickly (Chiappa et al, 2008). More importantly, when inspiratory loading is undertaken between two bouts of maximal cycling (a Wingate test), performance in the second cycle test has been shown to improve compared with when a passive recovery between the two cycle tests (Chiappa et al, 2009). Finally, research has also shown that trained inspiratory muscles are more effective consumers of lactate during both recovery and exercise (Brown et al, 2008, 2010).

Thus low-intensity inspiratory loading, especially of trained inspiratory muscles, may help to speed lactate clearance, thereby enhancing tolerance to subsequent exercise. In practical terms, the ideal load setting for 'cool-down' is equivalent to the lowest setting on most training devices (10–15 cmH$_2$O).

 Case study

Henry is a relatively active man of 67 with severe chronic obstructive pulmonary disease (COPD). During his youth he had enjoyed a wide range of activities, including competitive football, and more latterly hill walking. A moderately heavy smoker since his late teens (24 pack years), Henry was diagnosed with COPD at the age of 54. A history revealed that he had quit smoking in his early 40s in response to health education advertising, as well as the development of symptoms of exertional dyspnoea and a series of chest infections. His symptoms had continued to worsen over the next 10 years and he was finally diagnosed with COPD following spirometry in primary care. Pharmacotherapy was complex, consisting of two antibiotics, an anti-cholinergic, a β$_2$-agonist and corticosteroid.

A major contributory factor to Henry's disability was his susceptibility to chest infections, which resulted in at least

three exacerbations per year and an almost continuous underlying infection. Following a particularly severe bout of pneumonia at the age of 56 that resulted in a 4-week hospital stay, Henry reached an all-time low in both his mental state and his physical capacity. He was depressed, anxious and chronically fatigued. Henry also felt helpless and was unable to take part in even the most basic of activities; his wife helped him to dress and wash, and he was confined to the ground floor of their home. In short he felt that his 'life was over' and that he was now just in a 'downward spiral waiting to die'.

At discharge, Henry's chest physician felt that he had reached the end of the line in terms of pharmacotherapy options, but referred him to a specialist respiratory physiotherapist for breathing retraining. In particular, there was a need to regain some respiratory function so that Henry

Continued

Case study—cont'd

could recommence use of his dry-power inhaler (DPI) as he disliked using a nebulizer and was unable to coordinate a metered-dose inhaler.

The physiotherapist began outpatient treatment with some basic breathing retraining exercises and inhaler technique coaching. After the first two sessions Henry's inspiratory muscle strength was assessed and found to be very low (48 cmH$_2$O), he was shown how to use a pressure threshold inspiratory muscle trainer, and the physiotherapist explained that daily training would reduce his dyspnoea and should enable him to start using his favoured DPI. Initially, the training device was set to the lowest load and Henry was asked to undertake 30 breaths twice daily at home. He returned to see the physiotherapist after 1 week and reported that he was finding the training a challenge, but that he already felt that he could cope with an increase in the training load as 30 continuous breaths felt manageable, and he was keen to progress. On this visit, the load was set to 50% of Henry's inspiratory mouth pressure. Henry also received some further breathing retraining exercises and inhaler technique practice. On his visit 1 week later, Henry reported that the new [50%] setting had made 30 breaths impossible in one set, but that by the end of the week he had completed 30 breaths continuously for the first time. Henry's frame of mind appeared much improved and he reported he felt he was finally doing something that 'put him the driving seat'. Henry's next appointment was 1 month later, and in the intervening period he was instructed to increase the training load by small amounts every time he exceeded 30 breaths in two successive training sessions.

At his 6-week appointment Henry was visibly more vigorous and cheerful. His inspiratory muscle strength had increased by 48% and his peak inspiratory flow rate was now sufficient for him to use his favoured DPI. He reported that he was now able to wash and dress himself, that he was also able to use the upper floor of his home, and that he had taken his first recreational walk in a nearby park with his grandchildren. Henry's training load was now 65% of his inspiratory muscle strength, and he was keen to continue the training on a daily basis. Six weeks later, Henry returned for his fourth appointment (12 weeks after commencing IMT), walking freely and without the frequent bouts of dyspnoea and coughing that had punctuated his gait previously. He reported that for the first time in more then 10 years he felt he was free from a chest infection and had virtually no cough; spirometry revealed his FEV$_1$ (forced expiratory volume in 1 second) had increased from 24% of predicted at baseline to 38%, and his inspiratory muscle strength had improved by a further 27% (to 84 cmH$_2$O). He also reported that, since his previous appointment, he was sleeping better, was able to walk on an incline and had taken a series of short walks with his grown-up son on the moorland near his home. He was overjoyed with the improvements, which at discharge he had thought were impossible. At this, his final outpatient appointment, Henry was advised to move to maintenance IMT (training every other day) and given the 'all clear' to join an exercise class for the over-60s at his local leisure centre. Henry was also provided with a programme of 10 Functional IMT exercises to do at home, and scheduled for 6 monthly appointments.

REFERENCES

Aagaard, P., Simonsen, E.B., Andersen, J.L., et al., 2000. Neural inhibition during maximal eccentric and concentric quadriceps contraction: effects of resistance training. J. Appl. Physiol. 89, 2249–2257.

ATS/ERS, 2002. ATS/ERS Statement on respiratory muscle testing. Am. J. Respir. Crit. Care Med. 166, 518–624.

Aznar-Lain, S., Webster, A.L., Canete, S., et al., 2007. Effects of inspiratory muscle training on exercise capacity and spontaneous physical activity in elderly subjects: a randomized controlled pilot trial. Int. J. Sports Med. 28, 1025–1029.

Beckerman, M., Magadle, R., Weiner, M., et al., 2005. The effects of 1 year of specific inspiratory muscle training in patients with COPD. Chest 128, 3177–3182.

Black, L.F., Hyatt, R.E., 1969. Maximal respiratory pressures: normal values and relationship to age and sex. Am. Rev. Respir. Dis. 99, 696–702.

Bosnak-Guclu, M., Arikan, H., Savci, S., et al., 2011. Effects of inspiratory muscle training in patients with heart failure. Respir. Med. 105, 1671–1681.

Brown, P.I., Sharpe, G.R., Johnson, M.A., 2008. Inspiratory muscle training reduces blood lactate concentration during volitional hyperpnoea. Eur. J. Appl. Physiol. 104, 111–117.

Brown, P.I., Sharpe, G.R., Johnson, M.A., 2010. Loading of trained inspiratory muscles speeds lactate recovery kinetics. Med. Sci. Sports Exerc. 42, 1103–1112.

Cader, S.A., de Souza Vale, R.G., Zamora, V.E., et al., 2012. Extubation process in bed-ridden elderly

intensive care patients receiving inspiratory muscle training: a randomized clinical trial. Clinical Interventions in Aging 7, 437–443.

Cahalin, L.P., Semigran, M.J., Dec, G.W., 1997. Inspiratory muscle training in patients with chronic heart failure awaiting cardiac transplantation: results of a pilot clinical trial. Phys. Ther. 77, 830–838.

Casali, C.C., Pereira, A.P., Martinez, J.A., et al., 2011. Effects of inspiratory muscle training on muscular and pulmonary function after bariatric surgery in obese patients. Obes. Surg. 21, 1389–1394.

Cavalheri, V., Camillo, C.A., Brunetto, A.F., et al., 2010. Effects of arm bracing posture on respiratory muscle strength and pulmonary function in patients with chronic obstructive pulmonary disease. Rev. Port. Pneumol. 16, 887–891.

Chatham, K., Ionescu, A.A., Nixon, L.S., et al., 2004. A short-term comparison of two methods of sputum expectoration in cystic fibrosis. Eur. Respir. J. 23, 435–439.

Chiappa, G.R., Roseguini, B.T., Alves, C.N., et al., 2008. Blood lactate during recovery from intense exercise: impact of inspiratory loading. Med. Sci. Sports Exerc. 40, 111–116.

Chiappa, G.R., Ribeiro, J.P., Alves, C.N., et al., 2009. Inspiratory resistive loading after all-out exercise improves subsequent performance. Eur. J. Appl. Physiol. 106, 297–303.

Copestake, A.J., McConnell, A.K., 1995. Inspiratory muscle training reduces exertional breathlessness in healthy elderly men and women. In: International Conference on Physical Activity and Health in the Elderly. University of Sterling, Scotland, p. 150.

Correa, A.P., Ribeiro, J.P., Balzan, F.M., et al., 2011. Inspiratory muscle training in type 2 diabetes with inspiratory muscle weakness. Med. Sci. Sports Exerc. 43, 1135–1141.

Dall'Ago, P., Chiappa, G.R., Guths, H., et al., 2006. Inspiratory muscle training in patients with heart failure and inspiratory muscle weakness: a randomized trial. J. Am. Coll. Cardiol. 47, 757–763.

de Jong, W., van Aalderen, W.M., Kraan, J., et al., 2001. Inspiratory muscle training in patients with cystic fibrosis. Respir. Med. 95, 31–36.

Demoule, A., Verin, E., Montcel, S.T., et al., 2008. Short-term training-dependent plasticity of the corticospinal diaphragm control in normal humans. Respir. Physiol. Neurobiol. 160, 172–180.

Dronkers, J., Veldman, A., Hoberg, E., et al., 2008. Prevention of pulmonary complications after upper abdominal surgery by preoperative intensive inspiratory muscle training: a randomized controlled pilot study. Clin. Rehabil. 22, 134–142.

Edwards, A.M., Maguire, G.P., Graham, D., et al., 2012. Four weeks of inspiratory muscle training improves self-paced walking performance in overweight and obese adults: a randomised controlled trial. J. Obes. 2012, 918202.

Enright, P.L., Kronmal, R.A., Manolio, T.A., et al., 1994. Respiratory muscle strength in the elderly. Correlates and reference values. Cardiovascular Health Study Research Group. Am. J. Respir. Crit. Care Med. 149, 430–438.

Enright, S., Chatham, K., Ionescu, A.A., et al., 2004. Inspiratory muscle training improves lung function and exercise capacity in adults with cystic fibrosis. Chest 126, 405–411.

Fernandes, M., Cukier, A., Feltrim, M.I., 2011. Efficacy of diaphragmatic breathing in patients with chronic obstructive pulmonary disease. Chron. Respir. Dis. 8, 237–244.

Fregonezi, G.A., Resqueti, V.R., Guell, R., et al., 2005. Effects of 8-week, interval-based inspiratory muscle training and breathing retraining in patients with generalized myasthenia gravis. Chest 128, 1524–1530.

Fry, D.K., Pfalzer, L.A., Chokshi, A.R., et al., 2007. Randomized control trial of effects of a 10-week inspiratory muscle training program on measures of pulmonary function in persons with multiple sclerosis. J. Neurol. Phys. Ther. 31, 162–172.

Geddes, E.L., O'Brien, K., Reid, W.D., et al., 2008. Inspiratory muscle training in adults with chronic obstructive pulmonary disease: An update of a systematic review. Respir. Med. 102, 1715–1729.

Goldstein, R., De Rosie, J., Long, S., et al., 1989. Applicability of a threshold loading device for inspiratory muscle testing and training in patients with COPD. Chest 96, 564–571.

Gosselink, R.A., Wagenaar, R.C., Rijswijk, H., et al., 1995. Diaphragmatic breathing reduces efficiency of breathing in patients with chronic obstructive pulmonary disease. Am. J. Respir. Crit. Care Med. 151, 1136–1142.

Gosselink, R., De Vos, J., van den Heuvel, S.P., et al., 2011. Impact of inspiratory muscle training in patients with COPD: what is the evidence? Eur. Respir. J. 37, 416–425.

Griffiths, L.A., McConnell, A.K., 2007. The influence of inspiratory and expiratory muscle training upon rowing performance. Eur. J. Appl. Physiol. 99, 457–466.

Griffiths, L.A., McConnell, A.K., 2012. The influence of rowing-related postures upon respiratory muscle pressure and flow generating capacity. Eur. J. Appl. Physiol. Apr 24 [Epub ahead of print].

Hamilton, A.L., Killian, K.J., Summers, E., et al., 1996. Symptom intensity and subjective limitation to exercise in patients with cardiorespiratory disorders. Chest 110, 1255–1263.

Hart, N., Hawkins, P., Hamnegard, C.H., et al., 2002. A novel clinical test of respiratory muscle endurance. Eur. Respir. J. 19, 232–239.

Hawkes, E.Z., Nowicky, A.V., McConnell, A.K., 2007. Diaphragm and intercostal surface EMG and muscle performance after acute inspiratory muscle loading. Respir. Physiol. Neurobiol. 155, 213–219.

Heritier, F., Rahm, F., Pasche, P., et al., 1994. Sniff nasal inspiratory pressure. A noninvasive assessment of inspiratory muscle strength. Am. J. Respir. Crit. Care Med. 150, 1678–1683.

Hill, K., Jenkins, S.C., Philippe, D.L., et al., 2007. Comparison of incremental and constant load tests of inspiratory muscle endurance in COPD. Eur. Respir. J. 30, 479–486.

Hull, J., Aniapravan, R., Chan, E., et al., 2012. British Thoracic Society guideline for respiratory management of children with neuromuscular weakness. Thorax 67 (Suppl. 1), i1–40.

Hulzebos, E.H., Helders, P.J., Favie, N.J., et al., 2006a. Preoperative intensive inspiratory muscle training to prevent postoperative pulmonary complications in high-risk patients undergoing CABG surgery: a randomized clinical trial. J. Am. Med. Assoc. 296, 1851–1857.

Hulzebos, E.H., van Meeteren, N.L., van den Buijs, B.J., et al., 2006b. Feasibility of preoperative inspiratory muscle training in patients undergoing coronary artery bypass surgery with a high risk of postoperative pulmonary complications: a randomized controlled pilot study. Clin. Rehabil. 20, 949–959.

Hulzebos, E.H., Smit, Y., Helders, P.P., van Meeteren, N.L., 2012. Preoperative physical therapy for elective cardiac surgery patients. Cochrane Database Syst, Rev 11.

Inzelberg, R., Peleg, N., Nisipeanu, P., et al., 2005. Inspiratory muscle training and the perception of dyspnea in Parkinson's disease. Can. J. Neurol. Sci. 32, 213–217.

Johnson, P.H., Cowley, A.J., Kinnear, W.J., 1998. A randomized controlled trial of inspiratory muscle training in stable chronic heart failure. Eur. Heart J. 19, 1249–1253.

Johnson, M.A., Mills, D.E., Brown, D.M., et al., 2011. Inspiratory loading intensity does not influence lactate clearance during recovery. Med. Sci. Sports Exerc. 44 (5), 863–871.

Koessler, W., Wanke, T., Winkler, G., et al., 2001. 2 years' experience with inspiratory muscle training in patients with neuromuscular disorders. Chest 120, 765–769.

Koulouris, N., Mulvey, D.A., Laroche, C.M., et al., 1989. The effect of posture and abdominal binding on respiratory pressures. Eur. Respir. J. 2, 961–965.

Laoutaris, I., Dritsas, A., Brown, M.D., et al., 2004. Inspiratory muscle training using an incremental endurance test alleviates dyspnea and improves functional status in patients with chronic heart failure. Eur. J. Cardiovasc. Prev. Rehabil. 11, 489–496.

Leith, D.E., Bradley, M., 1976. Ventilatory muscle strength and endurance training. J. Appl. Physiol. 41, 508–516.

Lin, S.J., McElfresh, J., Hall, B., et al., 2012. Inspiratory muscle training in patients with heart failure: a systematic review. Cardiopulm. Phys. Ther. J. 23, 29–36.

Lomax, M., McConnell, A.K., 2009. Influence of prior activity (warm-up) and inspiratory muscle training upon between- and within-day reliability of maximal inspiratory pressure measurement. Respiration 78, 197–202.

Lomax, M., Grant, I., Corbett, J., 2011. Inspiratory muscle warm-up and inspiratory muscle training: separate and combined effects on intermittent running to exhaustion. J. Sports Sci. 29, 563–569.

Lotters, F., van Tol, B., Kwakkel, G., et al., 2002. Effects of controlled inspiratory muscle training in patients with

COPD: a meta-analysis. Eur. Respir. J. 20, 570–576.

Magadle, R., Bererar-Yanay, N., Weiner, P., 2002. The risk of hospitalization and near-fatal and fatal asthma in relation to the perception of dyspnea. Chest 121, 329–333.

Magadle, R., McConnell, A.K., Beckerman, M., et al., 2007. Inspiratory muscle training in pulmonary rehabilitation program in COPD patients. Respir. Med. 101, 1500–1505.

Martinez, A., Lisboa, C., Jalil, J., et al., 2001. Selective training of respiratory muscles in patients with chronic heart failure. Rev. Med. Chil. 129, 133–139.

McConnell, A.K., 2011. Breathe strong, perform better. Human Kinetics Publishers, Champaign IL.

McConnell, A.K., Copestake, A.J., 1999. Maximum static respiratory pressures in healthy elderly men and women: issues of reproducibility and interpretation. Respiration 66, 251–258.

McConnell, A.K., Griffiths, L.A., 2010. Acute cardiorespiratory responses to inspiratory pressure threshold loading. Med. Sci. Sports Exerc. 42, 1696–1703.

McConnell, A.K., Caine, M.P., Donovan, K.J., et al., 1998. Inspiratory muscle training improves lung function and reduces exertional dyspnoea in mild/moderate asthmatics. Clin. Sci 95, 4p.

McConnell, A.K., Romer, L.M., Weiner, P., 2005. Inspiratory muscle training in obstructive lung disease; how to implement and what to expect. Breathe 2, 38–49.

Minoguchi, H., Shibuya, M., Miyagawa, T., et al., 2002. Cross-over comparison between respiratory muscle stretch gymnastics and inspiratory muscle training. Intern. Med. 41, 805–812.

Moodie, L., Reeve, J., Elkins, M., 2011. Inspiratory muscle training increases inspiratory muscle strength in patients weaning from mechanical ventilation: a systematic review. Journal of Physiotherapy 57, 213–221.

O'Brien, K., Geddes, E.L., Reid, W.D., et al., 2008. Inspiratory muscle training compared with other rehabilitation interventions in chronic

obstructive pulmonary disease: a systematic review update. Journal of Cardiopulmonary Rehabilitation and Prevention 28, 128–141.

Padula, C.A., Yeaw, E., Mistry, S., 2009. A home-based nurse-coached inspiratory muscle training intervention in heart failure. Appl. Nurs. Res. 22, 18–25.

Padulo, J., Mignogna, P., Mignardi, S., et al., 2012. Effect of different pushing speeds on bench press. Int. J. Sports Med. 33, 376–380.

Paulin, E., Yamaguti, W.P., Chammas, M.C., et al., 2007. Influence of diaphragmatic mobility on exercise tolerance and dyspnea in patients with COPD. Respir. Med. 101, 2113–2118.

Plentz, R.D., Sbruzzi, G., Ribeiro, R.A., et al., 2012. Inspiratory muscle training in patients with heart failure: meta-analysis of randomized trials. Arq. Bras. Cardiol. 99, 762–771.

Rahn, H., Otis, A.B., Chadwick, L.E., et al., 1946. The pressure–volume diagram of the thorax and lung. Am. J. Physiol. 146, 161–178.

Romer, L.M., McConnell, A.K., 2003. Specificity and reversibility of inspiratory muscle training. Med. Sci. Sports Exerc. 35, 237–244.

Ross, E.Z., Nowicky, A.V., McConnell, A.K., 2007. Influence of acute inspiratory loading upon diaphragm motor-evoked potentials in healthy humans. J. Appl. Physiol. 102, 1883–1890.

Savci, S., Degirmenci, B., Saglam, M., et al., 2011. Short-term effects of inspiratory muscle training in coronary artery bypass graft surgery: A randomized controlled trial. Scand. Cardiovasc. J. 45, 286–293.

Sawyer, E.H., Clanton, T.L., 1993. Improved pulmonary function and exercise tolerance with inspiratory muscle conditioning in children with cystic fibrosis. Chest 104, 1490–1497.

Shoemaker, M.J., Donker, S., Lapoe, A., 2009. Inspiratory muscle training in patients with chronic obstructive pulmonary disease: the state of the evidence. Cardiopulmonary Physical Therapy Journal 20, 5–15.

Steier, J., Kaul, S., Seymour, J., et al., 2007. The value of multiple tests of respiratory muscle strength. Thorax 62, 975–980.

Sutbeyaz, S.T., Koseoglu, F., Inan, L., et al., 2010. Respiratory muscle training improves cardiopulmonary function and exercise tolerance in subjects with subacute stroke: a randomized controlled trial. Clin. Rehabil. 24, 240–250.

Thomas, M.J., Simpson, J., Riley, R., et al., 2010. The impact of home-based physiotherapy interventions on breathlessness during activities of daily living in severe COPD: a systematic review. Physiotherapy 96, 108–119.

Toigo, M., Boutellier, U., 2006. New fundamental resistance exercise determinants of molecular and cellular muscle adaptations. Eur. J. Appl. Physiol. 97, 643–663.

Tong, T.K., Fu, F.H., Eston, R., et al., 2010. Chronic and acute inspiratory muscle loading augment the effect of a 6-week interval program on tolerance of high-intensity intermittent bouts of running. J. Strength Cond. Res. 24 (11), 3041–3048.

Topin, N., Matecki, S., Le Bris, S., et al., 2002. Dose-dependent effect of individualized respiratory muscle training in children with Duchenne muscular dystrophy. Neuromuscul. Disord. 12, 576–583.

Tsao, H., Hodges, P.W., 2007. Immediate changes in feedforward postural adjustments following voluntary motor training. Exp. Brain Res. 181, 537–546.

Turner, L.A., Mickleborough, T.D., McConnell, A.K., et al., 2011. Effect of inspiratory muscle training on exercise tolerance in asthmatic individuals. Med. Sci. Sports Exerc. 43, 2031–2038.

Unal, O., Arslan, H., Uzun, K., et al., 2000. Evaluation of diaphragmatic movement with MR fluoroscopy in chronic obstructive pulmonary disease. Clin. Imaging 24, 347–350.

Van Houtte, S., Vanlandewijck, Y., Gosselink, R., 2006. Respiratory muscle training in persons with spinal cord injury: a systematic review. Respir. Med. 100, 1886–1895.

Volianitis, S., McConnell, A.K., Koutedakis, Y., et al., 1999. The influence of prior activity upon inspiratory muscle strength in rowers and non-rowers. Int. J. Sports Med. 20, 542–547.

Volianitis, S., McConnell, A.K., Jones, D.A., 2001a. Assessment of maximum inspiratory pressure. Prior submaximal respiratory muscle activity ('warm-up') enhances maximum inspiratory activity and attenuates the learning effect of repeated measurement. Respiration 68, 22–27.

Volianitis, S., McConnell, A.K., Koutedakis, Y., et al., 2001b. Specific respiratory warm-up improves rowing performance and exertional dyspnea. Med. Sci. Sports Exerc. 33, 1189–1193.

Weiner, P., Weiner, M., 2006. Inspiratory muscle training may increase peak inspiratory flow in chronic obstructive pulmonary disease. Respiration 73, 151–156.

Weiner, P., Azgad, Y., Ganam, R., et al., 1992. Inspiratory muscle training in patients with bronchial asthma. Chest 102, 1357–1361.

Weiner, P., Azgad, Y., Weiner, M., et al., 1995. Inspiratory muscle training during treatment with corticosteroids in humans. Chest 107, 1041–1044.

Weiner, P., Ganem, R., Zamir, D., et al., 1996. Specific inspiratory muscle training in chronic hemodialysis. Harefuah 130, 73–76, 144.

Weiner, P., Gross, D., Meiner, Z., et al., 1998a. Respiratory muscle training in patients with moderate to severe myasthenia gravis. Can. J. Neurol. Sci. 25, 236–241.

Weiner, P., Zeidan, F., Zamir, D., et al., 1998b. Prophylactic inspiratory muscle training in patients undergoing coronary artery bypass graft. World J. Surg. 22, 427–431.

Weiner, P., Waizman, J., Magadle, R., et al., 1999. The effect of specific inspiratory muscle training on the sensation of dyspnea and exercise tolerance in patients with congestive heart failure. Clin. Cardiol. 22, 727–732.

Weiner, P., Berar-Yanay, N., Davidovich, A., et al., 2000a. The perception of dyspnoea in patients with asthma, before and following treatment with inhaled glucocorticosteroids. Respir. Med. 94, 161–165.

Weiner, P., Berar-Yanay, N., Davidovich, A., et al., 2000b. Specific inspiratory muscle training in patients with mild asthma with high consumption of inhaled beta(2)-agonists. Chest 117, 722–727.

Weiner, P., Magadle, R., Beckerman, M., et al., 2002a. The relationship among inspiratory muscle strength, the perception of dyspnea and inhaled beta2-agonist use in patients with asthma. Can. Respir. J. 9, 307–312.

Weiner, P., Magadle, R., Massarwa, F., et al., 2002b. Influence of gender and inspiratory muscle training on the perception of dyspnea in patients with asthma. Chest 122, 197–201.

Weiner, P., Magadle, R., Beckerman, M., et al., 2004. Maintenance of inspiratory muscle training in COPD patients: one year follow-up. Eur. Respir. J. 23, 61–65.

West, C.R., Taylor, B.J., Campbell, I.G., et al., 2009. Effects of inspiratory muscle training in Paralympic athletes with cervical spinal cord injury. Med. Sci. Sports Exerc. 41, S31–S32.

Winkler, G., Zifko, U., Nader, A., et al., 2000. Dose-dependent effects of inspiratory muscle training in neuromuscular disorders. Muscle Nerve 23, 1257–1260.

Yamaguti, W.P., Claudino, R.C., Neto, A.P., et al., 2012. Diaphragmatic breathing training program improves abdominal motion during natural breathing in patients with chronic obstructive pulmonary disease: a randomized controlled trial. Arch. Phys. Med. Rehabil. 93, 571–577.

Website

www.physiobreathe.com.

Chapter | 7 |

Functional training of the respiratory muscles

THE RATIONALE FOR FUNCTIONAL TRAINING

As was discussed in Chapter 3 (section 'Non-respiratory functions of the respiratory muscles'), the role of the respiratory muscles extends far beyond that of driving the respiratory pump. This fact explains why most, if not all patients, find walking makes them more breathless than riding a stationary cycle ergometer. However, the contribution of the respiratory muscles to postural control (balance) and core stabilization is not addressed directly in a rehabilitation context. This is surprising because these non-respiratory roles have profound implications for how we *should* train these muscles to optimize their function and minimize the unpleasant symptoms that they generate. A detailed description of the trunk musculature and its non-respiratory roles can be found in Chapter 3. The current section will focus upon the specific rationale for functional training of the respiratory muscles.

The non-respiratory roles of the respiratory muscles are often brought into conflict with their role in breathing; the external manifestation of this conflict is dyspnoea that is disproportionate to the ventilatory demand of the activity. Similarly, in patients with abnormal respiratory mechanics, muscles that do not normally make a substantive contribution to breathing can become vital contributors to thoracic expansion. This helps to explain why patients become breathless during activities of daily living that engender only modest increases in ventilatory demand, such as dressing and hair washing.

Because of the multiple roles of the trunk muscles, respiratory muscle training cannot be optimized if it is delivered using an exclusively 'isolationist' model of training, i.e., if optimal function is to be achieved, the core stabilizing role of the diaphragm must be trained in the context of an activity that challenges core stability. Notwithstanding this, there remains a role for the isolated training of the 'Foundation' phase (see Ch. 6), which provides the foundation onto which functional training is built – in other words, an 'isolate, then integrate' approach to training.

The rationale for functional respiratory training is identical to the rationale for any kind of functional training. When functional conflicts occur within the muscular system, the risk of system failure can be mitigated by providing the muscles in question with reserve capacity (Foundation inspiratory muscle training: IMT), as well as by establishing specific neural activation patterns as routine through training (Functional IMT).

As was explained in Chapter 5, muscles respond to training in highly specific ways that limit the transferability of training benefits when the training stimulus is non-functional (e.g., an isolated leg extension is unlikely to improve walking performance). In functional training, muscles are subjected to forces during functional movements in order to develop the neuromuscular system in ways that are transferable to real-world activities. To date, a missing element from the functional training repertoire has been any consideration of the role of respiratory muscles (major trunk stabilizers and controllers) in functional movements, and vice versa.

As well as satisfying the demands of breathing, the trunk muscles are responsible for a wide range of movements during activities of daily living, e.g., flexion, extension, rotation, stabilization and so on. Ambulation involves continuous perturbation to postural control whilst simultaneously increasing the demand for breathing. These challenges are exacerbated still further if ambulation is combined with carrying, as the trunk must also be stabilized exerting a compressive influence on the thorax. The respiratory muscles must accommodate all of these functions simultaneously, a requirement that demands specific training.

Although it is commonplace to use functional training techniques in a clinical rehabilitation context, functional training movements are typically undertaken as brief, isolated exercises in which the ventilatory demand remains modest. Thus, these exercises rarely simulate the simultaneous challenge of elevated breathing and functional movement accurately; indeed, it is typical for therapists to seek actively to minimize conflicts between breathing and movement by coaching patients to synchronize breathing movements so that the actions of the inspiratory and expiratory muscles coincide with extension and flexion movements of the trunk. Unfortunately, whilst helpful, this synchronization is rarely achievable in everyday life, with the result that the patients may remain unable to deal with the conflicting requirements of breathing and movement.

In his book on low back disorders, Professor Stuart McGill rightly highlights the specific challenge that elevated ventilation represents to spine stability, as well as the increased risk that it poses for back injury (McGill, 2007). The therapeutic approach suggested by McGill is to undertake a range of stabilizing exercises (e.g., side bridge) immediately after an activity that raises ventilation, the idea being that the resultant hyperpnoea is superimposed on exercises that challenge the stabilizing musculature. The aim is to produce what McGill calls a 'grooved' pattern of muscle activation, similar to a rope running in a well-worn slot, so that breathing and stabilization take place simultaneously but without any compromise to either. Often, people cope with their inability to meet the conflicting demands on their respiratory muscles by holding their breath during exercises such as a side bridge. This is clearly a bad 'groove' to get stuck in.

The breathing challenge that is recommended in this chapter is not limited to raising ventilatory flow rate (as recommended by McGill); rather, the functional exercises that are recommended will also increase the requirement for inspiratory pressure (force) generation by the inspiratory muscles. These exercises involve breathing against an inspiratory load during functional movements. This is actually no different from using any external resistance during functional training (e.g., elastic resistance or dumbbell); its purpose is to challenge the neuromuscular system's ability to bring about controlled movements.

In addition to providing a stable platform, the respiratory muscles play an important role in postural control during brief perturbations to balance. A good example of this is the automatic, anticipatory activation of specific trunk muscles immediately before large arm movements (see Ch. 3). The role of the diaphragm in this type of postural control is pre-programmed ('grooved'); this is known because diaphragm activation *precedes* movements that destabilize the body (Hodges et al, 1997a; Hodges et al, 1997b). However, this automatic activation does not mean that the programme is not dynamic or adaptable; rather, the programme varies according to the movement parameters of the task and according to factors such as the prevailing postural conditions (stable or unstable), muscle fatigue, injury, pain and so on. For muscles that are involved in automatic anticipatory postural adjustments, such as the transversus abdominis, isolated specific training can normalize previously abnormal patterns of motor activation, i.e., restore a programme to normality ('flip the rope back into the groove') (Tsao & Hodges, 2008). In other words, isolated voluntary training of muscles involved in automatic anticipatory postural adjustments leads to improvement in complex automatic control strategies. The similarity of the diaphragm's role to that of the transversus abdominis makes it extremely likely that this effect is also present for the diaphragm. Therefore, isolated voluntary training of the diaphragm (the kind of training undertaken during Foundation IMT) most likely enhances its automatic functioning during complex movements. The implications of this pre-programmed role of the diaphragm also need to be considered, and they are incorporated within the guidance on functional training provided below.

Finally, on a practical note, any close-fitting clothing (e.g., bras, waistbands, corsets) will restrict breathing by impeding inspiratory (outward) thoracic and abdominal movements. This needs to be considered in the context of functional training. Patients undertaking their training in loose-fitting exercise clothing will find the benefits diminished when wearing their normal clothing if this is tight fitting, and may be disheartened as a result. It is possible to simulate restrictions imposed by clothing, and this is also addressed in the guidance on functional training provided below.

ASSESSING PATIENT NEEDS

This section will suggest some methods for assessing patients in order to select the most appropriate types of exercise to meet their specific needs. However, by way of an introduction, patient assessment is placed in the context of what has typically been done to assess patients prior to implementing Foundation IMT.

Historically, patients being considered for Foundation IMT have typically been assessed on the basis of their inspiratory muscle function, and specifically their maximal inspiratory pressure (MIP) (see Ch. 6, sections 'Patient selection' and 'Assessment of respiratory muscle function'). However, as was explained in Chapter 6, there are a number of reasons why MIP is not a good predictor of the likely benefits of Foundation IMT, and especially of Functional IMT. First, although reference values for MIP exist, the measurement is not straightforward to undertake, the equations have very poor predictive power (Enright et al, 1994; McConnell & Copestake, 1999) and the definition of 'weakness' is primarily statistical and not functional (Enright et al, 1994). Secondly, although patients with a $MIP < 60$ cmH_2O appear to show larger improvements than those with stronger inspiratory muscles (Lotters et al, 2002; Gosselink et al, 2011), those with stronger inspiratory muscles still show an improvement in breathlessness and exercise tolerance after IMT (Lotters et al, 2002). Thirdly, MIP takes no account of the demand side of the demand/capacity relationship of the inspiratory muscles; the closest functional correlates of dyspnoea are not indices of airway obstruction or gas exchange impairment, but rather inspiratory muscle function (O'Donnell et al, 1987; Killian & Jones, 1988) and the degree of lung hyperinflation (O'Donnell et al, 1998; Marin et al, 2001) – in other words, the relative load upon the inspiratory muscles. Finally, in the context of Functional IMT, MIP provides no insight into the conflicts that might exist between the respiratory and non-respiratory functions of the trunk muscles.

Accordingly, the use of functional, patient-centred indices would seem to be the most appropriate way to approach assessing the degree of functional overload of the inspiratory muscles, and thence the most appropriate approach to IMT. For severely incapacitated patients, Foundation IMT may be the most that can be achieved, but for those who are ambulatory, or have the potential to become so, functional training regimens can be developed. Since a functional approach has not been applied to date, there is no empirical evidence to guide the prescription of IMT based upon the demand/capacity imbalance principle. However, in order to 'get the ball rolling' in terms of generating functional, patient-centred indices of inspiratory muscle overload, one potential method is suggested below (see section 'Assessment of load/capacity imbalance'). Prior to this, the assessment of dyspnoea is described briefly; as dyspnoea is not only the primary correlate of load/capacity imbalance, it is also relatively easy to assess.

Assessment of dyspnoea

Dyspnoea can be assessed in three main contexts: (1) by reflection upon the type of everyday tasks that elicit dyspnoea, (2) by quantifying the severity of dyspnoea during exercise using a rating scale, and (3) by quantifying the severity of dyspnoea during loaded breathing using a rating scale. Each has their own pros and cons, and the best 'picture' of a given patient's limitations is probably obtained by using a combination of methods.

Reflexive assessment of dyspnoea

Of the many reflexive methods available, two of the most widely used and best supported by evidence are the Medical Research Council (MRC) Scale and the Baseline Dyspnoea Index (BDI) and Transition Dyspnoea Index (TDI) (BDI-TDI). Copies of these instruments can be found in Boxes 7.1 and 7.2A,B, respectively. These scales provide a useful insight into the limitations imposed upon everyday life by dyspnoea. In addition, the BDI-TDI allows changes to be monitored in response to interventions or disease progression.

Box 7.1 MRC scale

The original questionnaire contained over 60 questions (Fletcher et al, 1959), but an extract from the questionnaire has been used extensively over the past 50 years to assess the extent to which dyspnoea limits physical activity, i.e., the magnitude of the task that provokes dyspnoea. Patients select one from the following list of statements:
1. I get breathless only with strenuous exercise.
2. I get short of breath when hurrying on the level or up a slight hill.
3. I walk slower than people of the same age on the level because of breathlessness, or have to stop for breath when walking at my own pace on the level.
4. I stop for breath after walking 100 yards or after a few minutes on the level.
5. I am too breathless to leave the house.

In addition, patients can be quizzed regarding the specific movements and tasks that elicit dyspnoea, since this information will provide a guide to the type of functional exercises that address these deficits. For example, if patients identify hair brushing/washing as a task that specifically elicits dyspnoea, exercises that simulate this challenge can be selected. If, on the other hand, the patient reports feeling unsteady or off balance when they get out of breath, this may suggest that they have lumbopelvic dysfunction that can be addressed with specific exercises. The following is a list of suggested questions, which is by no means exhaustive:

- What activities cause you to get out of breath, e.g., gardening, drying after bathing?
- How long can you do the activity for before you stop or slow down?
- What position are you in when you get breathless, e.g., standing?
- How breathless are you when you sit/stand/walk/etc. (a rating scale can be used to quantify this)?
- What activities have you changed or stopped doing because of breathlessness, e.g., gardening?
- How have you modified your activities because of breathlessness, e.g., sit instead of stand, use a walking aid?
- Do you ever lose your balance when you are out of breath, or feel that you need to steady yourself?
- Do you get low back pain, or feel your back is weak, or unstable?

Assessment of dyspnoea during exercise

The most commonly used and well-validated scale for the assessment of dyspnoea during exercise is the Category Ratio scale created by Borg (1982, 1998). This is a general intensity scale with ratio properties that can be used to

Box 7.2A **Baseline Dyspnoea index***

Functional impairment

Grade	Symptoms
4	No impairment. Able to carry out usual activities and occupation without shortness of breath.
3	Slight impairment. Distinct impairment in at least one activity but no activities completely abandoned. Reduction, in activity at work or in usual activities, that seems slight or not clearly caused by shortness of breath.
2	Moderate impairment. Patient has changed jobs and/or has abandoned at least one usual activity due to shortness of breath.
1	Severe impairment. Patient unable to work and has given up most or all usual activities due to shortness of breath.
0	Very severe impairment. Unable to work and has given up most or all usual activities due to shortness of breath.
W	Amount uncertain. Patient is impaired due to shortness of breath, but amount cannot be specified. Details are not sufficient to allow impairment to be categorized.
X	Unknown. Information unavailable regarding impairment.
Y	Impaired for reasons other than shortness of breath. For example, musculoskeletal problem or chest pain.

Magnitude of task

Grade	Symptoms
4	Extraordinary. Becomes short of breath only with extraordinary activity such as carrying very heavy loads on the level, lighter loads uphill, or running. No shortness of breath with ordinary tasks.
3	Major. Becomes short of breath only with such major activities as walking up a steep hill, climbing more than three flights of stairs, or carrying a moderate load on the level.
2	Moderate. Becomes short of breath with moderate or average tasks such as walking up a gradual hill, climbing fewer than three flights of stairs, or carrying a light load on the level.
1	Light. Becomes short of breath with light activities such as walking on the level, washing, or standing.
0	No task. Becomes short of breath with light activities such as walking on the level, washing, or standing.

Grade	Symptoms
W	Amount uncertain. Patient's ability to perform tasks is impaired due to shortness of breath, but amount cannot be specified. Details are not sufficient to allow impairment to be categorized.
X	Unknown. Information unavailable regarding limitation of magnitude of task.
Y	Impaired for reasons other than shortness of breath. For example, musculoskeletal problem or chest pain.

Magnitude of effort

Grade	Symptoms
4	Extraordinary. Becomes short of breath only with the greatest imaginable effort. No shortness of breath with ordinary effort.
3	Major. Becomes short of breath only with effort distinctly submaximal, but of major proportion. Tasks performed without pauses unless the task requires extraordinary effort that may be performed with pauses.
2	Moderate. Becomes short of breath with moderate effort. Tasks performed with occasional pauses and requiring longer to complete than the average person.
1	Light. Becomes short of breath with little effort. Tasks performed with little effort or more difficult tasks performed with frequent pauses and requiring 50–100% longer to complete than the average person might require.
0	No effort. Becomes short of breath at rest, while sitting or lying down.
W	Amount uncertain. Patient's ability to perform tasks is impaired due to shortness of breath, but amount cannot be specified. Details are not sufficient to allow impairment to be categorized.
X	Unknown. Information unavailable regarding limitation of magnitude of effort.
Y	Impaired for reasons other than shortness of breath. For example, musculoskeletal problem or chest pain.

*Mahler DA, Weinberg DH, Wells CK et al, 1984. The measurement of dyspnea: Contents, interobserver agreement, and physiologic correlates of two new clinical indexes. Chest 85; 751–758.

quantify either breathing or limb effort independently, as well as concurrently within the same exercise test (Borg et al, 2010). A copy of the instrument and instructions for its use can be found in Boxes 7.3 and 7.4 respectively. Typically, the scale is presented to the participant periodically during exercise, and they report their perception verbally or by pointing at the scale. This enables symptom profiles to be generated, as well as isolated ratings at specified intensities of exercise. Furthermore, participants can be asked to exercise to a specified level of perceived effort for the purposes of exercise training, or to compare physical capacity between individuals.

Box 7.2B Transition Dyspnoea Index*

Change in functional impairment

Grade	Symptoms
−3	Major deterioration. Formerly working and has had to stop working and has completely abandoned some of usual activities due to shortness of breath.
−2	Moderate deterioration. Formerly working and has had to stop working or has completely abandoned some of usual activities due to shortness of breath.
−1	Minor deterioration. Has changed to a lighter job and/or has reduced activities in number or duration due to shortness of breath. Any deterioration less than preceding categories.
0	No change. No change in functional status due to shortness of breath.
+1	Minor improvement. Able to return to work at reduced pace or has resumed some customary activities with more vigour than previously due to improvement in shortness of breath.
+2	Moderate improvement. Able to return to work at nearly usual pace and/or able to return to most activities with moderate restriction only.
+3	Major improvement. Able to return to work at former pace and able to return to full activities with only mild restriction due to improvement of shortness of breath.
Z	Further impairment for reasons other than shortness of breath. Patient has stopped working, reduced work, or has given up or reduced other activities for other reasons. For example, other medical problems, being 'laid off' work, etc.

Change in magnitude of task

Grade	Symptoms
−3	Major deterioration. Has deteriorated two grades or greater from baseline status.
−2	Moderate deterioration. Has deteriorated at least one grade but fewer than two grades from baseline status.
−1	Minor deterioration. Has deteriorated less than one grade from baseline. Patient with distinct deterioration within grade, but has not changed grades.
0	No change. No change from baseline.
+1	Minor improvement. Has improved less than one grade from baseline. Patient with distinct improvement within grade, but has not changed grades.
+2	Moderate improvement. Has improved at least one grade but fewer than two grades from baseline.
+3	Major improvement. Has improved two grades or greater from baseline.
Z	Further impairment for reasons other than shortness of breath. Patient has reduced exertional capacity, but not related to shortness of breath. For example, musculoskeletal problem or chest pain.

Change in magnitude of effort

Grade	Symptoms
−3	Major deterioration. Severe decrease in effort from baseline to avoid shortness of breath. Activities now take 50–100% longer to complete than required at baseline.
−2	Moderate deterioration. Some decrease in effort to avoid shortness of breath, although not as great as preceding category. There is great pausing with some activities.
−1	Minor deterioration. Does not require more pauses to avoid shortness of breath, but does things with distinctly less effort than previously to avoid breathlessness.
0	No change. No change in effort to avoid shortness of breath.
+1	Minor improvement. Able to do things with distinctly greater effort without shortness of breath. For example, may be able to carry out tasks somewhat more rapidly than previously.
+2	Moderate improvement. Able to do things with fewer pauses and distinctly greater effort without shortness of breath. Improvement is greater than preceding category, but not of major proportion.
+3	Major improvement. Able to do things with much greater effort than previously with few, if any, pauses. For example, activities may be performed 50–100% more rapidly than at baseline.
Z	Further impairment for reasons other than shortness of breath. Patient has reduced exertional capacity, but not related to shortness of breath. For example, musculoskeletal problem or chest pain.

*Mahler DA, Weinberg DH, Wells CK, Feinstein AR, 1984. The measurement of dyspnea: Contents, interobserver agreement, and physiologic correlates of two new clinical indexes. Chest 85, 751–758.

Box 7.3 **Borg CR-10***

0	Nothing at all	'No P'
0.3		
0.5	Extremely weak	Just noticeable
1	Very weak	
1.5		
2	Weak	Light
2.5		
3	Moderate	
4		
5	Strong	Heavy
6		
7	Very strong	
8		
9		
10	**Extremely strong 'Max P'**	
11		
⇓		
•	Absolute maximum	Highest possible

*© Gunnar Borg (Borg, 1998; Borg et al, 2010).

Box 7.4 **Borg CR-10 scale instructions***

Basic instruction: 10, 'Extremely strong – Max P', is the main anchor. It is the strongest perception (P) you have ever experienced. It may be possible, however, to experience or to imagine something even stronger. Therefore, 'Absolute maximum' is placed somewhat further down the scale without a fixed number and marked with a dot '•'. If you perceive an intensity stronger than 10, you may use a higher number.

Start with a *verbal expression* and then choose a *number*. If your perception is 'Very weak', say 1; if 'Moderate', say 3; and so on. You are welcome to use half values (such as 1.5, or 3.5 or decimals, for example, 0.3, 0.8, or 2.3). It is very important that you answer what *you* perceive and not what you believe you ought to answer. Be as honest as possible and try not to overestimate or underestimate the intensities.

Scaling perceived exertion: We want you to rate your perceived (P) exertion, that is, how heavy and strenuous the exercise feels to you. This depends mainly on the strain and fatigue in your muscles and on your feeling of breathlessness or aches in the chest. But you must only attend to your subjective feelings and not to the physiological cues or what the actual physical load is.

1	is 'very light' like walking slowly at your own pace for several minutes.
3	is not especially hard; it feels fine, and it is no problem to continue.
5	you are tired, but you don't have any great difficulties.
7	you can still go on but have to push yourself very much. You are very tired.
10	this is as hard as most people have ever experienced before in their lives.
•	this is 'Absolute maximum', for example, 11 or 12 or higher.

*Borg G, 1998. Borg's Perceived Exertion and Pain Scales. Human Kinetics, Champaign, IL, pp. 44–52.

Assessment of dyspnoea during loaded breathing

The Borg CR-10 can also be used during a loaded breathing task to assess breathing effort perception and its response to training (Weiner et al, 2000; Magadle et al, 2002; Weiner et al, 2003; Beckerman et al, 2005). Typically, participants breathe against a series of fixed-pressure threshold loads corresponding to unloaded breathing, and 5, 10, 20 and 30 cmH$_2$O. After breathing against each load for 1 minute, participants provide an intensity rating using the Borg CR-10. Ideally, the test should be discontinuous such that each rating is discrete, independent of other ratings and unaffected by accumulated inspiratory muscle fatigue; randomization of load presentation is also recommended. The test is susceptible to differences in breathing pattern, so use of a breathing pacer is advisable (a breathing pacer App can be obtained at www.physiobreathe.com/apps).

No published data are currently available to define normal ranges for this test, but ratings of effort are inversely proportional to inspiratory muscle strength (MIP), and the test also exhibits excellent sensitivity to changes in MIP following IMT (Weiner et al, 2000; Magadle et al, 2002; Weiner et al, 2003;Beckerman et al, 2005). Since no normative data exist currently, it is recommended that practitioners/clinics develop their own methods and normative data for identifying patients with abnormally high ratings of dyspnoea. Notwithstanding the lack of published normative data, a look-up chart can be found in Figure 7.1 (see also section 'Assessment of load/capacity imbalance', below). It should also be noted that some patients with

asthma may have abnormally low ratings (Kikuchi et al, 1994), which is a contraindication for IMT (see Ch. 6, section 'Contraindications').

Assessment of load/capacity imbalance

The look-up chart in Figure 7.1 can be used to assess the extent to which there is a functional imbalance between the combined, intrinsic and extrinsic loading of the inspiratory muscles and the capacity of the inspiratory muscles to deliver inspiratory pressure. The chart is based upon unpublished data collected from normal individuals and

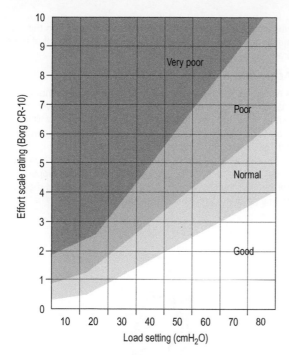

Figure 7.1 Load/capacity imbalance chart. Chart for assessing the extent of functional imbalance between the combined intrinsic and extrinsic loading of the inspiratory muscles, and the capacity of the inspiratory muscles to deliver inspiratory pressure. After breathing against a given load for 60 seconds, the participant rates their effort using the Borg CR-10 scale. Good = no imbalance and above average inspiratory muscle function. Normal = no imbalance with normal inspiratory muscle function. Poor = imbalance such that intrinsic and extrinsic inspiratory loading exceeds inspiratory muscle capacity. Very poor = large imbalance such that intrinsic and extrinsic inspiratory loading exceeds inspiratory muscle capacity considerably.
(The chart is based on unpublished data from McConnell and colleagues.)

those with respiratory disease by McConnell and colleagues over the course of two decades. To undertake the test, the participant breathes against one to three inspiratory loads using the methods described in the section 'Assessment of dyspnoea during loaded breathing', above. The resulting Borg CR-10 rating can then be compared with the rating classifications on the chart.

FUNCTIONAL TRAINING EXERCISES

The remainder of this chapter is devoted to a description of a range of functional inspiratory muscle training (IMT) exercises. Two approaches can be taken to the selection

of exercises for a particular patient: (1) use a generic set of around 10 exercises that provides a holistic set of benefits (some suggested workout protocols are provided at the end of this chapter), and (2) create a bespoke set of exercises based upon specific patient weaknesses, e.g., situations and tasks that are particularly challenging for the patient. A combination of these two approaches probably represents an optimal solution.

Underlying principles

Functional IMT should be preceded by a 6-week period of Foundation IMT, and the development of good diaphragm breathing technique (see Ch. 6). When embarking upon the Functional phase of training, it is important to ensure that patients have good technique and exercise form, before adding *any* resistances. Start patients off by performing each exercise with nothing more than a focus on maintaining slow, deep diaphragmatic breathing throughout. Using an external breathing pacer that provides an auditory cue (obtainable via www.physiobreathe.com/apps) can be very helpful for supporting this process, as well as during the functional exercises themselves. Next add an external resistance to inhalation using an inspiratory muscle-training device (IMTD) set on its minimum load. Gradually increase the load on the IMTD over a period of a few weeks until it reaches the prescribed level for the exercise. See Box 7.5 for guidance regarding abdominal bracing and achieving a neutral spine position, as well as the sections on breath control and load setting in Chapter 6. In addition, consider incorporating IMT into interval training, drills or circuits; the IMT can be introduced into the recovery phase of interval training, or it can be a separate station during a drill or circuit.

Before using these exercises, be sure to note the following principles:

- The limb resistances imposed using cords or bands should be low to begin with, but they can be increased as the training progresses. Don't be too ambitious with the resistance, which is intended primarily to create a postural challenge to the trunk, not to create a resistance-training stimulus to the limbs.
- Ensure elastic resistances are under tension at the start of the exercise (see the previous point for guidance on resistance level).
- For exercises involving hand weights, if these are not available they can be substituted with other items such as cans of food or bags loaded with heavy items.
- For exercises that incorporate abdominal bracing (see section 'Tips for Bracing and Posture'), add the IMTD only once patients able to force their diaphragm into the braced abdominal compartment.
- The compressive effects of tight clothing can be simulated by wrapping elastic resistance bands around the appropriate areas of the trunk (Fig. 7.3).

Box 7.5 **Tips for bracing and posture**

Bracing

Many of the exercises in this chapter involve an abdominal bracing. Bracing requires co-contraction of muscles that bring about opposing movements. For example, co-contraction of the arm muscles involves simultaneous, forceful contraction of the elbow flexor (biceps) and extensor (triceps) such that the muscles are contracted but the arm neither flexes nor extends (i.e., there is a static contraction of both muscles). This same principle can be applied to the muscles of the abdomen such that they form a stiff, stabilizing corset around the abdomen. The muscle fibres in the multiple layers of the abdominal wall run obliquely across one another, like plywood, forming an extremely strong, yet flexible, cylinder.

Correct bracing requires some practice, and the best place to start is learning how to activate the main compressive muscle, the transversus abdominis. The failure to automatically activate the transversus abdominis is associated with low back pain, but learning how to activate this muscle voluntarily has been shown to restore its automatic function in stabilizing the spine. Reconnecting with the transversus abdominis can be achieved by practising drawing in the anterior abdominal wall toward the spine. The objective is to maximize the reduction in waist girth during this manoeuvre, when this occurs correctly the rectus abdominis and pelvic floor inevitably become involved. Once patients can draw in successfully, they need to practise activating the transversus abdominis and accompanying abdominal muscles using a bracing contraction – one in which the trunk volume changes very little, yet the muscles are contracted forcefully.

Initially, this should be practised with maximal effort, but as patients become more adept at activating the muscles involved the intensity can be reduced, and they will be able to feel (literally) the supportive corset that the manoeuvre creates around the abdomen.

Keep in mind that the use of the term *bracing* in this book is not intended to imply the adoption of a rigid, inflexible trunk. Instead, it implies a focus on the core muscles as a seat of strength and stability. Moderate co-contraction of the abdominal-stabilizing muscles is the objective, and not inflexible rigidity of the abdominal compartment. The only exceptions to this are static exercises that specifically require trunk rigidity (e.g., planking).

Breathing during abdominal bracing

Inhaling will feel more difficult during abdominal bracing because the downward movement of the diaphragm is opposed by the raised pressure and increased stiffness of the abdominal compartment. Patients will need to work hard to overcome this extra resistance without releasing the brace, but this resistance is providing a very potent training stimulus – not only to the diaphragm but also to the muscles of the abdominal wall. This is because the diaphragm movement increases the pressure inside the abdominal compartment, requiring all of the muscles to contract more forcefully to maintain the brace. In fact, when bracing is performed with maximal effort, this is an excellent exercise in its own right. Diaphragm breathing should be practised during abdominal bracing in the seated or standing position before incorporating it into other exercises. For exercises that involve bracing, add the IMTD only when the patient is able to force their diaphragm into the braced abdominal compartment without losing control of the brace.

Achieving a neutral spine

A neutral spine position is also referred to throughout this chapter; this describes a position in which the pelvis is level, with neither a forward nor a backward tilt (Fig. 7.2). Forward tilt accentuates lumbar lordosis, and backward tilt does the opposite. Both of these produce undesirable loading on the spine.

You can get a feel for this by standing with your back against a wall. If your heels, buttocks, and shoulder blades (upper portion, not the tips) are touching the wall, your pelvis should be in a neutral position.

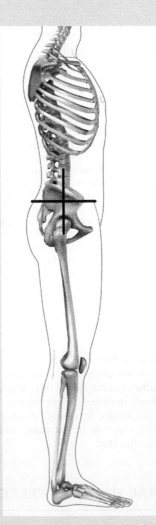

Figure 7.2 Neutral spine position; the pelvis is level. *(From McConnell AK, 2011. Breathe strong, perform better. Human Kinetics, Champaign, IL, with permission.)*

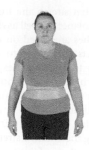

Figure 7.3 Position of elastic resistance to simulate tight-fitting clothing.

The exercises have been designed specifically to minimize the requirement for special equipment. Below is a list of the equipment used, as well as potential alternatives:

Ideal equipment	Alternative equipment
Inspiratory muscle training device	Pursed lips with braced trunk
Swiss ball	Chair with balance cushion
Balance cushion	Close foot stance
Dumbbells (1–10 kg)	Canned food, small sand bags
Small medicine ball (2–10 kg)	Canned food, medium sand bags
Step	Stairs
Elastic resistance band or cord	
Exercise mat	Carpeted area
Bounceable ball	
Small shopping bag	
Chair with and without arms	

Where an IMTD is used during an exercise, the loads to be used will be graded as 'light' or 'moderate'. These correspond to the following 'repetition maximum' and maximal inspiratory pressure (MIP) percentage settings:

- *Light:* equivalent to the 50- to 100-repetition maximum (20–40% of MIP, or an effort rating of 2 to 3 on the Borg CR–10 scale)
- *Moderate:* equivalent to the 20- to 40-repetition maximum (50–60% of MIP, or an effort rating of 4 to 6 on the Borg CR-10 scale).

The exercises are grouped into four sections: (1) trunk strength and lumbopelvic stabilization exercises, (2) dynamic trunk activation exercises, (3) postural control exercises, and (4) pushing and pulling exercises. Each section is subdivided into exercises with 'Easy', 'Moderate' and 'Difficult' classifications. Within each of these classifications, the challenge can be increased progressively, and this is described as appropriate. *It is essential that clinical judgement is applied at all times* in relation to the suitability of any given exercise for any given patient. For example, the 'Difficult' stretches shown below would be entirely unsuitable for a patient with osteoporotic kyphosis.

During most exercises that involve rhythmic movements, there is a requirement to *swap breathing phases halfway through a set*, i.e., to switch from inhaling whilst overcoming a resistance (concentric phase) to exhaling. This can be achieved easily by pausing between repetitions and adding half a breath cycle. For example, for a bicep curl, at the end of a series of repetitions where inhalation occurs during the concentric phase, pause with the hands raised, exhale and then inhale as the resistance is lowered (eccentric phase). In this way, the inhalation is switched from the concentric to the eccentric phase of the movement.

Individual workouts should be preceded by *stretching and mobilizing* exercises (see below). An individual workout should consist of around 10 exercises, with an even mix from each of the four sections. Patients should undertake these functional workouts at least three times per week. On other days, Foundation IMT should be undertaken once daily (at least 3 days per week). The difficulty of the exercises should be increased progressively; firstly by adding resistances, and then by progressing through moderate and difficult classifications. It is also good to vary the exercises from time to time to introduce new challenges.

Some suggested workout protocols are provided at the end of this chapter, and video clips of all exercises are available at www.physiobreathe.com.

Stretching and mobilizing

Developing range of movement is as important for the thorax as it is for any other part of the body. However, the trunk and rib cage are often overlooked when it comes to these activities, despite the fact that these areas include numerous muscles, their attachments, and associated connective tissue (e.g., the rib cage). The rib cage is potentially a huge source of resistance to inhalation, especially in restrictive diseases such as kyphoscoliosis. Any resistance to thoracic expansion increases the work of breathing and the associated perception of breathing effort. The exercises below are grouped into sets of 'Easy', 'Moderate' and 'Difficult' exercises that stretch the trunk in the anterior, posterior and lateral planes, as well as during rotation. Easy and moderate stretches are based on those of Minoguchi et al (2002). These sets can be used to stretch and mobilize the rib cage in order to free-up rib expansion and reduce breathing effort. Each movement should be sustained at maximum range of movement for around 30 seconds.

Diaphragm breathing can be practised during the stretches. In particular, the tension in the trunk muscles that is created during the anterior stretch over a Swiss ball provides a useful resistance for the diaphragm to work against.

Easy

Easy stretching and mobilizing exercises are performed seated on a chair, in the sequence:

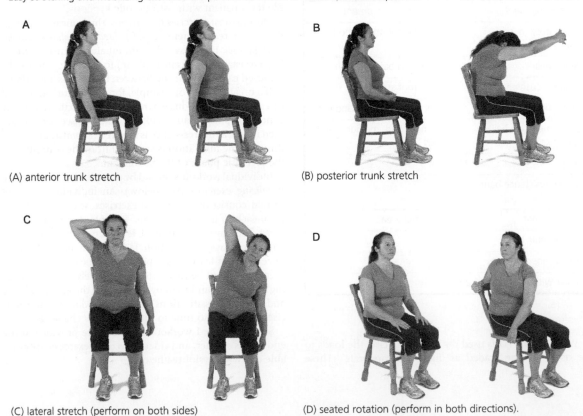

(A) anterior trunk stretch

(B) posterior trunk stretch

(C) lateral stretch (perform on both sides)

(D) seated rotation (perform in both directions).

Moderate

Moderate stretches and mobilizing exercises are performed standing on both feet, in the sequence:

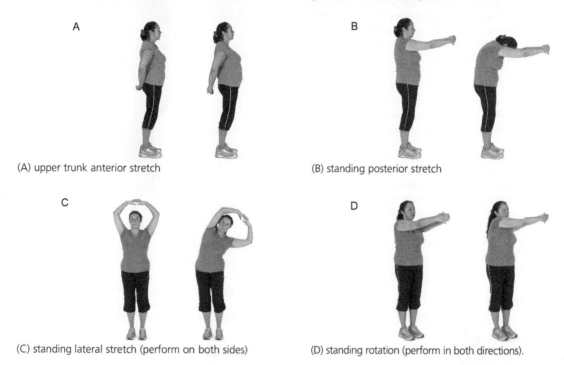

(A) upper trunk anterior stretch

(B) standing posterior stretch

(C) standing lateral stretch (perform on both sides)

(D) standing rotation (perform in both directions).

Difficult

Difficult stretches and mobilizing exercises are performed over a Swiss ball, on hands and knees, then lying down, in the sequence:

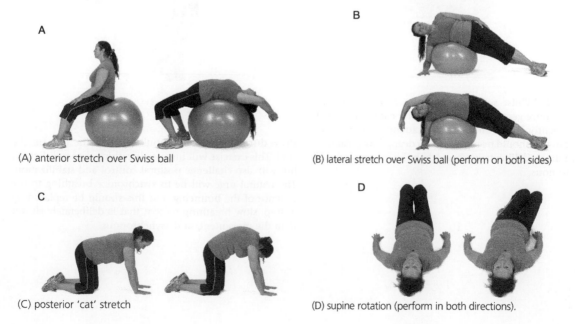

(A) anterior stretch over Swiss ball

(B) lateral stretch over Swiss ball (perform on both sides)

(C) posterior 'cat' stretch

(D) supine rotation (perform in both directions).

Breath control

As was described in Chapter 6, developing breath control is a skill that can and should be practised, because it maximizes breathing efficiency and minimizes the distracting influence of dyspnoea. This can be practised in situations where breathing demand / distress is high; under these conditions, patients should be encouraged to practise deep, slow breath control, and to slow their breathing frequency as much as they can tolerate (a breathing pacer App can be obtained at www.physiobreathe.com/apps). Keeping breathing calm and relaxed under stressful conditions can help to minimize stress and anxiety, and build a sense of mastery.

In addition, below are three further exercises that can help overcome the urge to synchronize breathing with the cadence of movement, which is almost always too high. The exercises involve high-cadence body movements, during which the patient should practise deep, slow, controlled breathing that is deliberately *not* synchronized with movement (a breathing pacer App can be obtained at www.physiobreathe.com/apps).

Swiss ball bounce

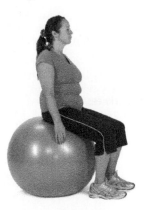

Procedure: Whilst seated on a Swiss ball, the patient should bounce gently up and down. The natural urge will be to synchronize breathing to the cadence of the movement, but this should be replaced by a deep, slow breathing pattern that is deliberately slower than the movement, and asynchronous.

Marching on the spot

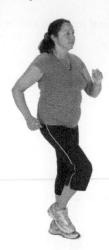

Procedure: The patient should march on the spot at a challenging but manageable pace. This exercise will also increase breathing demand, and is therefore more difficult than the Swiss ball bounce. The natural urge will be to synchronize breathing to the cadence of the movement, but this should be replaced by a deep, slow breathing pattern that is deliberately slower than the movement, and asynchronous.

Ball bounce on the spot

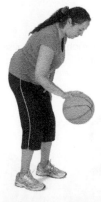

Procedure: The patient should bounce the ball on the spot. This exercise will increase breathing demand slightly, but will also challenge postural control and stabilization. The natural urge will be to synchronize breathing to the cadence of the bouncing, but this should be replaced by a deep, slow breathing pattern that is deliberately slower than the movement, and asynchronous.

Trunk strength and lumbopelvic stability exercises

As was described in Chapter 3, an association has been found between respiratory problems and low back pain. For example, epidemiological data suggest that back pain is more prevalent in women with disorders of continence and respiration than in those without (Smith et al, 2006). Furthermore, physiological data show that the postural function of the diaphragm, abdominal and pelvic floor muscles is reduced by incontinence (Deindl et al, 1994) and respiratory disease (Hodges et al, 2000). Accordingly, it is reasonable to suggest that lumbopelvic stability is impaired in people with respiratory problems, and that correcting this deficit will be beneficial for patients' back pain as well as their dyspnoea. Typical responses in people who are unable to accommodate the simultaneous demands of both stabilization and breathing are either to suspend breathing or to seek stability from an external support, e.g., wall, furniture or walking aid. Thus, training patients so that they are able to accommodate the demands of stabilization and breathing simultaneously should enhance their functional capacity during a wide range of daily activities.

The exercises below are graded, but in all instances training should commence without any resistance to breathing. During the initial phase of training, the focus should be upon maintaining, deep, slow, controlled breathing throughout. Once this can be achieved, the IMTD can be added to the exercise.

Plank

Benefits: This is a 'bread-and-butter' core exercise for developing trunk strength and lumbopelvic stability. It engages the entire trunk- and pelvic-stabilizing musculature including the diaphragm. This exercise builds 'inner strength', facilitating the ability to maintain pelvic stability in the face of large posturally challenging movements of the legs, such as walking and stair climbing. Combining this stabilizing exercise with a breathing challenge ensures that both functions can be performed without compromise to either.

IMTD loading level: light to moderate
Duration: 15 to 60 seconds
Sets: 3

Procedure: Adopt the starting position shown above for the selected level of difficulty. If using an IMTD, this should be held in the mouth, without using the hands. Once in position, brace the abdominal muscles (maximally) and breathe slowly and deeply at around 12 breaths per minute throughout the exercise. If using an IMTD, inhale forcefully through the IMTD before exhaling slowly and fully for about 4 seconds (breathing rate should be around 12 per minute). Ensure maintenance of a completely straight bodyline and do not allow flexion at the hip or abdomen.

Variations: To add difficulty, do any of the following: raise one straight leg off the floor and move it toward the ceiling, bring one knee toward the elbow on the same side of the body (as if climbing a rock face), or bring one knee in and underneath the body toward the opposite elbow. As the leg is raised, inhale forcefully through the IMTD before exhaling slowly as it is lowered. Repeat using the opposite leg. Swap breathing phases between sets so that the exhalation occurs as the leg is lifted.

Easy　　　　　　　　　　　　**Moderate**

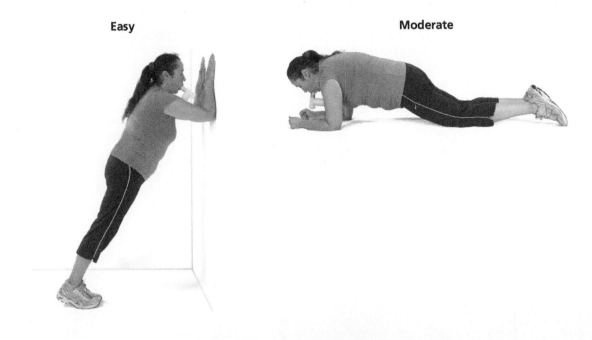

Difficult

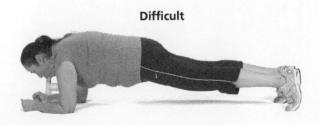

Side bridge

Benefits: This is another 'bread-and-butter' core exercise for developing trunk strength and lumbopelvic stability. It engages the entire trunk- and pelvic-stabilizing musculature including the diaphragm, as well as the back extensors. Superimposing the requirement for increased breathing effort onto this exercise helps ensure that the challenge of keeping the trunk stiff does not lead to a failure to maintain deep, controlled breathing.

    IMT loading level: light to moderate
    Duration: 15 to 60 seconds
    Sets: 2 or 3 per side

Procedure: Adopt the starting position shown for the selected level of difficulty. If using an IMTD, this should be held in the mouth without using the hands. Once in position, brace the abdominal muscles (maximally) and breathe slowly and deeply at around 12 breaths per minute throughout the exercise. If using an IMTD, inhale forcefully through the IMTD before exhaling slowly and fully for about 4 seconds (breathing rate should be around 12 per minute). Ensure maintenance of a completely straight bodyline and do not allow flexion at the hip or abdomen.

Variations: To add difficulty, raise the top arm and / or leg towards the ceiling. As the limb is raised, inhale forcefully through the IMTD before exhaling slowly as it is lowered. Swap breathing phases between sets so that the exhalation occurs as the leg is lifted.

Easy

Moderate

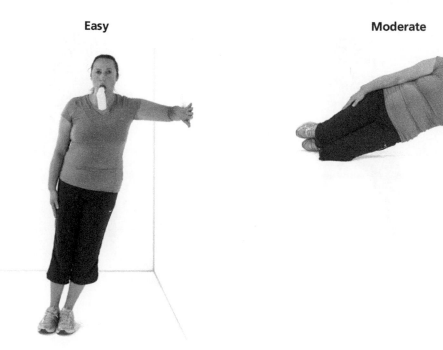

Difficult

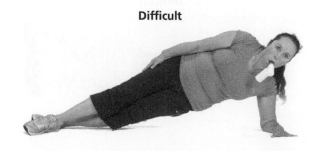

Bridge

Benefits: This exercise helps to develop balance between the posterior and anterior muscles of the trunk. When undertaken with a leg lift, the exercise challenges the ability to maintain pelvic alignment (if the unsupported hip drops towards the floor, the deep stabilizers are weak).

> **IMT loading level:** light to moderate
> **Duration:** 15 to 60 seconds
> **Sets:** 3

Procedure: Adopt the starting position shown for the selected level of difficulty. If using an IMTD, this should be held in the mouth without using the hands. Once in position, brace the abdominal muscles (maximally) and breathe slowly and deeply at around 12 breaths per minute throughout the exercise. If using an IMTD, inhale forcefully through the IMTD before exhaling slowly and fully for about 4 seconds (breathing rate should be around 12 per minute). Ensure maintenance of a completely straight bodyline and do not allow flexion at the hip or abdomen.

Variations: To add difficulty, raise a straightened leg as high as possible (there is a tendency to sag in the middle or tilt to one side). As the leg is raised, inhale forcefully through the IMTD before exhaling slowly as it is lowered. Repeat using the opposite leg. Swap breathing phases between sets so the exhalation occurs as the leg is lifted.

Easy

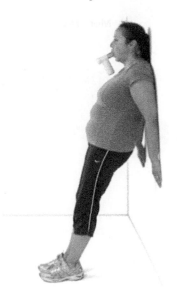

Moderate

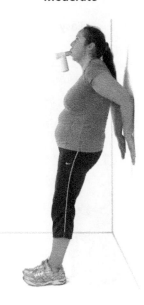

Difficult

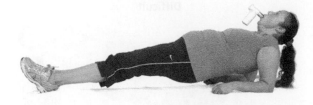

Plank with lower body instability

Benefits: This is a slightly more advanced version of the plank in which a postural control dimension is added to the exercise so that trunk stabilization must be maintained under conditions of instability. Because the lower body is the unstable section, the emphasis is on the pelvic stabilizers. This exercise helps to develop control over the linkage between movements of the upper and lower body.

IMT loading level: light to moderate
Duration: 15 to 60 seconds
Sets: 2 or 3

Procedure: Adopt the starting position shown above for the selected level of difficulty. If using an IMTD, this should be held in the mouth, without using the hands. Once in position, brace the abdominal muscles (maximally) and breathe slowly and deeply at around 12 breaths per minute throughout the exercise. If using an IMTD, inhale forcefully through the IMTD before exhaling slowly and fully for about 4 seconds (breathing rate should be around 12 per minute). Ensure maintenance of a completely straight bodyline and do not allow flexion at the hip or abdomen.

Variations: To add difficulty, move the ankles or knees closer together or gently rotate the ball sideways, controlling its movement with the trunk muscles.

Easy

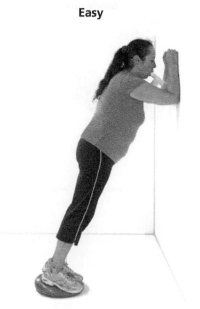

Moderate

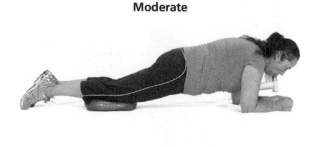

Difficult

This can be performed with the shins on a Swiss ball or with the toes on a balance cushion (on a chair, or floor). Some patients may find it more comfortable to take their weight onto their elbows than onto their hands.

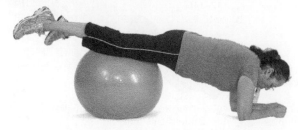

Plank with upper body instability

Benefits: This is a slightly more advanced version of the plank in which a postural control dimension is added to the exercise so that trunk stabilization must be maintained under conditions of instability. Because the upper body is the unstable section, the emphasis is on the trunk stabilizers. This exercise helps to develop control over the linkage between movements of the upper and lower body.

> **IMT loading level:** light to moderate
> **Duration:** 15 to 60 seconds
> **Sets:** 2 or 3

Procedure: Adopt the starting position shown for the selected level of difficulty. If using an IMTD, this should be held in the mouth, without using the hands. Once in position, brace the abdominal muscles (maximally) and breathe slowly and deeply at around 12 breaths per minute throughout the exercise. If using an IMTD, inhale forcefully through the IMTD before exhaling slowly and fully for about 4 seconds (breathing rate should be around 12 per minute). Ensure maintenance of a completely straight bodyline and do not allow flexion at the hip or abdomen.

Variations: To add difficulty, move the elbows closer together or gently rotate the ball sideways, controlling its movement with the trunk muscles.

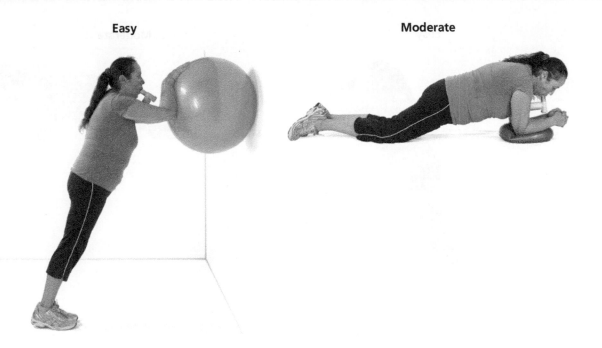

Easy　　　　　　　　　　　　**Moderate**

Difficult

A less challenging version of this exercise can be achieved using a balance cushion placed on a chair.

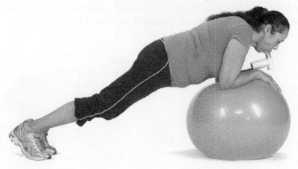

Gluteal bridge

Benefits: This is a good exercise for the gluteals and hamstrings, as well as the trunk and deep pelvic stabilizers. It challenges the ability to breathe effectively during hip extension.

> **IMTD loading level:** light to moderate
> **Duration:** 15 to 60 seconds
> **Sets:** 3

Procedure: Adopt the starting position shown for the selected level of difficulty. If using an IMTD, this should be held in the mouth without using the hands. Once in position, brace the abdominal muscles (maximally) and breathe slowly and deeply at around 12 breaths per minute throughout the exercise. If using an IMTD, inhale forcefully through the IMTD before exhaling slowly and fully for about 4 seconds (breathing rate should be around 12 per minute). In the Easy and Difficult versions, ensure maintenance of a completely straight bodyline and do not allow flexion at the hip or abdomen.

Variations: To add difficulty to the Difficult version, raise one foot off the floor and straighten the leg in line with the rest of the body; hold for 5 seconds. Alternate the raised leg for the duration of the exercise. If the pelvis tilts towards the floor when weight is taken off one foot, this indicates that the deep stabilizers are weak.

Easy

Lean back, controlling the body weight using the gluteals and hamstrings.

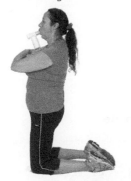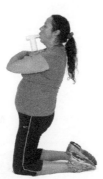

Moderate

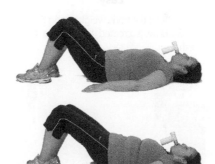

Difficult

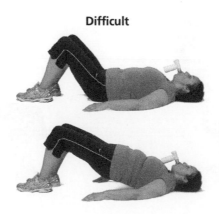

Gluteal bridge with upper body instability

Benefits: This is a slightly more advanced version of the gluteal bridge in which a postural control dimension is added to the exercise. Because the upper body is the unstable section, the emphasis is on the trunk stabilizers. This exercise helps to develop control over the linkage between movements of the upper and lower body.

> **IMTD loading level:** light to moderate
> **Duration:** 15 to 60 seconds
> **Sets:** 3

Procedure: Adopt the starting position shown above for the selected level of difficulty. If using an IMTD, this should be held in the mouth without using the hands. Once in position, brace the abdominal muscles (maximally) and breathe slowly and deeply at around 12 breaths per minute throughout the exercise. If using an IMTD, inhale forcefully through the IMTD before exhaling slowly and fully for about 4 seconds (breathing rate should be around 12 per minute). In the Easy and Difficult versions, ensure maintenance of a completely straight bodyline and do not allow flexion at the hip or abdomen.

Variations: To add difficulty to the Moderate and Difficult versions, raise one foot off the floor and straighten the leg in line with the rest of the body; hold for 5 seconds. Alternate the raised leg for the duration of the exercise. If the pelvis tilts towards the floor when weight is taken off one foot, the deep stabilizers are weak. Be careful to maintain a straight bodyline and to keep the hips level.

Easy

Lean back, controlling the body weight using the gluteals and hamstrings. Instability is created by rotating the shoulders back and forth.

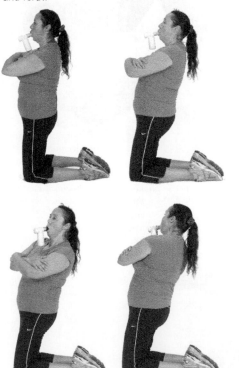

Moderate

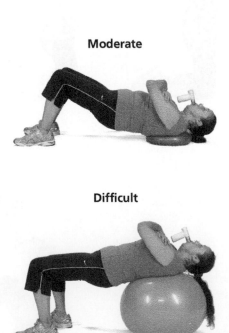

Difficult

Gluteal bridge with lower body instability

Benefits: This is a slightly more advanced version of the gluteal bridge in which a postural control dimension is added to the exercise. Because the lower body is the unstable section, the emphasis is on the pelvic stabilizers. This exercise helps to develop control over the linkage between movements of the upper and lower body.

IMTD **loading level:** light to moderate
Duration: 15 to 60 seconds
Sets: 3

Procedure: Adopt the starting position shown for the selected level of difficulty. If using an IMTD, this should be held in the mouth without using the hands. Once in position, brace the abdominal muscles (maximally) and breathe slowly and deeply at around 12 breaths per minute throughout the exercise. If using an IMTD, inhale forcefully through the IMTD before exhaling slowly and fully for about 4 seconds (breathing rate should be around 12 per minute). In the Easy and Difficult versions, ensure maintenance of a completely straight bodyline and do not allow flexion at the hip or abdomen.

Variations: To add difficulty, raise one foot off the support and straighten the leg in line with the rest of the body; hold for 5 seconds. Alternate the raised leg for the duration of the exercise. If the pelvis tilts towards the floor when weight is taken off one foot, the deep stabilizers are weak. Be careful to maintain a straight bodyline and to keep the hips level.

Easy   **Moderate**

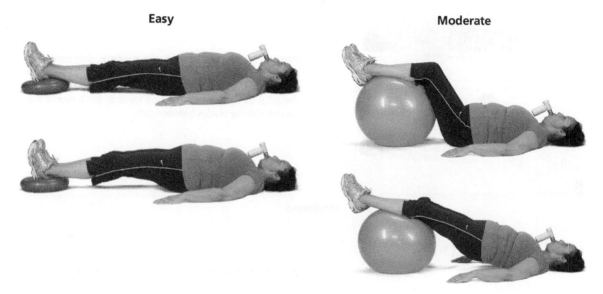

Difficult

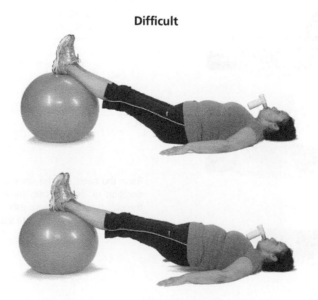

Leg raise

Benefits: This exercise challenges the pelvic and low back stabilizers during hip flexion. As with other exercises in this sub-section, it challenges the ability to maintain lumbopelvic stability without suspending breathing.

IMTD loading level: light to moderate
Duration: 15 to 60 seconds
Sets: 2 or 3

Procedure: Adopt the starting position shown above for the selected level of difficulty. If using an IMTD, this should be held in the mouth without using the hands. Once in position, brace the abdominal muscles (maximally) and breathe slowly and deeply at around 12 breaths per minute throughout the exercise. If using an IMTD, please follow the instructions regarding breathing pattern for each level of difficulty. Push the back towards the floor, but concentrate on maintaining a neutral spine (it may help to place the fingers under the small of the back). For Moderate and Difficult versions, raise the feet about 15 to 20 cm (6 to 8 inches) off the floor and brace the abdominal corset muscles (maximally).

Variations: To add difficulty, extend duration, add ankle weights or move the legs in a continuous scissor action, breathing steadily throughout.

Easy

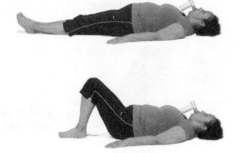

With the feet lightly in contact with the floor, slide both heels towards the buttocks and return immediately to the start position with a controlled cadence. Inhale forcefully through the IMTD as the heels are moved towards the buttocks and swap breathing phases between sets.

Moderate

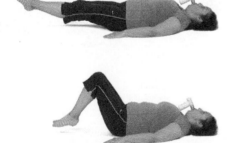

With the feet off the floor, bring both heels towards the buttocks and return immediately to the start position with a controlled cadence. Inhale forcefully through the IMTD as the heels are moved towards the buttocks and swap breathing phases between sets.

Difficult

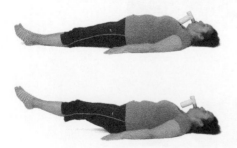

Raise the heels off the floor and maintain elevation for the duration of the exercise. Inhale forcefully and continuously through the IMTD before exhaling slowly and fully for about 4 seconds (the breathing rate should be around 12 per minute).

Braced curl-up

Benefits: During this exercise, the rectus abdominis and other expiratory muscles pull the ribs downwards in an expiratory movement. Developing the ability to inhale under these conditions will enhance the ability to breathe in situations where the body movements and breathing are out of phase in terms of the actions required of the respiratory muscles, i.e., inhaling during non-respiratory activation of expiratory muscles.

　IMT loading level: light to moderate
　Duration: 15 to 60 seconds
　Sets: 3 to 6

Procedure: Adopt the starting position shown; this is the same for all levels of difficulty. If using an IMTD, this should be held in the mouth without using the hands. Once in position, brace the abdominal muscles (maximally). Curl up and raise the shoulders off the floor 8 to 10 cm (3 to 4 inches), curling into the brace and keeping the neck position neutral (don't allow the chin to rest on the chest). While in the 'up' position, take three to six rapid, but deep and forceful inhalations through the IMTD. Maintain the up position for long enough to complete the required number of breath repetitions. Make sure the brace is maintained during the up phase. Then relax, release the brace and rest the shoulders on the floor for no more than 2 or 3 seconds before repeating (15 to 30 seconds up, 2 or 3 seconds down).

Variations: To add difficulty, take the feet off the floor and pulse them up and down a few centimetres. Here are two other alternatives: keep one leg extended, either resting on the floor or raised 2 to 3 inches (swap legs between sets); extend one leg and the opposite arm, raising them off the floor in time with the inhalations (swap limbs between sets).

All versions

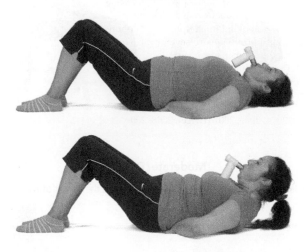

Seated hip extension

Benefits: This exercise requires activation of the trunk-stabilizing muscles to prevent toppling backwards. The muscles involved exert compressive forces on the chest wall and abdomen, which must be overcome during inhalation.

> **IMT loading level:** moderate to high
> **Duration:** 30 breath repetitions
> **Sets:** 1

Procedure: Adopt the starting position shown. If using an IMTD, this should be held in the mouth without using the hands. Once in position, brace the abdominal muscles (moderately). Ensure that the hips are extended as far as is comfortable so that the shoulders are behind the hips. Rest the hands on the thighs, or fold the arms across the chest. Once in position inhale forcefully through the IMTD, completing the 30 repetitions continuously.

Variations: To add difficulty, clasp a small disk weight or dumbbell to the chest, or extend alternate legs at the knee to generate a postural challenge.

Easy

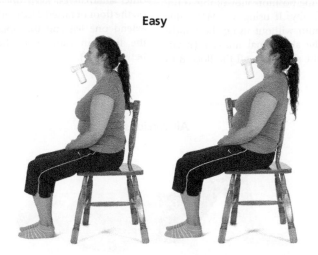

Moderate / Difficult

The distinction between Moderate and Difficult is the extent of hip extension.

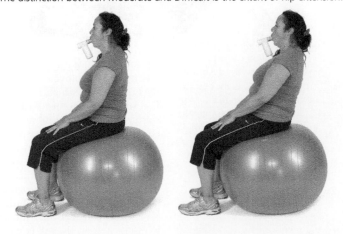

Reverse curl

Benefits: During this exercise, compressive (expiratory) forces are exerted on the rib cage and abdomen. The exercise therefore develops the ability to inhale under these conditions, which will enhance the ability to breathe in situations where the body movements and breathing are out of phase in terms of the actions required of the breathing muscles, i.e., inhaling during non-respiratory activation of expiratory muscles.

    IMTD loading level: light to moderate

    Duration: 10 to 15 repetitions

    Sets: 2 to 4

Procedure: Adopt the starting position shown for the selected level of difficulty. If using an IMTD, this should be held in the mouth without using the hands. Once in position, brace the abdominal muscles (maximally). For specific guidance see the description for each version.

Variations: To add difficulty, resist the pelvic tilt using the hands (Moderate) or elastic resistance bands looped across the hips and anchored to the floor using the hands (Easy and Difficult).

Easy

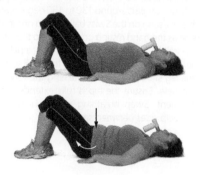

Tilt the pelvis posteriorly (see arrows), inhaling forcefully through the IMTD with each posterior tilt (swap breathing phases between sets, exhaling during the tilt).

Moderate

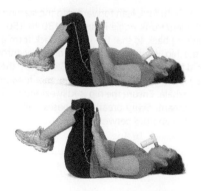

Raise the hips off the floor far enough for the thighs to touch the hands (the hands should be a stationary target), inhaling forcefully through the IMTD with each lift (swap breathing phases between sets, exhaling during the tilt).

Difficult

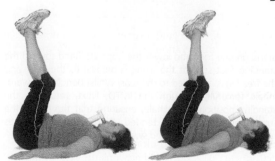

Raise the hips and lower back off the floor, keeping the legs straight and inhaling forcefully through the IMTD with each lift (swap breathing phases between sets, exhaling during the tilt).

Hip extension

Benefits: This exercise challenges core stabilization in all three planes of movement, as well as engaging the gluteals and hamstrings and encouraging full hip extension. The ability to extend at the hip is essential for efficient ambulation and is impaired in patients who use walking aids.

IMTD loading level: light
Duration: 8 to 12 repetitions
Sets: 2 (one on each side)

Procedure: Adopt the starting position shown for the selected level of difficulty. If using an IMTD, this should be held in the mouth without using the hands. Once in position, adopt a neutral spine alignment and brace the abdominal muscles (moderately). For specific guidance see the description for each version.

Variations: To add difficulty, add resistance to the leg (Easy and Moderate), or hold a dumbbell (Difficult).

Easy

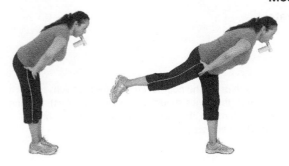

Standing on both feet, lean forward into the starting position so that the leg/trunk angle is around 130 to 150 degrees and one or both hands are resting on the Swiss ball. Extend one leg back (on the same side as the hand resting on the ball) so that the leg and back form a straight line. As the hip is extended, inhale forcefully through the IMTD. Hold the hip extension for 3 to 5 seconds, then return to the leg start position (maintaining the forward flexed trunk) and exhale. Ensure the hip is fully extended at the end of the movement. Swap breathing phases halfway through the set, and swap sides between sets.

Moderate

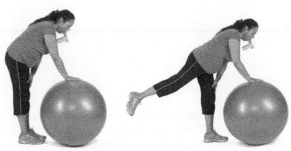

Standing on both feet, lean forward into the starting position so that the leg/trunk angle is around 130 to 150 degrees. Extend one leg back so that the leg and back form a straight line. As the hip is extended, inhale forcefully through the IMTD. Hold the hip extension for 3 to 5 seconds, then return to the leg start position (maintaining the forward flexed trunk) and exhale. Ensure the hip is fully extended at the end of the movement. Swap breathing phases halfway through the set, and swap sides between sets.

Difficult

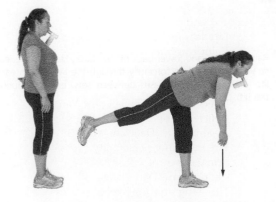

Stand on one foot and lower the opposite hand toward the standing foot so that the trunk is parallel to the floor and the free leg is extended to the rear. Whilst bending forward, inhale forcefully through the IMTD. Next, return to the standing position and exhale, ensuring that the hip of the supporting leg is fully extended. Swap breathing phases halfway through the set and swap sides between sets.

Superman

Benefits: This exercise is a bread-and-butter exercise for promoting healthy, 'grooved' muscle activation patterns whilst ensuring that this can be combined (automatically) with breathing. It involves the deep pelvic stabilizers, the extensors of the hip and lumbar spine as well as the transversus abdominis. This exercise places a particular emphasis on developing lumbopelvic stability.

IMTD loading level: moderate
Duration: 10 to 20 repetitions
Sets: 2 to 4 (1 to 2 on each side)

Procedure: Adopt the starting position shown above for the selected level of difficulty. If using an IMTD, this should be held in the mouth without using the hands. Once in position, adopt a neutral spine alignment and brace the abdominal muscles (moderately). For specific guidance see the description for each version.

Variations: To add difficulty, wrist and ankle weights can be used. Also pause in the extended position to 'draw' a square in the air with the hand and foot, inhaling against the IMTD as this is done.

Easy

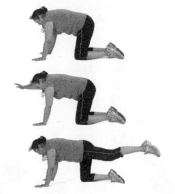

There are always three points of contact with the floor in this version of the exercise, and the moving limb is changed during a series of 4 sets. Lift one limb until it is horizontal. As the limb moves toward the horizontal position, inhale against the IMTD. Pause for 1 or 2 seconds and commence a slow, controlled exhale as the limb is brought back towards the starting position (swap breathing phases between sets). Do not allow the limb to touch the floor; instead immediately return it to the horizontal position and inhale. Ensure that the back remains flat and the shoulders level. Complete the required number of repetitions as a continuous set before swapping limbs.

Moderate

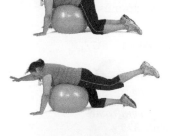

Supported by a Swiss ball, lift the right hand and left knee off the floor and extend the arm and leg until both are horizontal. As the arm and leg move toward the horizontal position, inhale against the IMTD. Pause for 1 or 2 seconds and commence a slow, controlled exhalation as the hand and knee are brought back towards the starting position (swap breathing phases between sets). Do not allow the hand and knee to touch the floor; instead, immediately return the arm and leg to the horizontal position and inhale. Ensure that the back remains flat and the shoulders level. Complete the required number of repetitions as a continuous set before swapping sides.

Difficult

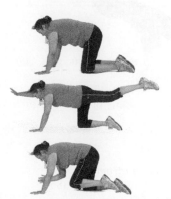

Lift the right hand and left knee off the floor and extend the arm and leg until both are horizontal. As the arm and leg move toward the horizontal position, inhale against the IMTD. Pause for 1 or 2 seconds and commence a slow, controlled exhalation as the hand and knee are brought back towards the floor (swap breathing phases between sets). Do not allow the hand and knee to touch the floor; instead bring them together under the body, and then immediately return the arm and leg to the horizontal position and inhale. Ensure that the back remains flat and the shoulders level. Complete the required number of repetitions as a continuous set before swapping sides.

Ski squats with leg lift

Benefits: This exercise challenges the ability to keep the hips level, and it puts emphasis on the development of strength in the lumbopelvic stabilizers. The added breathing challenge helps ensure that forceful breathing does not jeopardize pelvic stability.

> **IMTD loading level:** moderate
> **Duration:** 15 to 60 seconds
> **Sets:** 2 or 3

Procedure: Adopt the starting position shown for the selected level of difficulty. If using an IMTD, this should be held in the mouth without using the hands. Once in posi- tion, adopt a neutral spine alignment and brace the abdom- inal muscles (maximally). Extend one knee and inhale forcefully through the IMTD before exhaling slowly and fully for about 3 seconds, whereupon the starting position is resumed (the breathing rate should be around 15 per minute). Be careful not to allow the hip to drop to the unsupported side. Repeat with the opposite leg, alternating for as many repetitions as possible.

Variations: To add difficulty, deepen the squat, place a Swiss ball between the back and the wall or stand on a balance cushion. The repetitions can also be undertaken continuously on the same leg, swapping legs between sets.

Easy	Moderate

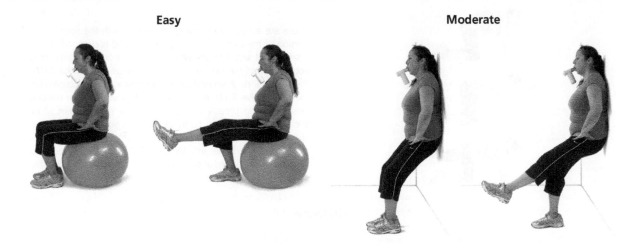

Difficult

Increase difficulty by depending the squat.

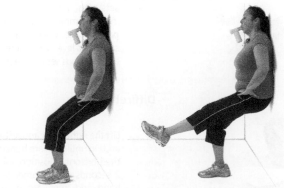

Bent leg deadlift

Benefits: This exercise has been described as 'the best core exercise of them all', because it is such a great challenge to the entire lumbopelvic-stabilizing system as well as to the trunk (from ankles to shoulders). This exercise is a staple of weight training, but carries a high risk of injury if not performed with good style. A common fault is losing the flat-back posture, and this can occur if the drive to breathe overwhelms the ability to maintain the braced position. By using a manageable resistance and imposing a breathing challenge simultaneously, the dual demands that these challenges impose can be accommodated.

IMTD loading level: light to moderate
Duration: 10 repetitions
Sets: 2 sets separated by 30 to 60 seconds of rest

Procedure: Adopt a starting position appropriate to the level of difficulty, i.e., bring the hands closer to the ankles for greater difficulty. If using an IMTD, this should be held in the mouth, without using the hands. Once in position, adopt a neutral spine alignment and brace the abdominal muscles (maximally). As the hips are extended, inhale forcefully through the IMTD and exhale when returning to the starting position. Alternate this pattern between sets so that the exhalation occurs during hip extension. Concentrate on not allowing the brace to release during either phase of breathing. Also concentrate on maintaining good lifting form and extending fully at the hip (rolling the shoulders back can help with this).

All versions

Difficulty is graded according to the height from which the resistance is lifted.

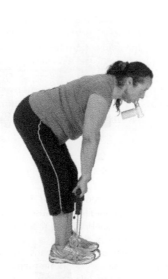
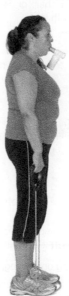

Dynamic trunk activation exercises

Arm resistance

Benefits: The exercises are all designed to train the ability of the trunk to move and control a resistance imposed via the upper limbs without the need to suspend breathing. These types of challenges engage the diaphragm and transversus abdominis in a feed-forward manner that is intended to stiffen the trunk. Although this mechanism is good for stability, it impedes breathing. These exercises therefore develop the ability to manage the demands of dynamic trunk loading without impairing breathing.

> **IMTD loading level:** moderate
> **Duration:** 10 repetitions (for each arm)
> **Sets:** 4

Procedure: Difficulty is graded primarily according to posture, which can be: (1) seated, (2) standing on two feet, or (3) standing on one foot. Difficulty can also be graded according to the size of the resistance being moved in the hands; the exercise can commence with no resistance. Adopt the starting position appropriate to the level of difficulty. If using an IMTD, this should be held in the mouth without using the hands. Once in position, adopt a neutral spine alignment and brace the abdominal muscles (moderately). As the hand resistance is overcome, inhale forcefully through the IMTD and exhale when returning to the starting position. Arm movements should ideally be unilateral to maximize the postural challenge created. Alternate the breathing pattern between sets so that the exhalation occurs as the resistance is overcome.

Stance variations

Easy

Perform exercises seated on a chair or Swiss ball. Add difficulty by lifting one leg or both legs.

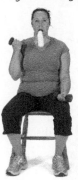

Moderate

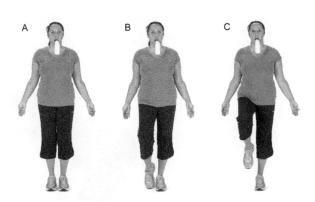

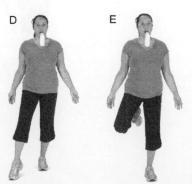

Difficult

Perform exercises whilst standing on one leg. Add difficulty by tapping with one heel on the floor or standing on a balance cushion.

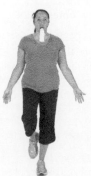

Perform exercises in a standing position with the following posture variations: (A) standing on two feet with close stance, (B) standing on one leg with toe providing support, (C) marching on the spot, (D) tapping the ground with the toe, moving it 'round the clock', and (E) with rhythmic knee flexion.

Arm movement variations

These can be performed with any of the stance variations. The arm movements can be undertaken without any resistance, or with the added challenge of an elastic resistance band or hand weight. Unless a single resistance is held in both hands (e.g., halo), arm movements can be bilateral (less challenging) or unilateral (more challenging).

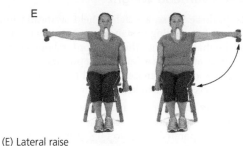

(E) Lateral raise

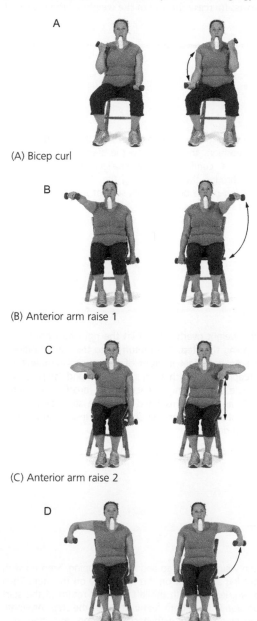

(A) Bicep curl

(B) Anterior arm raise 1

(C) Anterior arm raise 2

(D) Anterior arm raise 3

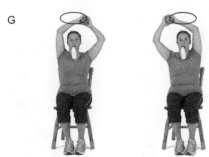

(F) Side swing (swing the weight to each side in turn, maintaining control at all times)

(G) Halo (move the weight around the head clockwise and then anticlockwise)

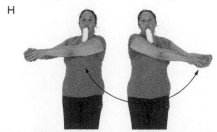

(H) Standing front swing (swing the weight from side to side across the front of the body, maintaining control at all times)

Rise with overhead weight

Benefits: In this exercise, a weight is held overhead whilst either moving from sitting to standing or stepping up. This is an exercise that combines the need for lumbopelvic and thoracic stabilization with a demand for postural control. It is a good 'compound' exercise that will be beneficial to a wide range of everyday activities.

IMT loading level: light to moderate
Duration: 15 repetitions
Sets: 2 sets separated by 30 to 60 seconds of rest

Procedure: Adopt the starting position shown above for the selected level of difficulty. If using an IMTD, this should be held in the mouth without using the hands. Once in position, adopt a neutral spine alignment and brace the abdominal muscles (moderately). For specific guidance see the description for each version.

Variations: Increase the size of the weight or the height of the step.

Easy

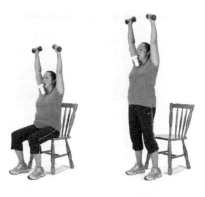

Place the weight overhead and rise from the seated to the standing position, then return to the start position. Stand and sit at a comfortable but challenging pace. Inhale forcefully through the IMTD during the stand phase (swap the breathing phase between sets so that the inhale occurs during the sitting phase).

Moderate

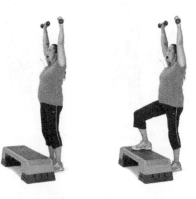

Place the weight overhead and lift the right foot onto the step, tapping the step. Then return it to the start position standing on both feet in front of the step. Alternate the lead 'stepping' leg with each repetition, and 'step' at a comfortable but challenging pace. Inhale forcefully through the IMTD as the foot is lifted onto the step (swap the breathing phase between sets so that the inhalation occurs on the step-down).

Difficult

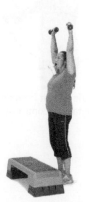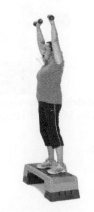

Place the weight overhead and begin stepping. Step up with the right leg and stand on this leg briefly on the step. Then step down, leading with the left leg, and return to the start position standing on both feet in front of the step. Alternate the lead stepping leg with each repetition, and step at a comfortable but challenging pace. Inhale forcefully through the IMTD during the step-up (swap the breathing phase between sets so that the inhale occurs on the step-down).

Squat with overhead resistance

Benefits: This exercise is more challenging than it appears, involving the quadriceps, gluteals, lumbopelvic stabilizers, upper back, shoulders and chest. By combining a body-weight squat with an additional challenge to the trunk (from the overhead resistance) and a breathing resistance, the exercise becomes more challenging than a conventional squat. This exercise enhances the ability to coordinate and control multiple actions involving large muscle groups.

  IMTD loading level: light to moderate
  Duration: 15 to 60 seconds
  Sets: 3 sets separated by 30 to 60 seconds of rest

Procedure: Adopt the starting position shown above for the selected level of difficulty. If using an IMTD, this should be held in the mouth without using the hands. Once in position, adopt a neutral spine alignment and brace the abdominal muscles (moderately). For specific guidance see the description for each version.

Variations: In addition to increasing duration, make the exercise more challenging by increasing cadence, squeezing a weight between the hands or standing on a large balance cushion.

Easy

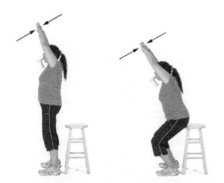

Perch with the buttocks resting on the edge of a stool, table or the back of a chair with feet shoulder-width apart. Place both hands above the head with one palm resting on the back of the other hand; press the hands together, ensuring that the brace and the hand pressure are maintained throughout the squat exercise. Stand up and then return to perching on the edge of the stool; try not to rest too heavily on the stool. Move at a comfortable but challenging pace, concentrating on maintaining hand pressure and squat style. Inhale forcefully through the IMTD during the sitting phase (exhale when standing up). Alternate this pattern between sets so that the exhalation occurs during the squat. Halfway through each set, swap hands so that the opposite hand is in front.

Moderate

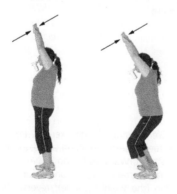

Standing upright with feet shoulder-width apart, place both hands above the head with one palm resting on the back of the other hand; press the hands together, ensuring that the brace and the hand pressure are maintained throughout the squat exercise. Squat to a knee angle of about 150 degrees (roughly a quarter-squat); then follow the instructions for the Easy version.

Difficult

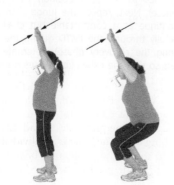

Standing upright with feet shoulder-width apart, place both hands above the head with one palm resting on the back of the other hand; press the hands together, ensuring that the brace and the hand pressure are maintained throughout the squat exercise. Squart to a knee angle of about 130 degrees (roughly a half-squat); then follow the instructions for the Easy version.

Bag pick-up

Benefits: This exercise simulates the everyday demands of picking up and carrying a bag of shopping, challenging both trunk stabilization and postural control. The former compresses the trunk, whereas the latter necessitates feed-forward activation of the diaphragm and transversus abdominis. Superimposing a controlled breathing demand upon these challenges facilitates the ability to meet them in daily life.

IMTD loading level: light to moderate
Duration: 15 to 60 seconds
Sets: 2 to 4 sets separated by 30 to 60 seconds of rest

Procedure: Adopt the starting position shown for the selected level of difficulty. If using an IMTD, this should be held in the mouth without using the hands. Once in position, adopt a neutral spine alignment and brace the abdominal muscles (moderately). For specific guidance see the description for each version.

Variations: In addition to increasing duration, make the exercise more challenging by swinging the arms, marching on the spot, adding periodic lowering and lifting of the weight.

Easy / Moderate

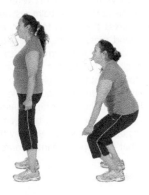

The Easy form of this exercise is without any weight, whereas the Moderate form requires a weight to be held in the reaching hand. Standing upright with feet shoulder-width apart and arms at the sides of the body, squat down as if to pick-up a heavy bag. The hand should reach down to a typical height for a bag handle (30 to 45 cm, or 12 to 18 inches); pause briefly in the squat position before returning to the start position and then reaching down on the opposite side for the next repetition (if using a weight, transfer this between the hands). Inhale forcefully through the IMTD during the reach-down phase (exhale when standing up). Alternate this pattern between sets so that the exhalation occurs during the active phase.

Difficult

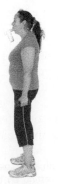 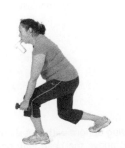

This is effectively a static lunge exercise. Begin by standing upright with feet together holding a weight in one or both hands, then step forward and drop down into the lunge as deeply as is comfortable (active phase) and reach forward with one hand (the weighted one); reverse the manoeuvre by pushing back to the start position with feet together (recovery phase). Next, repeat the lunge with the opposite leg, and continue at a comfortable but challenging pace. Inhale forcefully through the IMTD during the active phase (exhale during the recovery phase). Alternate this pattern between sets so that the exhalation occurs during the active phase.

Side crunch

Benefits: This lateral trunk flexion exercise involves not only the oblique muscles but also those of the rib cage. Developing these muscles is beneficial for activities that involve twisting or flexing the trunk. This exercise essentially compresses the rib cage so combining it with a breathing exercise that requires forceful inhalation will help to build the ability to inhale during movements that compress the chest.

IMTD loading level: moderate
Duration: 15 to 20 repetitions
Sets: 2 (1 on each side)

Procedure: Adopt the starting position shown for the selected level of difficulty. If using an IMTD, this should be held in the mouth without using the hands. Once in position, brace the abdominal muscles (moderately). For specific guidance see the description for each version.

Easy

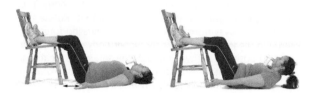

Lie supine on a mat with calves resting on a box or chair so that the hips and knees are bent at ~90 degrees. Flex the upper body to one side, reaching towards the box/chair and inhaling forcefully through the IMTD. Exhale when returning to the start position, then repeat on the same side. Swap breathing phases halfway through each set and swap sides between sets.

Moderate

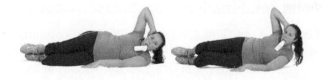

Lie on one side on a mat, with hips and knees bent at 90 degrees. Flex the upper body upwards, lifting the upper trunk off the mat and inhaling forcefully through the IMTD. Exhale when returning to the start position, then repeat on the same side. Swap breathing phases halfway through each set and swap sides between sets.

Difficult

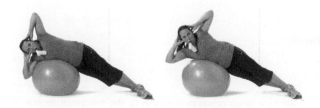

Position the trunk sideways on the ball with feet against a wall (one slightly in front of the other). Flex the upper body toward the wall, inhaling forcefully through the IMTD. Exhale when returning to the start position. Swap breathing phases halfway through each set and swap sides between sets.

Trunk lateral rotation

Benefits: This exercise involves the trunk rotators, which are responsible for controlling the counter-rotation of the shoulders during walking. Too much rotation will generate instability, inefficiency, and loss of balance. This exercise will help to develop the ability to control trunk movement, even when breathing demand is high, as well as overcoming the trunk compression that the rotation produces.

IMTD loading level: moderate
Duration: 15 to 20 repetitions
Sets: 2 (1 on each side)

Procedure: Adopt the starting position shown for the selected level of difficulty. If using an IMTD, this should be held in the mouth without using the hands. Once in position, brace the abdominal muscles (moderately). For specific guidance see the description for each version.

Easy

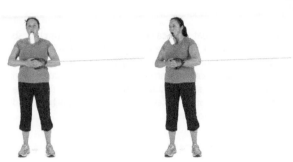

Stand or sit sideways to the resistance source. Fold the arms and hold the resistance in one hand, close to the body. The hips should remain facing forward throughout. Rotate the upper body away from the anchor point, inhaling forcefully through the IMTD. Exhale as the upper body returns to the starting position. Halfway through the set, swap breathing phases so that the exhalation occurs during the rotation away from the anchor point. On the second set, place the resistance on the opposite side of the body and repeat. Add difficulty by increasing the resistance or standing on a large balance cushion.

Moderate

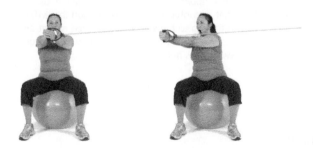

Kneel on the floor, or sit on a Swiss ball, sideways to the resistance source. The hips should remain facing forward throughout. Hold the resistance in both hands, at arm's length then follow the instructions for the Easy version.

Difficult

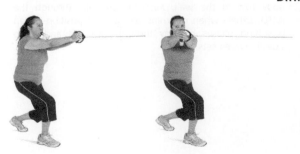

Adopt a lunge position, sideways to the resistance source. The hips should remain facing forward throughout. Then follow the instructions for the Easy version.

Trunk anti-rotation press

Benefits: This exercise requires the ability to resist a rotational force, which is as hard as actually generating rotational movement. The exercise is harder than it looks; watch out for asymmetry between sides and work to correct this.

IMTD loading level: moderate
Duration: 10 to 15 repetitions (each repetition is held for 3 to 5 seconds at the end position)
Sets: 2 or 4 (1 or 2 on each side)

Procedure: Adopt the starting position shown for the selected level of difficulty. If using an IMTD, this should be held in the mouth without using the hands. Once in position, brace the abdominal muscles (moderately). For specific guidance see the description for each version.

Variations: Vary the height of the resistance anchor to add upward and downward force to the lateral force.

Easy / Moderate

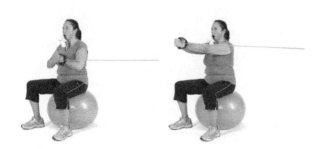

Adopt a seated position on a chair (Easy) or Swiss ball (Moderate) sideways to the resistance source, which can be an elastic cord/band, or a cable weight machine, providing resistance at shoulder height. With tension on the band, hold the band at mid-sternum level with both hands. Extend the handle directly forward in a straight line whilst resisting the increasing rotational force that is being applied to the outstretched arms. As the arms are extended forward, inhale forcefully through the IMTD, and hold this end position for 3 to 5 seconds. Exhale as the hands are brought back toward the chest. Without pausing, repeat the manoeuvre, swapping breathing phases halfway through the set so that the exhalation occurs as the hands extend forward.

Difficult

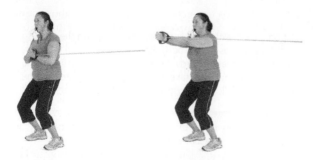

Assume a bilateral one-quarter squat position sideways to the resistance source. Then follow the instructions for the Easy/Moderate version. If it is too difficult to engage and maintain the abdominal brace, begin this exercise in a tall kneeling position.

Close arm dip

Benefits: The emphasis of this exercise is not the triceps (as it would be in a normal dip), but the complex of muscles around the shoulders that are responsible for pulling movements. These actions compress the thorax and therefore oppose inhalation.

Arms should remain close to the body to maximize scapular involvement and thoracic compression.

IMTD loading level: moderate
Duration: 10 to 15 repetitions (each repetition is held for 3 to 5 seconds at the end position)
Sets: 3

Procedure: Adopt the starting position shown for the selected level of difficulty. If using an IMTD, this should be held in the mouth without using the hands. Once in position, brace the abdominal muscles (moderately). For specific guidance see the description for each version.

Variations: Add weight on the lap.

Easy

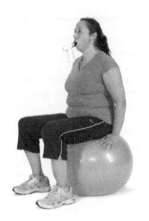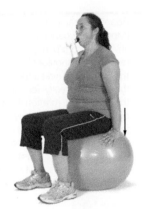

Sit on a chair or Swiss ball and place the hands next to the buttocks. Raise the buttocks off the chair/ball by pushing down and bringing the shoulder blades closer together. Inhale forcefully through the IMTD during the push, and hold this end position for 3 to 5 seconds. Exhale during the return to the relaxed sitting position. Without pausing, repeat the manoeuvre, swapping breathing phases halfway through the set so that the exhalation occurs during the push. Arms should remain close to the body to maximize scapular involvement and thoracic compression.

Moderate

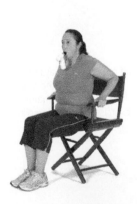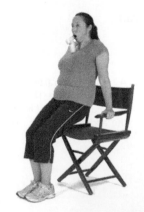

Sit on a chair with arms and place the hands on the arms so that they are close to the body. Keep the feet flat on the floor, close to the chair, to provide assistance. Push down on the arms of the chair to take the body weight through the hands. Then follow the instructions for the Easy version.

Difficult

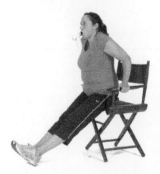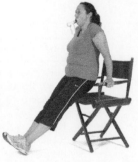

Sit on a chair with arms and place the hands on the arms so that they are close to the body. Move the heels away from the chair, with weight on the heels. Push down on the arms of the chair to take the body weight through the hands. Then follow the instructions for the Easy version.

Postural control exercises

Standing leg lift

Benefits: Standing on one leg is challenging for most people, but when breathing effort perturbs balance it can be virtually impossible. This exercise will develop the ability to dissociate the destabilizing influence of breathing from balance.

> **IMTD loading level:** moderate
> **Duration:** 30 to 60 seconds
> **Sets:** 2 to 4 (1 to 2 on each side)

Procedure: Adopt the starting position shown for the selected level of difficulty. If using an IMTD, this should be held in the mouth without using the hands. Once in position, brace the abdominal muscles (moderately) and breathe slowly and deeply at around 12 breaths per minute throughout the exercise. If using an IMTD, inhale forcefully through the IMTD before exhaling slowly and fully for about 4 seconds (breathing rate should be around 12 per minute). For specific guidance see the description for each version.

Variations: Stand on a balance cushion to add difficulty. Use an elastic resistance band tied around the ankle and anchored beneath the standing foot. Abduct the lifted leg.

Easy

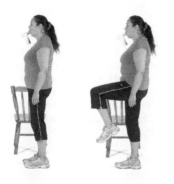

Stand next to a wall, mantlepiece, or piece of furniture that can provide support. Lift the foot furthest away from the support off the ground by bending the knee and hip. Then lower the leg, tapping the ground briefly before repeating the movement. Move at a comfortable but challenging pace, inhaling forcefully through the IMTD so that 5 to 6 deep breaths are completed in 30 seconds (10 to 12 in 60 seconds). Try to breathe *out of synch* with movements.

Moderate

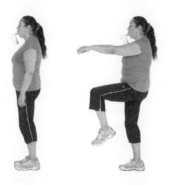

Lift one foot off the ground by bending the knee and hip; at the same time, raise the arm on the same side. Then lower the limbs, tapping the ground briefly before repeating the movement. Then follow the instructions for the Easy version.

Difficult

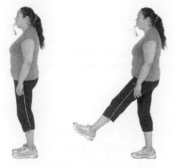

Lift one foot off the ground, flexing at the hip and keeping the leg straight. Then lower the leg, tapping the ground briefly before repeating the movement. Then follow the instructions for the Easy version.

Dumbbell running

Benefits: This exercise involves the entire trunk musculature, deltoids and biceps. It challenges the ability of the postural control system to maintain an upright posture. Most people find that they become much more breathless during walking and running activities than they do during cycling. This is because the postural control system is required to make continuous adjustments to posture during walking or running, which brings the breathing function into conflict with the postural function of these muscles. This exercise helps develop the ability to cope with external destabilizing forces that can cause loss of balance and breathlessness during ambulation.

IMT loading level: light to moderate
Duration: 30 to 60 seconds
Sets: 2 sets separated by 30 to 60 seconds of rest

Procedure: Adopt the starting position shown for the selected level of difficulty. If using an IMTD, this should be held in the mouth without using the hands. Once in position, brace the abdominal muscles (moderately). For specific guidance see the description for each version.

Variations: To add difficulty, stand on a balance cushion.

Easy

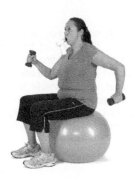

Sit on a chair or Swiss ball, with a light weight in each hand. Then pump the arms back and forth as if sprinting. Do this using a cadence that is challenging but comfortable (enough to disturb balance slightly). At the same time, inhale forcefully through the IMTD so that 5 to 6 deep breaths are completed in 30 seconds (10 to 12 in 60 seconds). Try to breathe *out of synch* with the arm movements.

Moderate

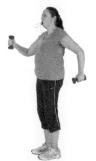

Stand upright with feet shoulder-width apart, knees bent slightly, and a light weight in each hand. Then follow the instructions for the Easy version.

Difficult

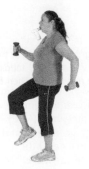

Stand upright on one leg with the knee bent slightly, and a light weight in each hand. Then follow the instructions for the Easy version.

Resisted front raise

Benefits: Simply flinging the arms away from the body requires feed-forward activity of the diaphragm and transversus abdominis to maintain balance. In situations where breathing demand is high, there is a direct conflict between the requirements for breathing and the requirements for postural control – and breathing always wins (see Ch. 1). This exercise helps to develop the ability to meet both of those demands comfortably, without compromising either. The benefits will be translated into a myriad of everyday activities where the demands of postural control and breathing are high (e.g., walking on uneven ground). Resistance can be generated using a weight or elastic resistance band. A weight is preferable, because it acquires momentum during movement.

IMT loading level: light to moderate
Duration: 15 to 60 seconds
Sets: 2 to 4 sets separated by 30 to 60 seconds of rest

Procedure: Adopt the starting position shown for the selected level of difficulty. If using an IMTD, this should be held in the mouth without using the hands. Once in position, brace the abdominal muscles (moderately). For specific guidance see the description for each version.

Variations: In addition to increasing duration, or the size of the resistance, this exercise can be made more challenging by increasing cadence, using a balance cushion, or adopting a split stance (one foot in front of the other, shoulder-width apart).

Easy

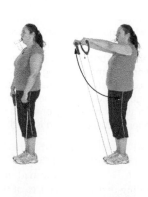

Stand upright with feet shoulder-width apart, knees bent slightly and a weight in both hands or holding each end of an elastic resistance (anchored under the feet). Swing the arms forward and upward, finishing with them at shoulder height. Do this with a cadence that is challenging but comfortable (enough to be slightly off balance). At the same time, inhale forcefully through the IMTD so that 5 to 6 deep breaths are completed in 30 seconds (10 to 12 in 60 seconds). Be careful not the rock back on the heels and to maintain complete control of the resistance at *all* times.

Moderate

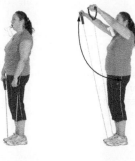

Follow the instructions for the Easy version, but raise the hands just above shoulder height.

Difficult

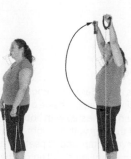

Follow the instructions for the Easy version, but raise the hands above the head.

Step-up/down

Benefits: This exercise involves the lumbopelvic stabilizers, as well as the hip, knee and ankle extensors. Stepping is an activity that causes many people to become breathless. This is not only because stepping is metabolically hard work, but also because it requires the respiratory muscles to be engaged simultaneously in active postural control. This exercise develops the ability to deal with these dual demands.

> **IMT loading level:** light to moderate
> **Step height:** 15 to 30 cm (6 to 12 inches)
> **Duration:** 30 to 60 seconds
> **Sets:** 2 to 4 sets separated by 30 to 60 seconds of rest

Procedure: Adopt the starting position shown for the selected level of difficulty. If using an IMTD, this should be held in the mouth without using the hands. Once in position, brace the abdominal muscles (moderately). For specific guidance see the description for each version.

Variations: In addition to increasing duration or step height, the exercise can be made more challenging by increasing cadence, or using hand weights.

Easy

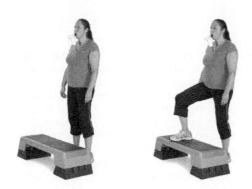

Stand upright with hands by the sides or crossed on the chest (try not to use the arms to assist with balance). Step up with the right foot, placing it on the step briefly before returning to the start position. Alternate the leg with each repetition, moving at a comfortable but challenging pace. Inhale forcefully through the IMTD as the leg is lifted, and exhale as it is lowered (swap breathing phases between sets so that the exhalation occurs as the leg is lifted).

Moderate

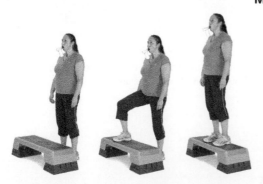

The procedure is as for Easy, but progresses so that the finish position is standing on top of the step. Step down backwards with the same lead leg.

Difficult

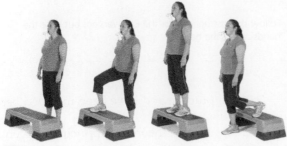

The procedure is as for Easy, but progresses so that the finish position is standing on opposite side of the step. Step up with the right leg, stand on the step with both feet, then step down the other side of the step with the right leg. Turn through 180 degrees to face the step and repeat. If using stairs, turn through 180 degrees when standing on the stair, and again for the next repetition.

Sit-stand

Benefits: Sitting and standing doesn't just require adequate strength in the hip and knee extensors, it also requires good core stability and postural control. Typically, people inhale just before rising, and perform a weak Valsalva to produce stability and stiffness in the trunk and pelvis. This exercise will reduce the reliance upon this pneumatic pressure for stability, replacing it with good neuromuscular strength and coordination.

IMT loading level: light to moderate
Duration: 10 to 15 repetitions
Sets: 2 to 4 sets separated by 30 to 60 seconds of rest

Procedure: Adopt the starting position shown for the selected level of difficulty. If using an IMTD, this should be held in the mouth without using the hands. Once in position, brace the abdominal muscles (moderately). For specific guidance see the description for each version.

Easy

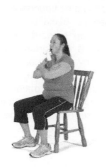
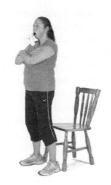

Begin in a seated position with the arms folded across the chest. Rise to the standing position as swiftly as possible, then return immediately to the seated position (under control) and repeat. Inhale forcefully through the IMTD when rising; exhale when sitting (swap breathing phases between sets so that the exhalation occurs when rising).

Moderate

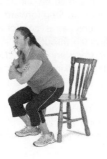
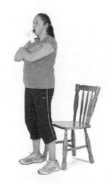

As for the Easy version, but instead of full sitting the buttocks should touch the chair only momentarily.

Difficult

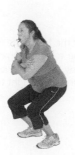
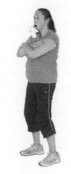

As for the Moderate version, but without any chair and with a smooth, fluid transition between the sit and stand phases.

217

Lunge

Benefits: This exercise challenges the ability to maintain postural control during a compound exercise that involves large muscle groups. It will develop the capacity to breathe effectively during movements that require forceful activation of large muscle groups.

IMT loading level: light to moderate
Duration: 10 to 15 repetitions
Sets: 2 to 4 sets separated by 30 to 60 seconds of rest

Procedure: Adopt the starting position shown for the selected level of difficulty. If using an IMTD, this should be held in the mouth without using the hands. Once in position, brace the abdominal muscles (moderately). For specific guidance see the description for each version.

Easy

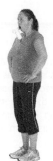
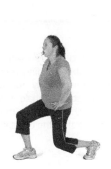

This is a static lunge exercise, which can be undertaken with support if necessary. However, it should be undertaken with hands on hips for maximum benefit. Begin by standing upright with feet together, then step forward and drop down into the lunge as deeply as is comfortable (active phase) then reverse the manoeuvre by pushing back to the start position with feet together (recovery phase). Next, repeat the lunge with the opposite leg and continue at a comfortable but challenging pace. Inhale forcefully through the IMTD during the active phase (exhale during the recovery phase). Alternate this pattern between sets so that the exhalation occurs during the active phase.

Moderate

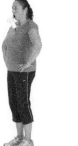
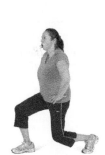

This is a dynamic lunge exercise that should be undertaken with hands on hips for maximum benefit. Step forward and drop down into the lunge as deeply as is comfortable (active phase) then bring the trailing leg through and stand upright again with feet together (recovery phase). Next, step forward with the opposite leg, walking forward with large, deep steps, punctuated by standing. Alternate the leading leg with each repetition, and step at a comfortable but challenging pace. Inhale forcefully through the IMTD during the active phase (exhale during the recovery phase). Alternate this pattern between sets so that the exhalation occurs during the active phase.

Difficult

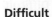
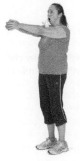
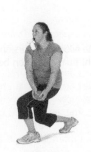

The procedure is the same as for the Moderate version, but also involves holding and moving a weight that is held at arm's length in front of the body. At the lowest point of the lunge, rotate the shoulders and the weight to the same side as the leading leg.

Pushing and pulling exercises

Upright chest press

Benefits: The chest press requires the ability to transform the trunk into a stable platform, but doing so places huge demands on the ability of the trunk muscles to carry out their breathing function (because the muscle actions tend to compress the rib cage). This exercise will help develop the coordinated action of the trunk stabilization and control musculature during the press movement. Undertaking this exercise in an unstable standing position and with a breathing challenge will improve the ability to coordinate the stabilizing and breathing actions of the trunk during an exercise that compresses the rib cage. This transforms a simple chest press into a core exercise that is highly functional.

IMTD loading level: light to moderate
Duration: 10 repetitions
Sets: 2 sets separated by 30 to 60 seconds of rest

Procedure: Adopt the starting position shown for the selected level of difficulty. If using an IMTD, this should be held in the mouth without using the hands. Once in position, brace the abdominal muscles (moderately). For specific guidance see the description for each version.

Variations: Add difficulty by using only one arm at a time, which creates additional rotational and postural challenges.

Easy

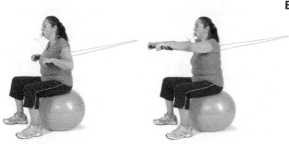

A resistance band should be anchored at its middle, at chest height. Facing away from the anchor point in a seated position (chair or Swiss ball), hold opposite ends of the band in each hand. Press the hands away from the body, and inhale forcefully through the IMTD throughout the movement (exhale as the hands return to the starting position). Swap breathing phases between sets so that the exhalation occurs during the press. Concentrate on not allowing the brace to release during either phase of breathing.

Moderate

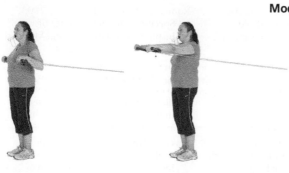

As for the Easy version, but instead of sitting adopt a standing position with feet shoulder-width apart and knees bent very slightly. A closer stance can be used to add difficulty.

Difficult

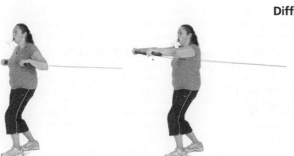

As for the Easy version, but instead of sitting adopt a standing position with one foot ~30 cm (~12 inches) in front of the other; feet should be approximately shoulder-width apart with knees bent slightly. A closer stance can be used to add difficulty.

Shoulder press

Benefits: This exercise is good for postural control, and it involves the trunk musculature, shoulders and triceps. As with the chest press, the shoulder press requires the ability to transform the thorax into a stable platform. This places huge demands on the ability of the trunk muscles to carry out their breathing function because this action stiffens the trunk (making inhalation more challenging). This exercise will help develop the coordinated action of the trunk stabilization and control musculature during the shoulder-press movement. An unstable standing position and a breathing challenge improve the ability to coordinate the stabilizing and breathing actions of the trunk. This transforms the exercise into a core exercise that is highly functional.

IMTD loading level: light to moderate
Duration: 10 repetitions
Sets: 2 sets separated by 30 to 60 seconds of rest

Procedure: Adopt the starting position shown for the selected level of difficulty. If using an IMTD, this should be held in the mouth without using the hands. Once in position, brace the abdominal muscles (moderately). For specific guidance see the description for each version.

Variations: The exercise can also be undertaken using hand weights. Add difficulty by using only one arm at a time, which creates an additional postural challenge.

Easy

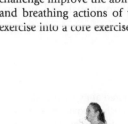
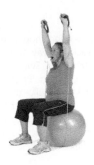

A resistance band should be anchored at floor level. Seated above the anchor point (chair or Swiss ball), hold one end of the band in each hand. Press the hands above the head, and inhale forcefully through the IMTD throughout the movement (exhale the hands return to the starting position). Swap breathing phases between sets so that the exhalation occurs during the press. Concentrate on not allowing the brace to release during either phase of breathing. Also concentrate on maintaining good lifting form and a neutral spine.

Moderate

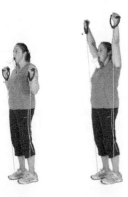

As for the Easy version, but instead of sitting adopt a standing position with feet shoulder-width apart. A closer stance can be used to add difficulty.

Difficult

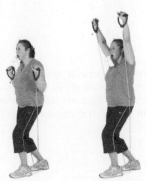

As for the Easy version, but instead of sitting adopt a standing position with one foot ∼30 cm (∼12 inches) in front of the other; feet should be approximately shoulder-width apart with knees bent slightly. A closer stance can be used to add difficulty.

Resisted pull

Benefits: This exercise is good for postural control, and it involves the back, shoulder and biceps muscles. Any action that compresses the rib cage creates a challenge to breathing, which is precisely what pulling movements impose. The use of a low anchor point for the resistance creates a postural challenge that pulls the body downwards as well as forwards. Undertaking the exercise in an unstable, upright position transforms it into a functional core activity. The single-arm version of the exercise also adds a rotational challenge that will train the trunk rotators.

IMTD loading level: light to moderate
Duration: 10 repetitions
Sets: 2 sets separated by 30 to 60 seconds of rest

Procedure: Adopt the starting position shown for the selected level of difficulty. If using an IMTD, this should be held in the mouth without using the hands. Once in position, brace the abdominal muscles (moderately). For specific guidance see the description for each version.

Variations: Add difficulty by using only one arm at a time, which creates additional rotational and postural challenges.

Easy

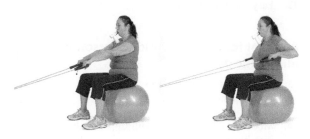

A resistance band should be anchored at floor height. Facing the anchor point in a seated position (chair or Swiss ball), hold one end of the band in each hand. Pull the hands towards the abdomen, and inhale forcefully through the IMTD throughout the movement (exhale as the hands return to the starting position). Swap breathing phases between sets so that the exhalation occurs during the pull. Concentrate on not allowing the brace to release during either phase of breathing.

Moderate

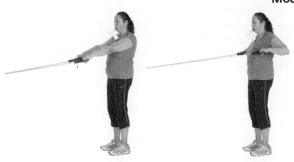

As for the Easy version, but instead of sitting adopt a standing position with feet shoulder-width apart. A closer stance can be used to add difficulty.

Difficult

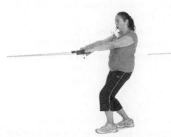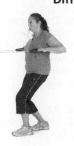

As for the Easy version, but instead of sitting, adopt a standing position with one foot about 30 cm (12 inches) in front of the other; feet should be approximately shoulder-width apart with knees bent slightly. A closer stance can be used to add difficulty.

Suggested workout protocols

Protocol one: ambulatory patient with moderate chronic obstructive pulmonary disease (COPD) and breathlessness during activities with arms overhead

1. Easy stretch set   184
2. Swiss ball bounce   186
3. Easy plank   188
4. Easy bridge   190
5. Easy seated hip extension   198
6. Easy bent leg deadlift   203
7. Seated lateral raise   204 and 205
8. Seated halo   204 and 205
9. Easy rise with overhead weight   206
10. Easy bag pick-up   208
11. Easy sit/stand   217
12. Easy shoulder press   220

Protocol two: ambulatory patient with heart failure and low back pain

1. Easy stretch set   184
2. Marching on the spot   186
3. Easy plank   188
4. Easy bridge   190
5. Braced curl-up   197
6. Easy seated hip extension   198
7. Easy superman   201
8. Seated bicep curl   204 and 205
9. Seated anterior raise 2   204 and 205
10. Easy squat with overhead resistance   207
11. Easy close arm dip   212
12. Easy sit/stand   217
13. Easy upright chest press   219

Protocol three: active patient with neuromuscular disease and a history of falls

1. Moderate stretch set   185
2. Swiss ball bounce   186
3. Moderate plank   188
4. Moderate gluteal bridge   193
5. Moderate seated hip extension   198
6. Moderate bent leg deadlift   203
7. Standing front swing   205
8. Standing halo   204 and 205
9. Moderate bag pick-up   208
10. Moderate trunk lateral rotation   210
11. Moderate dumbbell running   214
12. Moderate resisted front raise   215
13. Easy shoulder press   220

Protocol four: healthy older person with idiopathic dyspnoea

1. Moderate stretch set   185
2. Ball bounce on the spot   186
3. Moderate plank   188
4. Moderate gluteal bridge with upper body instability   194
5. Moderate gluteal bridge with lower body instability   195
6. Braced curl-up   197
7. Moderate reverse curl   199
8. Moderate bent leg deadlift   203
9. Standing side swing   204 and 205
10. Standing halo   204 and 205
11. Moderate rise with overhead weight   206
12. Moderate bag pick-up   208
13. Moderate trunk lateral rotation   210
14. Difficult sit/stand   217
15. Moderate chest press   219
16. Moderate resisted pull   221

REFERENCES

Beckerman, M., Magadle, R., Weiner, M., et al., 2005. The effects of 1 year of specific inspiratory muscle training in patients with COPD. Chest 128, 3177–3182.

Borg, E., Borg, G., Larsson, K., et al., 2010. An index for breathlessness and leg fatigue. Scand. J. Med. Sci. Sports 20, 644–650.

Borg, G.A., 1982. Psychophysical bases of perceived exertion. Med. Sci. Sports Exerc. 14, 377–381.

Borg, G., 1998. Borg's Perceived Exertion and Pain Scales. Human Kinetics, Champaign, IL.

Deindl, F.M., Vodusek, D.B., Hesse, U., et al., 1994. Pelvic floor activity patterns: comparison of nulliparous continent and parous urinary stress incontinent women. A kinesiological EMG study. Br. J. Urol. 73, 413–417.

Enright, P.L., Kronmal, R.A., Manolio, T.A., et al., 1994. Respiratory muscle strength in the elderly.

Correlates and reference values. Cardiovascular Health Study Research Group. Am. J. Respir. Crit. Care Med. 149, 430–438.

Fletcher, C.M., Elmes, P.C., Fairbairn, A.S., et al., 1959. The significance of respiratory symptoms and the diagnosis of chronic bronchitis in a working population. Br. Med. J. 2, 257–266.

Gosselink, R., De Vos, J., van den Heuvel, S.P., et al., 2011. Impact of inspiratory muscle training in patients with COPD: what is the evidence? Eur. Respir. J. 37, 416–425.

Hodges, P.W., Butler, J.E., McKenzie, D.K., et al., 1997a. Contraction of the human diaphragm during rapid postural adjustments. J. Physiol. 505 (pt 2), 539–548.

Hodges, P.W., Gandevia, S.C., Richardson, C.A., 1997b. Contractions of specific abdominal muscles in postural tasks are affected by respiratory maneuvers. J. Appl. Physiol. 83, 753–760.

Hodges, P.W., McKenzie, D.K., Heijnen, I., et al., 2000. Reduced contribution of the diaphragm to postural control in patients with chronic airflow limitation. In: Proceedings of the Thoracic Society of Australia and New Zealand. Melbourne, Australia.

Kikuchi, Y., Okabe, S., Tamura, G., et al., 1994. Chemosensitivity and perception of dyspnea in patients with a history of near-fatal asthma. N. Engl. J. Med. 330, 1329–1334.

Killian, K.J., Jones, N.L., 1988. Respiratory muscles and dyspnea. Clin. Chest Med. 9, 237–248.

Lotters, F., van Tol, B., Kwakkel, G., et al., 2002. Effects of controlled inspiratory muscle training in patients with COPD: a meta-analysis. Eur. Respir. J. 20, 570–576.

Magadle, R., Berar-Yanay, N., Weiner, P., 2002. The risk of hospitalization and near-fatal and fatal asthma in relation to the perception of dyspnea. Chest 121, 329–333.

Mahler, D.A., Weinberg, D.H., Wells, C.K., et al., 1984. The measurement of dyspnea. Contents, interobserver agreement, and physiologic correlates of two new clinical indexes. Chest 85, 751–758.

Marin, J.M., Carrizo, S.J., Gascon, M., et al., 2001. Inspiratory capacity, dynamic hyperinflation, breathlessness, and exercise performance during the 6-minute-walk test in chronic obstructive pulmonary disease. Am. J. Respir. Crit. Care Med. 163, 1395–1399.

McConnell, A.K., 2011. Breathe strong, perform better. Human Kinetics, Champaign, IL.

McConnell, A.K., Copestake, A.J., 1999. Maximum static respiratory pressures in healthy elderly men and women: issues of reproducibility and interpretation. Respiration 66, 251–258.

McGill, S., 2007. Low back disorders, second ed. Human Kinetics Europe Ltd, Champaign, IL.

Minoguchi, H., Shibuya, M., Miyagawa, T., et al., 2002. Cross-over comparison between respiratory muscle stretch gymnastics and inspiratory muscle training. Intern. Med. 41, 805–812.

O'Donnell, D.E., Sanii, R., Anthonisen, N.R., et al., 1987. Effect of dynamic airway compression on breathing pattern and respiratory sensation in severe chronic obstructive pulmonary disease. Am. Rev. Respir. Dis. 135, 912–918.

O'Donnell, D.E., Lam, M., Webb, K.A., 1998. Measurement of symptoms, lung hyperinflation, and endurance during exercise in chronic obstructive pulmonary disease. Am. J. Respir. Crit. Care Med. 158, 1557–1565.

Smith, M.D., Russell, A., Hodges, P.W., 2006. Disorders of breathing and continence have a stronger association with back pain than obesity and physical activity. Aust. J. Physiother. 52, 11–16.

Tsao, H., Hodges, P.W., 2008. Persistence of improvements in postural strategies following motor control training in people with recurrent low back pain. J. Electromyogr. Kinesiol. 18, 559–567.

Weiner, P., Berar-Yanay, N., Davidovich, A., et al., 2000. Specific inspiratory muscle training in patients with mild asthma with high consumption of inhaled beta(2)-agonists. Chest 117, 722–727.

Weiner, P., Magadle, R., Beckerman, M., et al., 2003. Comparison of specific expiratory, inspiratory, and combined muscle training programs in COPD. Chest 124, 1357–1364.

Website

www.physiobreathe.com.

Glossary

Abdominal cavity Space below the diaphragm that contains the abdominal viscera

Abdominal viscera Organs contained within the abdomen (including the liver, stomach, bowel)

Afferent nerve Sensory nerve carrying impulses towards the brain

Anastomoses Communications between blood vessels that enables arterial blood to be diverted to different regions of the tissue

Alveoli Small air sacs of the lungs that carry out exchange of oxygen and carbon dioxide between the air and the blood

Apnoea Cessation of breathing

Atelectasis Collapse of a small portion of the lung.

Autonomic nervous system Involuntary branch of the peripheral nervous system controlling functions such as heart rate, blood pressure, perspiration, pupillary dilation

Biopsy A small sample of tissue

Body mass index (BMI) A method of quantifying an individual's weight that relates weight to height: $BMI - weight\ (kg)/height^2\ (m^2)$

Breathing pattern The combination of respiratory flows, volumes and the timing of breaths

Bronchoconstriction Narrowing of the airways caused by contraction of muscles encircling the airways. Narrowing occurs in susceptible individuals in response to 'triggers' such as allergens and exercise

Bronchodilator Medication that dilates the airways

Cadence The frequency of limb movement, e.g., pedalling rate

Capillaries Tiny blood vessels that carry blood to the tissues of the body, including the lungs and muscles

Concentric muscle contraction A contraction during which the muscle gets shorter, e.g., lifting a dumbbell during a bicep curl

Cor pulmonale Failure of the right side of the heart caused by chronically raised pressure within the pulmonary circulation (pulmonary hypertension) and right ventricle of the heart

Dead space (V_D) The volume of the lungs that does not contribute to exchange of oxygen and carbon dioxide because it contains no alveoli, e.g., the trachea and other large airways. It is therefore 'wasted' breathing

Duty cycle The proportion of a breath that was inhalation, i.e., inspiratory duration divided by total breath duration $(T_I/[T_I + T_E])$

Dyspnoea Breathlessness, shortness of breath

Eccentric muscle contraction A contraction during which the muscle gets longer, e.g., lowering a dumbbell during a bicep curl

Efferent nerve Motor nerve carrying impulses away from the brain

Elastic work of breathing The work that is done by the inspiratory muscles to overcome the elastic properties of the lung and chest wall, which tend to deflate it

End-expiratory lung volume (EELV) The volume of air remaining in the lungs at the end of a normal exhalation. This value changes depending upon the conditions, e.g., it becomes smaller during exercise

Entrainment The synchrony between movement and breathing during exercise

Foundation training The initial phase of training lasting 4 to 6 weeks during which the foundations of inspiratory muscle strength, power and endurance are laid

Hypertrophy The increase in muscle fibre size (cross-sectional area) following training. This is due to an increase in the amount of protein within muscle cells, and not to an increase in the number of cells

Hyperpnoea Increase in minute ventilation in proportion to metabolic demand

Hyperinflation Breathing at an elevated lung volume such that EELV is higher than the relaxation volume of the lungs

Hyperventilation Overbreathing relative to metabolic demand

Inflammation A sign of cell damage that is associated with swelling and redness of the tissues, e.g., a nettle sting. The damage can be due to chemicals that irritate the cells, as well as mechanical trauma to cells

Inspiratory muscle training device (IMTD) A device that imposes a resistance-training stimulus upon the breathing muscles. The use of a pressure threshold product is recommended

Inspiratory capacity (IC) The difference between end-expiratory lung volume (EELV) and total lung capacity. This is the volume available to expand tidal volume

Ischaemia Inadequate blood supply to a tissue

Lactate threshold An intensity domain during exercise that results in an elevated concentration of the metabolite lactate in the blood. Further increases in exercise intensity above this level result in a progressive increase in the lactate concentration and are therefore non-sustainable

Locomotion Movement of the body such as walking running, cycling, rowing, swimming, skiing, etc.

Locomotor muscles Muscles used in locomotion, e.g., leg muscles in walking and cycling

Lung parenchyma Lung tissue

Maximal oxygen uptake ($\dot{V}O_{2max}$) The maximal amount of oxygen uptake measured at the mouth. It corresponds to the maximal ability to transport and utilize oxygen during a test of increasing intensity (also known as maximal oxygen consumption, aerobic capacity)

Maximum voluntary ventilation (MVV) The maximum amount of air that can be moved in and out of the lungs during a specific period (normally 15 seconds). It provides an index of the peak power output of the breathing pump

Maximum sustainable ventilatory capacity (MSVC) The maximum amount of air that can be moved in and out of the lungs during a sustained period of hyperventilation. It provides an index of the endurance of the breathing pump

Metabolism The cellular process of deriving energy from fuels such as carbohydrates. This can be aerobic (with oxygen) or anaerobic (without oxygen). Anaerobic metabolism can result in the production of lactic acid, which is also known as lactate in exercise biochemistry. The accumulation of lactic acid in the blood has been linked to the development of fatigue

Metabolic equivalent of the task (MET) The energy cost for oxygen consumption (VO_2) of an activity expressed as a ratio of a reference VO_2. This reference value is equivalent to resting VO_2 and is conventionally 3.5 millilitres of oxygen per minute per kilogram body mass ($ml \cdot min^{-1}.kg^{-1}$). The MET is therefore an index of the relative intensity of an activity.

Metaboreflex A reflex response to signals generated by metaboreceptor activation, which normally results in an increase in heart rate and blood pressure

Metaboreceptors Receptors within muscles that detect the by-products of metabolism (metabolites)

Minute ventilation ($\dot{V}_E$) The rate of air flow per minute. It is the product of tidal volume and breathing frequency

Orthopnoea Dyspnoea associated with a supine posture

Oxidative capacity The capacity to utilize oxygen to generate energy from fuel such as carbohydrates. This increases in response to endurance training

Oxygen uptake ($\dot{V}O_2$) The uptake of oxygen by the body measured at the mouth

Passive diffusion The passive process by which molecules move from an area of high concentration to an area of lower concentration, e.g., oxygen moving from the alveoli into the lung capillaries

Peak inspiratory flow rate The maximal inspiratory flow achieved during a maximal inspiratory effort

Placebo A treatment condition that is ineffective, but appears to the research participants to be a real treatment, e.g., a tablet that is made from sugar and not real medication. This manages the participants' expectations so that the placebo group also believe they will improve

Pulmonary circulation The blood supply to the lungs

Relaxation volume Lung volume at which all forces acting on the lungs are in equilibrium and the respiratory muscles are relaxed. In normal lungs this state is associated with an alveolar pressure of zero

Residual volume (RV) The volume that remains in the lungs at the end of a maximal exhalation. This is a fixed volume that only changes in response to disease and ageing

Tachypnoea Rapid breathing rate

Thoracic cavity Space above the diaphragm occupied by the lungs and heart (bounded by the rib cage)

Tidal volume (V_T) The volume of each breath

Time to the limit of tolerance (T_{lim}) The time taken to reach a point where the participant is no longer able to sustain the task. This varies according to the severity of the task

Trunk musculature Comprises the muscles of the thoracic and abdominal compartments, including those considered primarily to be respiratory muscles, e.g., the diaphragm

Unmyelinated Nerve lacking an outer, electrically insulating layer of myelin (myelin sheath)

Warm-up Prior activity of the muscles. This activity need not result in an increase in muscle or body temperature, but is a generic term for any prior activity

Wingate test Named after the Wingate Institute in Israel, this is a maximal sprint on a cycle ergometer lasting 30 seconds. The object is to generate the maximum amount of power

Zone of apposition The portion of the diaphragm that rests against the inside of the lower rib cage (because of the muscle's natural dome shape)

Index

NB: Page numbers in *italics* refer to boxes, figures and tables.

Index

O

Obesity
  exercise limitation, 81
  inspiratory muscle training (IMT),
    outcomes, *162*
  respiratory muscle function, changes,
    66–67
  respiratory muscle training (RMT),
    functional responses, 118–119
Obstructive sleep apnoea (OSA), 64, 65
  inspiratory muscle training (IMT),
    outcomes, *162*
  respiratory muscle function, changes,
    71–72
  respiratory muscle training (RMT),
    functional responses, 122–123
Optimization model, control of exercise
    hyperpnoea, 23–24
Overhead weight exercise, rise with, 206
Overload training stimulus, 135–137
Oxygen
  maximal uptake, 48–49
  O_2 transport, 15–17, *15, 16, 17*, 48
  O_2 usage, 48
  uptake efficiency slope (OUES),
    113–115
Oxygen transport, 15–17, *15, 16, 17*

P

Parenchymal pull, airways, 27
Parkinson's disease (PD), 66, 118
Parturition, 71
Passive flow resistance devices, 141, *142*
Peak inspiratory flow rate, 160
  see also Inspiratory flow rate
Pediatric Evaluation of Disability
    Inventory (PEDI), 66
Pelvic floor muscles, 85
Perfusion, gas exchange, 13–15,
    13, 14
Peripheral chemoreceptors, 22–23, *23*
Peripheral muscle myopathy, in chronic
    obstructive pulmonary disease
    (COPD), 76
Peripheral proprioceptors/
    metaboreceptors, 21–22
Physiology *see* Respiratory system,
    anatomy/physiology
Plank exercise, 188
  lower body instability, 191
  upper body instability, 192
Pneumothorax, 152
Positive end-expiratory pressure (PEEP),
    58, 71, 75
Positive end-inspiratory pressure
    (PEEP$_i$), 29

Posterior cricoarytenoid (PCA) muscle,
    9, 83
Post-operative pulmonary complications
    (PPC), 70
Post-polio syndrome, 66, 116, 117
Postural stability, 83
Posture
  control, 83, 84, 213–218
  foundation inspiratory muscle
    training (IMT), 152–153
  role of trunk muscles, 83–85
Pregnancy
  exercise limitation, 83
  inspiratory muscle training (IMT),
    outcomes, *162*
  respiratory muscle function, changes,
    71
Pressure threshold devices, 143
Pressure-volume relationship, lungs, *30,
    32, 32*
Proprioceptors, peripheral, 21–22
Pulmonary arterial hypertension (PAH)
  exercise limitation, 78–80
  respiratory muscle function, changes,
    64
Pulmonary circulation, 14–15
  blood flows/pressures, *13*
  diffusion, O_2 transport, 47
Pulmonary vasculature, 13
  vascular resistance (PVR), 14
Pushing/pulling exercise, 219–221

R

Radial traction, 22
Red blood cells (RBCs) (erythrocytes),
    15, 17–18, *18*, 50–51
Rehabilitation programme, foundation
    inspiratory muscle training
    (IMT), 166, 167–168
  incorporating RMT, 167–168, *168*
  pre-rehabilitation using IMT, 167
Renal failure, 69
  inspiratory muscle training (IMT),
    outcomes, *162*
  respiratory muscle training (RMT),
    functional responses, 120
Renshaw cells, 24
Repetition failure, foundation
    inspiratory muscle training
    (IMT), *157*, 165
Repetition maximum (RM) principle,
    164, 183
Residual volume (RV), 30
Resistance breathing, *104*
Resistance training, inspiratory muscles,
    138–140
  equipment, 141–143

expiratory muscle (EMT), 100–101
inspiratory muscle (IMT), 99–100,
    100, 101
Respiratory acidosis, 20
Respiratory alkalosis, 19
Respiratory controller, 38
  afferent input, 20–22
Respiratory disease
  exercise limitation, 75–78
  muscle function, changes, 58–63
  respiratory muscle training (RMT),
    functional responses, 108–113
Respiratory muscle training devices,
    141–143, *142*
Respiratory muscle training (RMT),
    methods, 135–148
  equipment, 141–143, *142*
  forms/outcomes, 138–141
  general principles, 135–138
  merits/limitations, *142*, 143
  treatment pathway, 149–150
Respiratory muscle training (RMT),
    responses, 37–40, 97–102
  disease-specific, functional, 108–123
  functional adaptations, 97–98,
    99–102, *99*
  healthy people, 102–108
  structural adaptations, 97–99
Respiratory muscles, 57–96
  breathing mechanics, changes, 57–72
  exercise limitation, role in, 72–83
  fatigue (RMF), healthy people, 73, 74
  function, assessment, 57–72, 158–161
  innervation, levels, *65*
  non-respiratory functions, 83–85
  training rationale, 85
Respiratory pump muscles, 6, *7*
  functional properties, 8–9
  mechanical properties, 31–33, *32, 33*
Respiratory system, anatomy/
    physiology, 3–36
  acid-base balance, 18–20, *19*
  breathing
    control, 20–24, *21*
    mechanics, 24–33
  carbon dioxide transport, 15, 17–18,
    17, 18
  dyspnoea/breathing effort, 33–35
  gross structure, 9–10, *9, 10, 11*
  oxygen transport, 15–17, *15,
    16, 17*
  thoracic structure/function, 3–10
  see also Gas exchange
Respiratory system training adaptations,
    51
Restrictive chest wall disorders
  exercise limitation, 77–78
  inspiratory muscle training (IMT),
    outcomes, *162*

232

Printed and bound by CPI Group (UK) Ltd, Croydon, CR0 4YY

03/10/2024

01040369-0001